Answers from the Family Doctor

370 Questions Patients Ask Most

Allan Bruckheim, M.D.

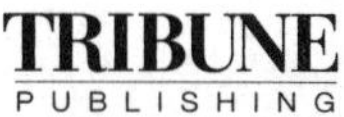
TRIBUNE PUBLISHING

c/o Contemporary Books
Two Prudential Plaza
Suite 1200
Chicago, Illinois 60601-6790

Edited by Anthony F. Serowik
Text design by Joy Dickinson
Illustrations by Dana Fasano

Every effort has been made to ensure the accuracy of this book. It should, however, be used for informational purposes only. This book is in no way intended to replace or supersede qualified medical care. The authors and publisher disclaim any liability resulting from the use of this book.

TRIBUNE PUBLISHING
Editorial Director:
George C. Biggers III
Managing Editor: Dixie Kasper
Senior Editor: Kathleen M. Kiely
Production Manager: Ken Paskman
Designers: Bill Henderson,
Eileen M. Schechner,
Joy Dickinson

Printed in the United States

FIRST EDITION

Library of Congress Cataloging-in-Publication Data

Bruckheim, Allan H.
Answers from the family doctor : 370 questions patients ask most / Allan H. Bruckheim
p. cm.
Includes index.
ISBN 1-56943-006-3
1. Medicine, Popular — Miscellanea. I. Title.
RC82.B78 1993
610—dc20 93-37715
CIP

Contents

This book is dedicated to
the world's best
support team,
my family:
Debbie and Robert,
and their daughters
Jackie and Dani;
Andrea and Andrew,
and their son Brandon;
Lori and Walter;
and the inspirational
leader of the pack,
my beloved wife,
Joyce.

Preface

When I undertook the authorship of a nationally syndicated health column, I thought it might be a noble task to try to increase the understanding of medicine among individuals whom I considered patients in a national "practice." Certainly the modern practice of medicine is complex: confusing to the people who are in need of care and often difficult for the caregiver to explain. I thought that providing simple descriptions of the processes of diagnosis and the courses of treatment would serve to expand on explanations offered by personal physicians. The questions I anticipated would be easy to answer, I thought, considering my resources: shelves full of up-to-date textbooks and daily mail filled with medical journals that provide all the latest information on research and health care.

To be sure, such simple questions are contained in the incredible amount of mail that fills my mailbox, but there is also much more: cries for help where none exists, screams of rage over the failure of medication or surgery to correct an illness or reduce the pain, criticism and complaints; side by side with suspicions about the health-care system as it exists today and suggestions on how to make it all work better. Frankly, I am amazed that such revelations, such intimacies, such confidences are shared with me, but the never-ending flood of letters has convinced me that there is a real need for authoritative information that deals head-on with medical issues.

Over time, the column has taken on a life of its own, and it now controls my life. Each question to be answered is chosen carefully, to provide information that is useful to as many people as possible. I strive to be upbeat, as well as interesting, and each answer is carefully researched. New challenges are met with additional study; and the impression that each answer I give serves as the beginning of someone's quest for knowledge preoccupies my thoughts.

Now, a new philosophy has taken hold, and serves as the inspiration for all the effort I put into writing the responses. This philosophy is built upon my own experience in practice, the lessons I have learned in teaching medical students, and the apparent needs of you, my readers.

The questions and answers selected for this book are based upon the same principles that inspire the column. It is important for you to appreciate these principles so you can fully profit from the information the answers provide and, most importantly, from the attitudes they promote, to gain the most from your health care. Consider each of the following principles as you read this book, and make them part of your thinking as you seek the knowledge you need in order to make the proper decisions about your own health care:

- The best choices in medical care depend upon a full understanding of the benefits and risks of any course of therapy.
- One of the best methods of obtaining the knowledge you need is to question the physician who knows the most about your condition and the care you are to have.
- You have the right to have your questions answered in a manner and in a language you can understand easily.
- There is a huge quantity of information in written form available to you, if only you can find the source. Once the source is found, by researching libraries and even telephone books for government agencies, it is your responsibility to request the material you need.
- There is little in medicine that is totally black or white. When the path is unclear, seek a second or even a third opinion about important decisions.
- Though the task is sometimes great, the outcome is worth the effort. The difference between the best decision and the worst one is often the difference between a cure and living with a chronic condition.

And whether you believe this or not, the fact is that:

The things you fear the most seldom happen.

You will find an expression of these philosophies in all the answers in this book. Now it is up to you to make them yours, for all the good they can and will do for you.

Acknowledgments

The block of granite that forms the top of the Great Pyramid rests upon literally thousands of similar stones that form the base and support the pinnacle. So it is with life: Every achievement is accomplished only with the support of many who go unthanked and unrecognized. Often, it is because there are just so many to acknowledge that neither space nor the limitations of memory are equal to the task. However, let me try to identify some of the people in my life whose influences are woven into the fabric of my work.

First there were my parents, who toiled that I might learn and serve. Perhaps they always knew I would live in the spirit of their sacrifice.

Then there were my teachers and professors, leading, inspiring and demanding, shaping the form of the man to come with their own abrasiveness and skill.

Next came my professional colleagues, who shared experience and knowledge — dedicated individuals who believed in the principles of caring and responsibility.

My patients committed to me the health of their minds and bodies, and bestowed upon me their confidence and trust. They taught me more than books, and showed me that more than science was needed to heal and comfort.

My students, inquiring and relentless in their search for the ultimate answers, kept me young in my thinking and stoked the fires of my personal search for "why."

Some special individuals who encouraged me along the way, and helped mold the man that evolved from the boy, deserve special thanks:

Dr. Thomas Stern, mentor, teacher, inspired innovator and leader.

Mr. Lawrence Kennedy, friend, guide and advisor.

Dr. Alan Goldberg, who fills life with music, merriment and charm.

Dr. Henry Dobies, who always knew I really did know it all, but won't admit it, for fear my head will swell.

Mr. Robert Reed, who has never ceased to encourage and assist.

Ms. Elyce Small Goldstein, who assured me the book would come someday.

Ms. Evelyn Smith, who guided a neophyte author through the days of learning.

And finally and most sincerely, my deepest thanks to my editor Tony Serowik, who walked with me step by step, enduring the frustration and the pain, and now, hopefully, sharing the glow of achievement.

ALLAN H. BRUCKHEIM, M.D.

About Dr. Bruckheim

A practicing physician for more than 30 years, Dr. Allan H. Bruckheim is also a clinical associate professor in the Department of Family Medicine at the New York Medical College in Valhalla. He is a past president of the New York State Academy of Family Physicians and a former vice chair of the National Council of Patient Information and Education. In recognition of his efforts in patient education, Dr. Bruckheim has been honored with numerous awards, including the American Academy of Family Physicians' Presidential Award and the Vincent Downing Award for Excellence in Medical Communication. The Family Doctor, Dr. Bruckheim's contemporary medical information column, appears in newspapers nationwide and is available on CD-ROM.

1.

The Heart and Circulatory System

Nothing is less in our power than the heart, and far from commanding we are forced to obey.

JEAN-JACQUES ROUSSEAU
French philosopher (1712–78)

Whether we're consciously aware of the minute-by-minute efforts of our hearts or not, this single, relatively small organ controls our lives. More than once a second, it beats and pumps blood through our bodies, getting vital oxygen to the tissues and keeping us alive. At a typical rate of 72 beats per minute, the heart will beat 104,000 times in an average day in adults, and even more than that in children.

The heart is so important that for many years the legal definition of death was the stopping of the heartbeat. Its importance in health is mirrored by its importance in culture. For centuries, people believed the heart was the center of emotions, especially of love. We speak of having "heart-to-heart talks," of "setting our hearts on something," and, of course, of "broken hearts." In truth, the heart has nothing to do with emotions or feelings, which are controlled by the brain.

For many other body systems, there is duplication of the main organ, which provides two kidneys, two lungs or two eyes to the body, so that if one fails the other can take over the vital functions and do all the work necessary to keep us alive and well. But each of us has only one heart, so it pays to keep this important organ in the best possible working order. Yet heart disease is the leading cause of death in the United States, a sobering thought when we realize that most types of heart disease can be prevented.

Perhaps the most important first step in heart disease prevention is an understanding of just how the heart works, and how the arteries and veins play important roles in the function of the circulatory system. Another term that identifies this system, which you may see in more technical books, is the *cardiovascular system*.

The heart is one part of the cardiovascular system. ("Cardio" means heart and "vascular" refers to blood vessels.) Your heart is located between the lungs directly under the breastbone of your chest. The bottom tip of the heart tilts to the left, which is why we think of the heart as being on the left side of our chests. An adult heart is about the same size and shape as a man's clenched fist.

The heart is made of muscle, some of the strongest muscles in the body. It is hollow and divided into four chambers. The two top chambers are called *atria* (the singular is atrium) and the two lower chambers are called *ventricles*, with the right atrium connecting to the right ventricle and the left atrium connecting to the left ventricle. A thin wall between the atria and ventricles divides the heart in half. There are large blood vessels leading into the atria and large blood vessels leaving the ventricles. At the entrance and exit to each ventricle, there is a valve that prevents backflow of blood and keeps it moving in the right direction.

Blood flows through the heart in a pattern that supplies the entire body with oxygenated blood. Blood goes from the *superior* and *inferior vena cava*, the largest veins in the body, into the right atrium, where it is pumped into the right ventricle. The right ventricle then pumps the blood through the pulmonary arteries into the lungs, where the blood takes on its vital cargo of oxygen. Oxygenated blood then flows through the pulmonary veins into the left atrium, which pumps it into the left ventricle. The left ventricle, which is the largest and most powerful of the four heart chambers, then pumps the oxygenated blood through the aorta, which is the largest artery and biggest blood vessel in the body, to the rest of the body.

When the blood leaves the heart, it's carried through blood vessels called *arteries* to all the tissues of the body. As the arteries progress away from the heart, they divide like branches on a tree — each branch or division providing circulation to another part of the body. Each time they divide, the resulting arteries are smaller, until they dwindle in size to very small vessels that run through the body's tissues. In the tissues, the blood flows through microscopically tiny vessels called *capillaries*, where it gives up oxygen to the tissue cells. The capillaries then feed back into veins, which then conduct the blood flow back toward the heart, where the whole cycle starts again. Each time the heart beats, it pumps about 75 milliliters ($2\frac{1}{2}$ ounces) of blood into the aorta.

For the heart to pump blood through the entire body, it must put a great deal of force into each heartbeat. Arteries are strong and stretchy to withstand this pressure. Veins do not need to be as elastic, since by the time blood reaches them, the blood pressure is reduced. However, because the pressure is lower, veins have many small valves that prevent backflow of blood. For the veins in the legs, it's the action of the leg muscles that helps squeeze the veins with each muscle contraction, helping to push the blood back to the heart. It's another way in which exercise is beneficial to the circulatory system.

Blood pressure is the force provided by the pumping action of the heart necessary to propel the blood through the arteries. It is an important measure of cardiovascular health. If blood pressure is too low, it may mean that not enough oxygenated blood will reach the tissues. If blood pressure is too high, it can blow out a blood vessel, rupturing the wall and leading to stroke or death.

Blood pressure is measured with an instrument called a ***sphygmomanometer***, which is made up of an inflatable cuff and a pressure gauge. The normal pressure for a healthy adult is 120/80. The two numbers provide important information about the health of the circulatory system. The ***systolic pressure*** (or first number) indicates the maximum pressure in the system that is attained when the heart has contracted completely. The ***diastolic pressure*** (or lower number) indicates the pressure in the arterial system that is present between beats, when the heart takes its momentary rest.

A reading of more than 140/90 is considered high, and when repeated tests confirm this level or higher, a diagnosis of hypertension (or high blood pressure) is made, which should be treated to reduce it. Statistics have shown that individuals with consistently high blood pressure run a higher risk of both stroke and heart attack. This is the result of damage to the walls of the arteries caused by the constant elevated pressure. While these complications of hypertension are both serious and life-threatening, there are no symptoms of this elevated pressure. Thus, hypertension is often referred to as "The Silent Killer."

All parts of the body need the oxygen that blood carries, and the muscle tissue that forms the heart is no different. The heart does not get its oxygen from the blood passing through its chambers. Just as with any other organ or tissue in the body, the heart depends on its own arteries to provide the nutrients and oxygen it requires. These are called the ***coronary arteries***, so named for their crownlike appearance as they branch out from the aorta and circle the outer surface of the heart.

There are two major heart arteries: The right coronary artery supplies blood to the back (posterior) part of the heart, while the left coronary artery sends a branch to the front (anterior) section of the heart. These arteries are vital to the health of the heart. When blood flow through one of the coronary arteries is blocked for an extended time, the heart muscle can become deprived of oxygen. This lack of oxygen can cause the death of the cells that form the muscles of the heart. When this happens, it's called a *heart attack*.

A heart attack can occur when something — a blood clot, a narrow area, a plug of fatlike material — blocks a portion of one of the coronary arteries that supply the heart muscle with blood. Any condition that narrows the inside channel of the arteries is called *coronary artery disease*. When a portion of heart muscle dies, it reduces the heart's strength and its ability to pump precious blood to the body. The leading cause of coronary artery disease is *arteriosclerosis*, which is the hardening and blocking of blood vessels. Depending on the site of the blockage and the amount of muscle that dies, a heart attack can be extremely serious or relatively minor. You may hear the term *myocardial infarction* (sometimes simply abbreviated as *MI*) used by your physician when explaining a heart attack. This is the clinical term for heart attack.

Most heart attacks occur to people in their middle or later years, although they can occur at any time in life. When we are born, our blood vessels are healthy, open and clear of obstacles. As we age, the walls of the arteries become thickened, and deposits of fatty substances start to develop within the artery wall. The inner opening of the arteries begins to narrow. These deposits of fat create the condition called *atherosclerosis*. Depending upon the severity, they may block the heart's arteries completely. Although everyone has some degree of fatty buildup in their arteries, heart attacks occur only when the buildup completely blocks the arteries, or when a small blood clot that would not cause a problem in a healthy open artery gets jammed in a narrowed section and stops the flow of blood. A blood clot that causes a heart attack is called *coronary thrombosis*.

Atherosclerosis can develop silently; that is, with no symptoms until the day a heart attack occurs. In some people, however, narrowing of the coronary arteries causes recurring chest pain, called *angina pectoris*, or simply *angina*. This chest pain most often is felt during exercise or periods of emotional stress, but also may occur during rest. Angina generates a sensation of heaviness, pressure, burning or tightness in the chest and usually lasts only a few minutes, stopping when the activity is terminated or the emotional stress passes. Angina is not a heart attack, and many people who suffer with angina never develop a heart attack. However, in some cases, angina is merely a prelude to a real heart attack.

The root cause of atherosclerosis is *cholesterol*, a fatlike substance that is the main ingredient in the fatty plaques, or deposits, that develop within the artery walls. People who have high blood cholesterol levels are more likely to develop these trouble-provoking fatty clogs in their arteries. That is why much of the emphasis in preventive medicine is upon the dietary control of cholesterol. By reducing the amount of cholesterol in the diet, the amount of circulating cholesterol in the blood may also be reduced. The less cholesterol circulating in the blood, the less chance there is for it to become part of a plaque that clogs an important artery. The good news is that with proper management, cholesterol can be reduced to the point where the plaques also begin to become smaller and eventually disappear.

Questions and Answers

1. *I'm only a social drinker, one or two drinks at parties and the like, so don't think that I'm looking for permission to be an alcoholic. However, I keep hearing stories that alcohol is quite beneficial, especially in preventing heart attacks. But my wife says that's not proof enough. Does alcohol really help?*

In one manner or another, this question is asked many times, and I wish there were an absolute (pun intended!) answer to your question. Studies that span a period of more than 15 years, including a recently published article, all seem to show that moderate drinkers have less coronary artery disease than others.

That is good news about coronary artery disease, but the statistics do not consider the downside of drinking the same amount of alcohol, such as its connection with cancer and stroke. Nor do they include the number of people who start down the path of moderation and end up in serious difficulty.

The more than 20 million alcoholics in the United States today surely started with just a drink or two, and I would not be happy to think my words started anyone on that road. So let me put it this way: If you now have one or two alcoholic drinks a day, I think that is permissible. If you don't drink now, don't take this answer as permission to start.

2. ***I experience not only the pain that comes with angina attacks, but also the fear of what it means for my future. Would you please explain just what is meant by angina, and tell of its treatment? Your answer can do much to help me cope with my situation.***

A little information can remove the anxiety from angina. Angina pectoris is chest pain caused by poor blood supply to the muscles of the heart due to narrowed or clogged coronary arteries. When your heart is working harder than its blood supply can keep up with, the area of the heart that is short of oxygen reacts like any other overworked muscle and sends out pain messages. This pain usually makes a person stop and rest, which reduces the demand on the heart, and so the pain goes away.

If the blood supply becomes permanently cut off to a section of the heart, this is a myocardial infarction, or heart attack. Angina can lead to a myocardial infarction, but it can remain as a stable condition that does not get worse, without a true heart attack developing.

Most people with angina describe the pain as a squeezing or burning sensation or tightness of the chest. Some feel angina pain around the lower jaw, back of the neck or the middle of the back. They also may feel a sense of foreboding or doom. The pain is felt during exertion, such as walking or climbing stairs, during an emotional upset or after a heavy meal. The pain goes away quickly if you sit down and rest for a few minutes.

Angina is a serious condition, but it does not necessarily mean that a heart attack is imminent. (Angina pain that is prolonged may be a symptom of a heart attack.) Unfortunately, there is no good correlation between the amount of angina pain and the extent of heart disease.

After a complete and careful physical examination, cardiac angiography, in which X-rays are taken of your heart after an opaque dye has been injected into the coronary arteries, can provide a clear picture of the heart's blood supply.

Angina can be effectively treated with medications, including nitroglycerin or other nitrates, beta blocker agents and calcium channel blockers. These drugs are taken either regularly to limit the number and severity of attacks or when an angina attack starts. However, they do not cure the underlying condition. Angina also can be treated surgically with coronary bypass operations that replace the narrowed or clogged arteries.

3. ***I can tell that my heart doesn't always beat on time and seems to jump once in a while. I think there's a special name for that, but I would like to know why it happens.***

An irregular heartbeat is called an arrhythmia. There are many kinds, bearing different names and having different causes. Some are quite common, like a skipped beat or extrasystole, and do not have serious implications. Others require study for a precise diagnosis.

Your heartbeat is affected by many factors. Body temperature, exercise and emotional stress are just a few. Even things you eat can cause your heart rate to change. Stimulants like the caffeine in coffee, tea, chocolate and cola often have that effect. Internally, impulses and signals that travel along nerves from the spinal cord and brain to the heart can affect the rhythm, pace and power of the heartbeat.

If your heart is healthy, it speeds up and slows down daily to meet the needs of your body. There are, however, several heart conditions that may cause abnormal arrhythmias.

A heart attack, technically called myocardial infarction, often causes damage to heart tissue and may lead to arrhythmias. An irregular heartbeat is also common in patients with congestive heart failure, which is when the heart is not strong and does not pump enough blood through the body. Other heart diseases also can cause arrhythmias.

If you think you're having problems with arrhythmias, see a doctor. A simple test like an electrocardiogram will enable your physician to determine whether the arrhythmias you're having are commonplace or whether they require treatment.

4. *Would you please explain the surgical procedure known as angioplasty? My father's doctors are advising this operation for him, but we don't know enough about it. Please help us make a sound decision.*

Angioplasty is an effective treatment for coronary artery disease, where the coronary arteries — those blood vessels that bring nutrients to the heart itself — are partially or totally closed.

Angioplasty is accomplished by inserting a narrow balloon attached to a guiding catheter through the circulatory system to the affected coronary artery. The balloon is placed at the narrowest part of the artery and inflated at high pressure. The expansion of the balloon forces open the material that closed the artery, creating a wider channel for blood to flow through.

Benefits from angioplasty — as opposed to bypass surgery — are that it: does not require surgery; can improve the ability to exercise without heart-related pain; may increase the patient's so-called quality of life; can reduce pain caused by angina; requires a much shorter hospital stay than bypass surgery; and costs much less than bypasses.

Patients most likely to be considered for angioplasty include those: with coronary closings that have occurred within the past six months; who are also candidates for bypass surgery; who have closings in several separate parts of arteries — but not in major sections of those vessels.

Complications can happen during or after it; it is more dangerous for women, particularly for those over 65 years old who have had bypass surgery than for any other group; the arteries may close again at some point; and bypass surgery must be done if the angioplasty fails.

Nevertheless, angioplasty is a major advance in medicine. It gets safer and more practical as experience is gained in its applications.

5. ***Following a recent severe heart attack, my father developed an aneurysm in his heart. We've discussed the situation with his doctor, who is recommending surgery because of a gradual decline in Dad's condition. We have tried to study up on this condition but are becoming confused as we read of the same condition in the brain and aorta. Can you sort this out for our family?***

To start the sorting out process, let's define aneurysm. It comes from the Greek word that means "a widening," and, in fact, an aneurysm is a widening or sac formation in a weakened section of the wall of any artery, vein or the heart. Aneurysms occur most frequently in the portion of the aorta (the largest artery in the body) that passes through the abdomen. They're found less frequently in the heart, the major blood vessels of the chest and the brain.

In your father's case, a portion of the muscle of the heart died when he had his heart attack. The artery leading to this section of the heart wall had become blocked, probably by a blood clot, and the blood flow to the heart tissue stopped. Without the oxygen and nutrients carried by the blood, the heart tissue could not survive.

During the healing process, the dead heart muscle was replaced by a thin scar, without the necessary strength to contain the pressure that develops each time the heart contracts. It's probably this area that is now bulging outward with each beat, forming a sac or aneurysm. This, in turn, reduces the ability of the remaining heart muscle to perform the vital function of pumping the blood to the body. While the heart works harder to compensate, it uses more oxygen. If the supplies are inadequate, angina may develop or heart failure may rear its ugly head.

When the aneurysm is removed surgically, the efficiency of the heart is improved, angina disappears, and your father's general condition improves. Frequently, a cardiac artery bypass procedure is performed at the same time as the aneurysm is removed, to help improve the circulation to the heart.

In your reading, do not be confused by references to arterial aneurysms, where the walls of the vessels are weakened by progressive atherosclerosis, or to brain (or berry) aneurysms, which result from a congenital condition.

6. *When my doctor showed me the X-rays he had taken of my lower back, he pointed out some small white flecks, which he called "calcifications in the aorta." He said they probably didn't mean anything serious, but I want to be sure. Do you think they are serious?*

Many things can be seen when an X-ray is carefully studied that sometimes have no relation to the original reason for the study and may have no bearing on your state of health. The calcifications seen on your X-ray are the result of arteriosclerosis, frequently called "hardening of the arteries."

Although such a finding would require additional work-up and investigations in a man under the age of 45, it's considered a normal part of the aging process and may frequently be seen in older patients. As the arteries age, they weaken and develop plaques of atherosclerosis, in which calcium may be deposited over time. It's the accumulation of this calcium that created the small white flecks that were observed on the X-ray.

While there's no cause for alarm (and I'm sure that these flecks have nothing to do with your back problem), it would be wise to have a general checkup that might look at your overall condition and provide you with a further reassurance as to the insignificance of these findings.

7. *I'm confused about some terms used to explain heart trouble. I can't distinguish the difference between heart attack and MI. Are they the same thing? Can you please explain what causes a heart attack?*

Yes, these terms are used to describe the same problem and are often used interchangeably. The term heart attack is rather vague and is often misused and misunderstood.

A myocardial infarction (MI) starts with an obstruction in an artery that brings blood to the heart and results in the death of some of the heart muscle, which no longer can receive nourishment and oxygen. The obstruction can be caused by fatty deposits in the walls of the blood vessels or by injury to the walls of a hardened artery, which is followed by the formation of a blood clot.

This clot, in turn, reduces or cuts off completely the blood flow to the heart muscle, which then becomes injured and dies. The bigger the area that is without blood flow, the more severe the damage. The longer the blood flow is interrupted, the more damage that is caused. For this reason, heart attack victims who receive immediate medical attention have the best chance of recovery.

It's important that you know the symptoms of a heart attack and heed their warning. They may include pain or pressure in the center of the chest, often feeling like a belt is being tightened around the chest. Pain in the left arm, shoulder or jaw also may indicate a developing heart problem. Sweating, nausea, weakness, dizziness, shortness of breath or rapid heartbeats all should be promptly reported to your doctor.

The best treatments now available should be administered within the first half-hour of the attack. These medications can dissolve a newly formed clot and restore circulation to the suffering heart muscles.

8. ***I was told by my doctor that I'm mildly anemic. I started taking vitamins with iron, but after several weeks I'm still anemic. I now read that there is a type of bone marrow transplant that can be done. Do you think that I should ask to have this done to cure my anemia?***

Let me start with your anemia problem before I take this opportunity to discuss bone marrow transplantation. A mild anemia is not a serious condition, but a few weeks of multivitamin and iron supplements may not be sufficient time to see the problem resolved. Give yourself a chance. If the hemoglobin does not rise to desired levels, let your doctor take a few more tests to determine the cause of your particular anemia and prescribe some of the available remedies for the situation.

While you're correct in relating bone marrow to blood production, anemia is not one of the conditions for which bone marrow transplantation (BMT) is indicated. Bone marrow contains the special cells that form red blood cells (the kind that carry the hemoglobin) as well as white blood cells (WBCs) of several types and platelets (which play a major role in blood clotting). WBCs (neutrophils) belong to the immune system and provide the first line of defense against infections. Because the marrow produces so many cells, it's an area in which there is active and rapid growth, and the metabolism of the cells is high.

The main use of BMT is during the treatment of several types of cancer and leukemia. Both the chemicals used to fight the cancer and the radiation therapy that may form part of the treatment can damage the highly active bone marrow. Therefore the doses of both may sometimes be kept down to protect the sensitive marrow. These low doses may not always be totally effective against the cancer cells, whereas higher doses might do the complete job. In such cases, BMT becomes an important tool to replace active bone marrow.

Bone marrow for transplantation can come from one of three sources: It may come from the patient (autologous). It is removed (or harvested) before treatment starts, and stored until it is needed. Marrow from a twin is called syngeneic, while marrow from brothers, sisters or other family members or an unrelated donor is called allogeneic. The immunological makeup of the bone marrow must closely resemble that of the patient, a task that is not always easily accomplished. However, once the availability of a suitable supply is assured, the cancer treatment can be started.

During the days of chemotherapy and radiation therapy, the cancer cells are destroyed (one hopes), but the sensitive marrow cells also may be killed. In addition, the loss of the living marrow removes the body's own protection from infectious disease. The patient must be placed in protective isolation during this time and until the transplanted marrow has time to produce sufficient white cells to fight infection.

The marrow is placed into the body through intravenous catheters or tubes. Once in the bloodstream, these cells travel to the bone cavities where marrow normally grows and begin producing cells. This begins about 14 to 30 days following the transplantation. When the daily blood counts show that the circulating WBCs have reached sufficiently high levels, the patient may be discharged from the institution for continuing outpatient follow-up care.

9. ***Where did the term "blue blood" come from? It's a term a lot of people use, but no one seems to know where the expression originated. I know you like medical trivia questions, so I hope you can tell me.***

Blood vessels look blue when viewed through the skin, although they contain blood that is red. The lighter the skin, the more noticeable that blue shade is.

In the days of aristocrats and peasants, the peasants worked in the fields, becoming brawny and tanned, and the color of the blood vessels became obscured. Back at the palace, the aristocrats with white, translucent skin remained carefully protected from the sun's rays. It was easy to see their vessels as fine blue lines contrasting with the fairness of their skin.

Blue vessels meant blue blood to these folk, and thus aristocrats became known as Blue Bloods. The fact is their blood is no different from ours.

10. ***I bruise very easily, even when I haven't knocked myself or fallen. Except for being advised not to take aspirin, I have not gotten any satisfactory answers from any of the doctors I've seen. Can you help me?***

I'm not sure that my answer will please you any more than those of the other doctors, but I will be happy to tell you what I know about your situation. You're probably a sufferer of purpura simplex, the most common vascular bleeding disorder. It represents a situation where the vessels that carry the blood are more fragile than normal and break or rupture easily.

Most often we find this condition in women who complain of bruises on the thighs, buttocks and upper arms that seemingly have no cause. Sometimes the history may reveal that another family member has suffered from the same problem, but laboratory tests of the blood fail to show anything abnormal in the mechanisms that control clotting and coagulation.

There are no medications effective in controlling the condition, and because we know that aspirin and aspirin-containing medications can reduce the blood's clotting ability, many doctors advise avoiding this chemical, even in the absence of any real evidence that the bruising is caused by aspirin. The good news is that it is not at all a serious condition. Aside from producing some unsightly bruises, it will not affect your general health in any way.

11. ***What are the real facts about heart bypass surgery? I'm terrified of all surgery, but two doctors have already counseled me to seriously consider the operation. Couldn't I just take the right medications to correct my problem, without all the risks of surgery?***

Many factors help to determine if bypass surgery is appropriate in any case of heart disease: age, the specific anatomy of the patient's heart and the degree to which its functioning is impaired.

This form of surgery is now widely practiced and relatively low risk. Bypass surgery is usually appropriate if the symptoms of heart disease being experienced are life-threatening and significantly restrict your lifestyle, while not responding to medical therapy.

In most cases, the surgery relieves the painful angina experienced in heart disease, eliminating the need for medication to accomplish the same goal. Related emotional problems of anxiety, depression, fatigue and sleep problems also are alleviated. Bypass surgery is being performed on people in their 80s and 90s, with impressive long-term results. In one study comparing surgical vs. medical treatment for heart disease sufferers over 65 years of age, 62 percent of the surgical group were free of chest pain five years after treatment, while only 29 percent of the medical treatment group could make the same statement.

Coronary artery surgery also has been shown to increase a patient's life span. In another study, 88 percent of patients who underwent surgery were alive after four years, vs. 63 percent of a medical treatment group.

Several conditions fall under the heading of heart disease, and not all of them respond to bypass surgery. Cases of congestive heart disease do not respond to surgery as well as angina.

One major consideration in bypass surgery is how long the bypass grafts will remain open before narrowing occurs due to atherosclerosis. If the blood flow through these new, surgically implanted blood vessels becomes restricted, symptoms of angina can return and the individual again runs the risk of heart attack. According to studies, approximately 60 percent of these grafts are still effective 10 to 12 years after surgery.

If you're still undecided, ask your doctors to explain your condition and their recommended course of action in greater detail. If necessary, don't hesitate to seek a third opinion.

12. ***Although I have read of many types of tumors and cancers, I don't think I have ever heard of cancer of the heart. This would certainly be something that should receive study to increase knowledge of prevention. Could you discuss this?***

Though there is much to know about preventing cancer of the lungs and early detection of breast cancers for early treatment, there is a legitimate reason for little discussion of heart tumors. They are among the most uncommon tumors found in post-mortem examinations — in as little as 0.3 percent of them.

Primary tumors of the heart, which originate in the heart muscle itself, are for the most part benign tumors and do not spread to other parts of the body. The most commonly found growth is called a myxoma, or a tumor of the connective tissue.

The greatest danger with tumors growing in the heart is their ability to disrupt the flow of electrical impulses that control the rate and rhythm of the heartbeat. Myxomas also produce symptoms that include weight loss, fatigue, painful joints, fever and even a rash. When the tumors grow into the cavity of the heart, they also can interrupt the easy passage of blood through the heart.

While the study of any disease leads to knowledge that may help fight other illnesses, it's the major diseases, which affect many people, that receive the most attention, and that is as it should be.

13. *My increasing difficulty with breathing has been diagnosed as congestive heart failure. Now I face a whole bunch of tests and am worried that perhaps much of this is unnecessary. Do you think that a complete work-up is needed when the diagnosis is already worked out?*

Not only are your doctor's tests necessary, they may be critical in pinpointing your actual condition and saving your life. Congestive heart failure (CHF) can take either of two forms: a reduced level of cardiac performance not capable of meeting the needs of your body, or hypertension resulting from the aftereffects of a heart attack or chronic salt and water retention.

Chest radiography (standard X-rays) can uncover signs of hypertension and measure the amount of fluid retention taking place in the chest. The size and silhouette of the heart itself can be studied on the X-rays in order to diagnose specific types of heart disease.

Echocardiography uses sound waves to analyze the heart's function, particularly in cases where the organ is performing poorly. The activity within the different chambers of the heart can be studied individually, pinpointing the site of reduced function. The technology allows the doctor to compare the heart while pumping and at rest to determine its ejection fraction (which tells how much of the blood in the heart has been pumped out to the body). A lower-than-normal reading indicates that your heart has become weakened.

Refinements of the craft include two-dimensional echocardiography, in which the ultrasound beam reveals a cross section of the heart's activity, and doppler echocardiography to learn the blood flow rate. (Previously, a catheter had to be inserted into the heart to determine these findings.)

Based on preliminary findings, your doctor will determine which tests are appropriate to your situation. While follow-up tests may be called for to clarify a difficult diagnosis, they serve one purpose: to eliminate any doubt as to your best course of treatment, and to help assure your recovery.

14. *Is there such a thing as a clot dissolver? Would it be a good medicine to use if the patient were supposed to be having a heart attack? Is it very expensive?*

Yes, there are such medications. Technically, a heart attack occurs when one or more arteries that feed blood to the heart become blocked by a blood clot. The blood no longer can reach the heart muscle, and the cells die from lack of oxygen and nutrition. It's this dying process that provokes the pain of the heart attack.

Physicians attempt to break down that blockage and restore the flow of blood to the heart muscle by using medications called thrombolytics, or clot dissolvers. The sooner the medication is administered after the blockage, the less chance there is of damage to the heart muscle, and the size of the damaged area may be reduced.

This is a relatively new method of treating fresh heart attacks, and the rules are changing as time goes on. Although originally used only in the first few hours after the attack, the time limit is growing longer and longer as we find that patients may benefit from the medication as late as six to eight hours later.

And yes, it may be very expensive. The latest development in this area is a medication called a tissue plasminogen activator (TPA), which can effectively dissolve clots but may cost more than $2,000 for a single injection.

15. *Which is the more dangerous condition, fainting or syncope? My mother has had several fainting spells lately, which quickly passed. Her doctor told her she had syncope. I'm worried that this means something he is not telling her. I hope you can help me understand what may be wrong with mother.*

Syncope and fainting are the same. I could add the term swooning as well, for they all mean a sudden but temporary loss of consciousness. Syncope is not uncommon in older people, and it occurs when they have been sitting or lying down and then quickly stand up.

This causes the blood to pool in the lower parts of the body, reducing the amount of blood flowing to the brain. Since this decreases the amount of oxygen being carried to the brain, brain activity is altered and a loss of consciousness occurs. This usually results in the person dropping to the floor, and the head is once again on a level with the heart. Blood flow to the brain returns to normal and consciousness returns quickly.

For many people, that is the end of the episode with no damage done. However, when fainting episodes recur frequently, medical investigation is necessary to determine the cause, as the syncope may sometimes be a sign of problems with the heart.

Now to your mother's problem. Though fainting may occur as a result of emotional stress, coughing attacks, overexertion and heat exhaustion, it frequently is a result of a slowed or irregular heartbeat. Sometimes, lowered blood pressure can be brought about by certain prescription medication, such as diuretics and tranquilizers. Adjusting the dosage of a medication may rapidly reverse the situation.

Your mother may merely need to adjust the way she arises from a sitting position to put everything back in order. But she was wise to consult with her doctor. The only way to find out if information is being withheld from you is to ask the physician directly.

16. ***I've had a heart attack recently and I want to do all that's necessary to prevent another. However, my doctors' advice seems almost impossible to carry out, since it involves changing so many of the things I was doing before. Isn't there any simpler way to prevent heart attacks, a pill or something that is easier to swallow?***

I wish there were some simple way to prevent heart attacks or, for that matter, any disease or condition. I try to address these situations with only the knowledge gained from science, not mere wishful thinking. It may make my answer harder "to swallow," but at least you know where I'm coming from.

Your doctors are probably telling you that a variety of lifestyle changes are effective in reducing the chance of a recurrence of a heart attack. These changes include giving up tobacco, lowering your blood pressure, losing those extra pounds, changing your eating habits to lower your cholesterol and decrease the ratio of total cholesterol to the "good" high-density lipoprotein (HDL) in your blood, controlling stress and, finally, increasing your level of physical activity by starting an exercise program.

The evidence that reduction of such risk factors will reduce the chances of another heart attack, as well as the possibility of stroke or other cardiovascular disease, is quite clear. The problem is developing these actions into a program that you, as the patient, can accept and carry out. That means work on your part, which can be made easier if you develop the necessary attitudes and understand the reasons for each bit of advice.

Once you truly believe that the change in behavior will have a positive result for you, you must make a conscious decision to adopt that change and carry it through. When temptation comes knocking on your door, remember the importance of your newly adopted actions and resist.

While your physicians may counsel and advise you, and prescribe any medication necessary, the responsibility for lifestyle changes must be yours. I would be the last to tell you that this is all easy, but the importance of such actions is enormous. It all becomes clearer and simpler when you take a long, hard look at the alternative.

17. ***The doctor has diagnosed all my problems as relating to hardening of the arteries, and wants me to pay some real attention to lowering my cholesterol. I have my doubts that this diet is going to get me anywhere. Do you think it will do some good?***

Toward the end of World War I, a handful of European doctors noticed a decline in coronary heart disease. The same thing happened following World War II. Doctors speculated that this happy phenomenon was related to the relatively small amounts of meat and other fatty foods available because of wartime shortages.

Today, researchers using high-tech equipment are coming up with some pretty reliable evidence that people who lower their blood cholesterol levels with diet or drugs can stop heart disease in its tracks. For a small fraction of especially fortunate people, this kind of intervention even reverses the damage done, permitting partially blocked arteries to return toward normal.

The proof comes by way of contrast angiography, a method akin to X-ray, that allows us to view the coronary arteries. So far, the regression of coronary atherosclerosis has been documented in some 100 patients, and the disease has been stopped in many, many more.

The simplest and safest way to reduce blood cholesterol is via your diet. You will want to reduce not only the amount of cholesterol you take in, but also the amount of saturated fats. Beyond this, researchers find that a relatively high percentage of polyunsaturated fats in the diet helps keep blood cholesterol low. An ideal diet would consist mainly of cereals, legumes, fruits and vegetables, all rich in fiber. If you must have cheese, look for low-fat varieties; save regular cheese, meat, chocolate, candy and coconut for special occasions.

If diet doesn't do it, your doctor may want to prescribe a medication to lower your blood cholesterol level. Though many of these are extremely efficient, their mild side effects — constipation, heartburn, nausea, belching, bloating — probably will reinforce your resolve to stick to your diet! In addition, these drugs can be expensive, and we don't know the effects of their prolonged use.

To be fair, it must be said that some large studies have failed to show that diet reduces the incidence of coronary heart disease. But you will be pleased to know that researchers nonetheless estimate that for every 1 percent you reduce your blood cholesterol, you will reduce your risk of heart attack by 2 percent. Stay on that diet — you're on the right track.

18. ***I would like some information about hemochromatosis. Though I have finally been diagnosed as having this condition, no one I know has ever heard of it. Can you please tell me just how rare hemochromatosis is?***

Hemochromatosis is a genetic disease which, if left untreated, can advance to cirrhosis or liver cancer. It may be more common than was previously recognized. Recent studies in Europe, Australia and the United States show that it affects one in 300 people. It's most often found in people between the ages of 40 and 60, but it also has been detected in both younger and older people.

Diagnosis is often difficult because the disease can have a wide range of symptoms, or no symptoms at all. One of the most common signs is a bronze discoloration of the skin. Pituitary failure is not uncommon and may lead to atrophy of the testicles and loss of sex drive in males.

Because hemochromatosis is hereditary, people who have blood relatives with the disease may be at risk even if they have no symptoms. Screening tests to diagnose the disease include serum iron and total iron-binding capacity tests. If these results suggest the disease, a liver biopsy also may be useful.

Although there is no cure, hemochromatosis can be controlled. Treatment involves phlebotomy (removing blood to reduce the level of iron) on a weekly basis at first, and then every two to four months.

19. *My doctor suspects I suffer from an irregular heartbeat and wants to try something called "Holter monitoring" on me. Is this monitoring going to tell the doctor anything he doesn't know already? Frankly, I'm suspicious it's just another way for him to run his bill up.*

Holter monitoring is a standard medical technique used to help detect relationships between physical symptoms and cardiac irregularities. The technique has proven its worth in many situations, but has been found to be of little use in other cases.

Basically, a Holter monitor is a miniaturized, portable device attached to the body and designed to record an electrocardiogram over an extended period of time — from 24 hours on up. The advantages of having a daylong record of the heart's activity — and not just a brief reading from a visit to a doctor's office — are obvious.

Most units are equipped with an "event button" that the wearer can press when experiencing unusual sensations, such as lightheadedness or palpitations. The resulting cue mark on the tape is compared to the accompanying readings to see if any unusual heart activity took place at that time.

However, not all sensations experienced by the wearer correspond to actual changes in the heart's activity. The resulting recordings must be studied carefully by a trained technician in order to reveal relevant information.

Newer versions of the Holter monitor digitally summarize and store the highlights of the heart's activity, rather than keeping a total record on recording tape. These newer versions are less expensive but cannot provide as detailed information as the older units, and important details of the heart's activity may be omitted.

20. *If a chest pain can be either angina or a heart attack, does this mean they are both the same thing? I take nitroglycerin tablets for my angina. Is this all right? I don't want to be taking the wrong thing.*

Angina is chest pain caused by a lack of oxygen to the muscles of the heart. This occurs when there's a narrowing of the coronary arteries, which provide oxygen and nutrients to the heart muscles. This narrowing may be due either to a spasm of the artery walls or to atherosclerosis, which is the partial clogging caused by deposits of cholesterol.

Yes, angina may be related to a heart attack. In angina, the partial cutoff in blood supply to the heart usually reverses itself and the pain goes away; the heart muscle is not damaged. If the coronary arteries become completely closed off or blocked, then the area of the heart that no longer can receive oxygen or nutrients is permanently damaged and dies. And that is a heart attack.

Nitroglycerin tablets or preparations are commonly used to treat angina. If angina pain lasts more than 30 minutes and if taking nitroglycerin does not make the pain go away, get medical help immediately. Although angina may be a warning sign of a heart attack, many people who suffer from occasional angina never suffer a real attack. However, I'm sure you would agree that when in doubt the prudent action is to quickly obtain the medical care you may need.

21. ***Could you please discuss what doctors mean by an enlarged heart? It might be a good thing if it meant I were more generous, but I don't think my doctor believes that. Does it mean I have a tumor there?***

To answer the last part of your question first, it's doubtful that your doctor would use the term enlarged heart to describe a tumor. And tumors of the heart are fairly rare.

There is a difference between having a "big" heart and one that is enlarged. An enlarged heart first may be detected on physical examination, when the doctor finds that the beat of the heart is located farther out to the left side of the chest than it should be. A routine chest X-ray may confirm that first impression.

Basically the term enlarged heart may be used to describe two different situations. In one case, the muscles of the heart have become larger because of the work demanded from them. The walls of the chambers of the heart (essentially the ventricles that push the blood through the body and lungs) become thicker.

In the second case, the walls of these same chambers become weaker and thinner due to disease, perhaps of a heart valve, and become dilated (stretched outward). These conditions can be evaluated by electrocardiograms and other tests that help tell one from the other.

22. ***My physician says I have a heart murmur. He was very careful in examining me and taking all types of tests, including an electrocardiogram, and now assures me that I have nothing to worry about. I thought that murmurs were signs of heart disease. Could it be he's just being gentle with a 78-year-old man?***

Not at all. It sounds as if he has taken all the steps necessary to satisfy both you and himself of the reasons that provoke the sounds he detected.

Heart murmurs are merely sounds produced by the flow of blood through the chambers of the heart and around the valves of the heart that control the direction of blood flow. When the smooth flow is disturbed by changes in the structure of the heart or its valves, a turbulence is produced that generates a sound that can be heard through the stethoscope.

Not every murmur is caused by a serious disease or pathology. Many can occur with the changes in the heart configuration that age brings on and are not a cause for alarm. However, your family physician's reassurance is not based on chance or speculation, but on the test results that can be evaluated fully only when a complete examination and history have been accomplished.

The changes that affect the sounds your beating heart produces may occur in the lungs and chest wall as well as your heart, and may be affected by your posture. Some sounds can be heard more clearly when you're squatting or standing, as well as during deep inspiration and expiration.

It's only when all possibilities have been explored and carefully considered that a physician may reassure the patient, as in your case. He isn't just being nice, he has been careful, concerned and professional.

23. ***I'm a 44-year-old woman in reasonably good health, but a frequent chest pain prompted me to visit my doctor. The diagnosis of disease of my heart valves called a prolapse was both a surprise and a cause of anxiety. What are the implications of this heart disease for me? Will it require that I change my lifestyle?***

Mitral valve prolapse (MVP) is a common abnormality of one of the heart valves, the mitral valve. It's more common in women than in men, and can be found in 5 to 10 percent of our population. While most often discovered in adults, MVP may be a congenital situation, which means present at birth.

The mitral valve normally prevents the blood that goes into the heart from the lungs from flowing backward. The valve leaves are held in place by fine cords, and close each time the heart contracts.

If the valves are not formed properly or the cords are too long, the valves fail to close properly and some blood may leak backward. This causes a murmur or low sound to be produced, which along with the click of the improperly closing valves are the clues the physician hears when listening to your heart through the stethoscope.

Further tests with electrocardiogram, chest X-rays or echocardiogram (which uses sound waves to form a picture of the heart) may be used to confirm the diagnosis, although frequently the typical pattern of sounds and your general physical condition are enough to identify the condition.

In the majority of patients, MVP is not a serious condition. In fact, once the diagnosis has been confirmed and the patient is assured that no real dangers exist, the chest pain often disappears without additional treatment. Most patients are in no danger and have no symptoms. Even those patients who do have symptoms rarely have evidence of increasing heart damage.

Most probably, MVP will not require you to change your lifestyle or necessitate ongoing treatment. Only in the case of severe leakage is surgical repair considered. Your physician is in the best position to offer you personalized advice and consultation.

24. *Would you please give me a rundown of a condition called peripheral vascular disease? All I'm sure of is that it affects my arteries.*

Here is a case where the name of the condition does a fair job of describing its nature. The word peripheral applies to the outer portions of the body, thus the arms and legs.

Peripheral vascular disease (PVD) encompasses a number of long-term or chronic diseases of the arms or legs, which arise from the fact that the arteries that bring blood to these areas have become narrowed due to disease and fail to provide sufficient blood supply.

The most common cause of this narrowing is arteriosclerosis, which accounts for almost 95 percent of cases. Older people are the most common victims, as PVD usually strikes after the age of 50. Men are the sufferers six to seven times more frequently than women.

A high number of PVD patients are smokers (almost 90 percent), and about 25 percent of patients have diabetes. But our old enemies — high blood pressure, high cholesterol and high weight — do their share of the damage as well, causing arteriosclerosis not only in the peripheral arteries but in the vessels in the brain and heart as well.

The most common symptom of PVD is pain on effort, which grabs at the calves of the legs after a short stroll, but then eases up when the effort is stopped. Arms and legs feel cold, wounds take longer to heal and gangrene may develop in the final stages of the disease.

While your physician may prescribe medications to help the blood circulate and reduce cholesterol, there is much you must do for yourself. Smoking must go absolutely, and a regular walking program should be developed and carried out regularly. Good foot hygiene is a must: clean socks, comfortable shoes and attention to toenails, corns and calluses.

Surgical procedures exist to widen the arteries or replace those that are totally blocked, but you have a 75 percent chance of bringing the condition under control by following the advice offered by good medical care.

25. *What can you tell me about phlebitis? This situation has come up among some of my friends, and I'm worried. If phlebitis occurs in one vein, say on the leg, is it likely to occur in another place? What treatments are available for this condition?*

Phlebitis, or more precisely thrombophlebitis, is a condition in which a thrombus, or clot, forms in a vein. It's the second most common problem of the vein that brings a patient to a doctor's office. The first most common problem is varicose veins, which can be one of the factors that lead to thrombophlebitis. The clot can form on any of the many valves that exist within the vein, and most commonly occurs in the veins of the calf.

There are two types of phlebitis: deep vein thrombophlebitis (DVT), the more serious condition of the two, and superficial phlebitis. DVT may occur without any symptoms at all, or with variable combinations of pain, tenderness, swelling and discoloration. The superficial variety usually can be felt with the fingers and produces an inflammatory reaction. This is revealed by pain, tenderness, redness and warmth in the area.

Thrombophlebitis can be the result of any prolonged bed rest required by a chronic disease, such as heart failure, stroke or the trauma of an accident. Even a healthy person can fall victim to phlebitis after a long trip, during which the legs remain immobilized in a pendent position for a long time.

While deep vein thrombosis may lead to death due to the passage of the clot to the lungs, superficial thrombophlebitis usually provokes no serious complications. Therefore, the treatment of DVT is intense, using medications (heparin or coumadin) that prevent the blood from clotting.

By comparison, superficial phlebitis requires only reducing the discomfort. Hot soaks over the clot, plus nonsteroidal anti-inflammatory drugs (NSAIDs) are all that is necessary; neither hospitalization nor antibiotics are indicated.

The presence of a phlebitis in one leg is not usually associated with clots in any other part of the body, nor an indication that these clots may reoccur. However, if varicose veins are considered to be a part of the problem, the use of elastic stockings or even surgery may be considered.

26. ***Fifteen years ago, my husband was hospitalized and diagnosed with polycythemia, no cure. Since that time, he has had to have one unit of blood withdrawn four times yearly. They say bloodletting is the only solution to his problem. I would appreciate another opinion.***

Polycythemia vera is a disease in which all of the elements of the bone marrow grow at a more rapid rate than normal and in which we see an increase in the mass of the red blood cells and hemoglobin.

About 7 million people suffer from polycythemia vera. The average age at onset for patients is about 60 years old. The disease is seen more in males than in females. The complaints of these patients include fatigue, difficulty in concentration, headache, drowsiness and forgetfulness, and even dizziness. About half of them suffer from itchy skin, particularly after a hot bath.

Most patients' skin color is normal, but when the physician examines the vessels at the back of the eye, the veins are dark red and full, betraying the presence of a high level of red cells. In general, the spleen also is palpable on physical examination. In spite of all of this, however, some patients suffer from no symptoms at all.

All the textbooks stress that phlebotomy (bloodletting) is part of the management of every polycythemia patient. This relatively simple procedure keeps most patients symptom-free and maintains the levels of hemoglobin as well as the number of red cells within normal limits.

It's only when the condition cannot be controlled with occasional blood removals that other drugs are used in conjunction with phlebotomy. Most of these medications are still under study and are difficult to administer because they must be individualized for each patient.

27. ***My sister has a strange problem in which her fingers sometimes turn blue. She says it's called Raynaud's phenomenon. Her doctor has prescribed medication and has told her that she can help herself prevent some of the attacks. What can I encourage her to do and not to do?***

Raynaud's phenomenon is usually brought on by exposure to cold or by emotional stress. The typical patient is female, between the ages of 15 and 50 years old. An attack usually begins with one finger becoming very cold and sensitive. It may progress to the entire hand and even the other hand.

At first, the involved fingers may turn red, then blue. This results from an abnormal narrowing of the arteries and arterioles in the fingers. As a response to the cold stimulus, they're undergoing vasospasm, or contracting in a manner that diminishes the normal blood flow to the tissue.

Raynaud's disease may be differentiated from secondary Raynaud's phenomenon by affecting both sides of the body, being symptomatic for two years without becoming worse, and showing no evidence of underlying causes.

Raynaud's phenomenon often is associated with other problems, so it's imperative that the patient get a thorough examination. Diseases such as arthritis, systemic lupus erythematosus or scleroderma may be associated with this problem. In fact, any problem that affects the body's connective tissues, blood vessels, skin, tendons and joints may lead to a greater susceptibility to Raynaud's phenomenon.

In addition to medication, there are a lot of precautions your sister can take to limit her Raynaud's attacks. If she's a smoker, she must quit. Smoking is a contributing factor to this problem, because it tends to narrow the blood vessels. In her case, she is already suffering from an abnormal and exaggerated response to stimulation that narrows blood vessels. To continue this habit is to ask for the problems and complications that far outweigh any possible satisfaction gained from smoking.

Raynaud's patients should avoid drugs that cause blood vessels to narrow. Included on this list are birth control pills and some heart, blood and migraine headache drugs.

Above all, Raynaud's patients should keep warm. Extra precautions include keeping all rooms in their homes warm at all times, and using electric or thermal blankets, or a heated waterbed. Whenever removing food from a freezer, Raynaud's patients should use potholders or hand mitts. They should wash dishes and vegetables in tepid or warm water. They should wear gloves or mittens even on short trips outdoors, such as going to the mailbox. The best way to always remember the gloves is to have an extra pair near the door.

When going out in cold weather, Raynaud's patients should wear layered clothing. In addition to keeping the hands covered, they should make sure the wrists are covered and kept warm. And when taking walks, they should stay on the sunny side of the street.

28. *I don't understand all that I read and hear about risk factors. It would seem that some people are just made so they can't help but develop high blood pressure (HBP), while others change their ways and escape. I am at an age where all of this is suddenly most important to me and wonder if you could shed some light on the subject.*

Risk factors are the result of statistical analysis of the elements that are present in people who do show elevated blood pressures. The more risk factors present in your personal or family history, the greater the chance is that you, too, will develop the condition.

However, it's really not that cut and dried. Some people with many risk factors never develop any signs of blood pressure elevation, while others who seem free of identifiable factors have higher than normal readings.

It becomes simpler to understand when you divide the factors into two kinds: those you can't change (called uncontrollable risk factors) and those that may be lessened by actions that you can take (controllable risk factors).

In the uncontrollable category, there are four headings:

- Heredity. Present when your parents or other close members of your family have a history of high blood pressure.
- Race. For reasons that are still poorly understood, a higher percentage of black Americans develop HBP than white Americans.
- Sex. Women before menopause are slightly less at risk than men; after menopause they catch up quite rapidly.
- Age. The older you are, the greater your chances of developing HBP.

It's in the controllable category that you find the things you can do something about, and where the greatest educational emphasis is placed. Here there are seven headings:

- Weight. The more your weight exceeds the normal for your height, the greater the chance of HBP. Lowering your weight to normal actually can reduce your blood pressure.
- Alcohol consumption. Yes, I also have heard that a drink is good for the circulation and digestion, but statistics prove that regular, excessive drinking can increase blood pressure.
- Sodium. In some people who are sensitive to the amount of sodium they consume (present in table salt and other foods and medicines), blood pressure rises when salt is taken in excess of the body's needs.

- Smoking. The nicotine in tobacco smoke causes the small blood vessels in the body to squeeze down (contract), which results in increased blood pressure.

- Oral contraceptives. Some women are sensitive to this medication, which results in their developing HBP. Smoking and birth control pills together make for a very high risk factor.

- Repressed anger. People who hold a lot of anger inside and are constantly frustrated with their situations tend to have more heart and blood pressure problems.

- Sedentary lifestyle. When the heart, blood vessels and muscles are not exposed to regular exercise, they lose their tone and HBP may result. In addition, lack of activity contributes to weight gain.

With all the indications in the controllable category, it's easy to understand how some people manage to overcome their tendency to develop HBP and improve their odds. The payoff is not only a reduction in heart problems and an increased life span, but also a life that is more than a mere existence — a life that is enjoyable, rewarding and fun to live.

29. *What is a blood sed rate, and what is normal? What determines the rate, and how can it be changed? I'm eager to know about this mysterious condition and will appreciate any enlightenment.*

The sed rate, which is technically the erythrocyte sedimentation rate (ESR), measures the rate that red blood cells settle, or sediment, in an anti-coagulated sample of venous blood. There is little sedimentation in normal blood, because the red cells have only a slightly heavier density than the blood plasma.

The sed rate varies with the age and sex of the patient. It's also affected by smoking, pregnancy, menstrual cycle, abnormal red cell shapes and other factors. In normal men, the red cells drift down at a rate of between 1 and 13 millimeters (one-twenty-fifth and one-half inch) per hour. Women may show a rate of between 1 and 20 millimeters (one-twenty-fifth and four-fifths of an inch) per hour, and still be considered normal.

The test has been used to screen for numerous diseases, including infections and acute and chronic inflammations. It also can be used as a screening tool in patients with nonspecific problems or systemic disease.

Repeated ESR testing also may allow doctors to monitor disease activity, helping them to track the progress of a disease and determining whether things are getting better or worse by noting significant increases or decreases in the sed rate. For example, in such diseases as temporal arteritis and polymyalgia, a normal ESR is very rare, but repeated sed rate testing done over a period of time allows doctors to monitor disease progression.

It's important to realize that the ESR is merely a test, useful for evaluating and following various conditions. ESR is not a disease in and of itself. Although it was once an important study of great help in making a diagnosis for many patients, it's less so these days because of the development of so many new and more sensitive tests. Still, in some cases, it remains a very valuable tool.

30. ***I suffer from a sick sinus in my heart, which may mean that I must have a pacemaker put in to keep my heart beating. I need to know all I can about this. I thought sinuses were in your nose. Can you tell me about this sinus in my heart?***

Though the words are the same, the anatomical structures are quite different. Sinuses in the head are open spaces in the bones of the head. The sinus in the heart, called the sinus node, is made up of cells that are responsible for kicking off the nerve impulses that control the beat of your heart. These impulses travel along a conduction system within the heart and assure that the rhythm and sequence of the heart muscle contractions will propel the blood through the heart and thus through the entire body.

The sick sinus syndrome (SSS) is a condition in which the system of impulse formation and conduction fails to operate properly, slowing the heartbeat or reducing its effectiveness. It's most common in patients over the age of 60 and is the reason for placing about half of the permanent pacemakers in use in the United States. There are a number of diseases that can cause SSS, including situations where the blood flow to the heart is reduced, infections of the heart and rheumatic heart disease.

31. ***My mother has been taken to the hospital several times because her heart suddenly starts beating out of control. She called it "tack" something and said that her heartbeat was 200 times per minute. Could you please tell me more about this disease? What should she do?***

Your word "tack" comes from the Greek *tachy*, which means swift. The name of the medical condition is tachycardia, or the rapid beating of the heart.

Generally this term is applied to any heart rate of more than 100 beats per minute. There are many types of tachycardia, depending upon their cause, which is usually determined by carefully examining the heart and evaluating the electrocardiogram (ECG).

When the condition starts suddenly without warning, it's called paroxysmal. The patient may feel faint and weak but rarely passes out completely. The patient should lie down immediately and remain calm and quiet to offset the effects of a lowered blood pressure that may be present during the attack of this rapid heartbeat.

A number of techniques called vagal maneuvers may be attempted by trained personnel to break the rapid rhythm. The patient may attempt a forcible exhaling effort against a firmly closed mouth and glottis (part of the vocal apparatus) to increase the pressure in the chest area (Valsalva's maneuver), or the carotid sinus, located on the side of the neck, may be massaged.

I stress this should be attempted only by trained personnel while the heart is being monitored by an ECG. Frequently this is all that is required to restore the heartbeat to normal.

When these techniques are unsuccessful, various medications, including verapamil or edrophonium, may be used. Digoxin also may be used when emergency treatment fails. And it's possible to return the beat to normal using electrical stimulation (electrical cardioversion).

Although this condition may be seen in younger people with no evidence of heart disease, in older people arteriosclerotic cardiovascular disease may be present.

32. *I'm a Type A personality — I admit it. In fact, I enjoy the rushing and competitiveness. Unfortunately, a friend tells me I'm a good candidate for a heart attack. I can't believe this, especially since I feel so good.*

Some 20 years ago, Drs. Mayer Friedman and Ray Rosenman sketched out the Type A personality: someone who does many things at once, takes on too much work, moves quickly, hates waiting, can't relax, interrupts, angers easily and is competitive.

Ever since then, cardiology has never been the same. This seemingly definitive list has raised as many questions as it has answered: Why exactly would Type A behavior lead to heart attack? Do some Type A characteristics count more than others? And most important, is there any way a Type A person can change into a more relaxed Type B?

Researchers speculate that it's the high levels of the hormones adrenaline, cortisol and testosterone found in young Type A men that contribute over time to a narrowing of the coronary arteries. But this still is unproven. Another question mark is whether these hormone changes are a result of Type A behavior or a cause of it.

We now know more about which Type A characteristics count most heavily. Some studies show that hostility and anger are far more reliable predictors of heart disease than any other Type A characteristics. This is good news indeed for people like you who are competitive, hurried and so forth, without being angry. It may well be that Type A behavior has its good and its bad components.

Even Type A's who are angry may not be headed for heart trouble. Hostility has been linked with coronary artery disease in younger people only. The theory here is that the older, hostile Type A's are a hardy bunch who have avoided heart disease, while the more vulnerable people in their age group succumbed to it prematurely.

Finally, the best news: It's possible to change Type A behavior through counseling. Patients learn that hostility and anger are likely to be harmful to their hearts and are trained in heading off these negative emotions. Of course, if Type A behavior turns out to be the result of hormone imbalances or other physical causes, counseling will help only temporarily. Researchers are working to discover whether drugs can control Type A behavior, and a few early experiments have hinted that they can.

33. ***My legs look terrible, as they are crisscrossed with many unsightly varicose veins. I understand that a treatment is available that does not require surgery for the removal of the veins. Do you know of any such treatment? How does it work?***

I think you're alluding to a type of treatment called compression sclerotherapy, which is useful for treating superficial varicose veins.

A sclerosing solution is used to thicken the walls of the vein and obliterate it, causing it to collapse. The solution, composed of 3 percent sodium tetradactyl sulfate, is injected into the veins. Anywhere from three to ten injections can be made into each leg. After the injections, the leg is tightly bandaged. These bandages are removed only after the medication has had a chance to act.

If the varicose veins are small and not too prominent, many people are satisfied with the results obtained from surgical elastic stockings, which can control varicose veins in many individuals. Using these stockings properly — putting them on each morning while still in bed, when the veins have diminished during the night, and wearing them faithfully all day, every day — may be just enough to allow the veins to return to normal size and function. These stockings are frequently used after most types of treatments for varicose veins to help in healing and maintaining good results.

Incidentally, even with surgical stripping, where varicose veins are actually removed, between 33 and 45 percent of patients will need additional treatment using compressive sclerotherapy for residual or recurrent varicose veins. Although the cosmetic results in each of these procedures may not be all you desire, treatment can prevent the condition from progressing.

34. *My doctor says I have something called Wolfe-Parkinson-White syndrome. Could you please explain πthis for me, and also tell me how it will affect me? I'm a 58-year-old woman.*

It's amazing how many clinical practitioners retain the use of such names for medical conditions, but perhaps it's understandable when you know that the descriptive name for your condition is anomalous atrioventricular excitation. That is not much help either in trying to understand the meaning of a condition that, in many people, provokes no symptoms.

Wolfe-Parkinson-White syndrome (WPW) is the result of a congenital variation in the heart conduction system. Instead of the impulses passing through a junction point in the system called the A-V node, they bypass this control by using a second conduction pathway, which is not usually present in most people, and arrive at the ventricle of the heart before the normal impulses. This can provoke the abnormal beating of the heart.

The diagnosis is made by examining an electrocardiogram, which may have been taken during a routine annual examination, or was used to seek an explanation for an episode of rapid heartbeat (paroxysmal tachycardia), which can occur in about 10 percent of people with this syndrome.

Usually these episodes resolve themselves, and the condition is considered benign. When these abnormal rhythms continue, medication such as propranolol or procainamide can be used.

When the presence of another abnormal beat, atrial fibrillation, complicates the treatment of the disease, an operation to cut the abnormal pathway may be considered. However, the odds are all in your favor, with the chances being that this condition may never cause you any inconvenience at all.

35. ***I have been on medicine for my hypertension for a long time. It's a pill called a water pill, and my old doctor was satisfied with the results. I moved and changed physicians, and my new doctor advised me to use another medication, because these water pills raise cholesterol and could be bad for me. Do you have an opinion about this?***

I have opinions about most things, but unfortunately, according to my wife, they're not always correct. On the question of diuretics (a fancier name for water pills), however, there's much controversy and disagreement.

According to recent studies, it does seem clear that diuretics have a negative effect on fats (lipids) in the blood. They raise the level of cholesterol as well as increase the low density lipoprotein (LDL — the "bad one"), but they don't increase high density lipoprotein (HDL — the "good one"). In addition, diuretics seem to lower insulin sensitivity, which could increase the risk of developing diabetes in some individuals.

However, physicians with a favorable opinion about diuretics claim there is no proof that the effects on cholesterol remain true over the long haul, or that the changes in insulin sensitivity are clinically significant.

Many physicians believe that the newer medications for hypertension — beta blockers, calcium channel blockers and angiotensin converting enzyme inhibitors (ACE inhibitors for short) — are medications that should be used in the initial treatment of the condition. And there is good proof to support that position as well.

In individual cases, it's the patient's personal history and physical condition that may lead the physician to consider the use of one type of medication over the other. It may be unwise to use a diuretic in a patient who already has an elevated cholesterol, or is a diabetic depending upon insulin to manage that condition.

As in so many situations in medicine, it takes a complete knowledge of the patient and concern for his or her well-being to make a decision of this nature. Find out why your doctor is advising a change in a medication you seem to be satisfied with, and participate in the decision based upon your new knowledge.

2.

The Lungs and Respiratory System

That ever death should let life bear his name, where life hath no more interest but to breathe.

WILLIAM SHAKESPEARE
Titus Andronicus

Many people equate the lungs with the entire respiratory system, but nothing could be further from the truth. While they are the most important organ in this impressive system, the lungs could not perform their function without the respiratory system's other parts.

Anatomically, the structures of the respiratory system include the nose, the throat, the ***larynx***, the ***bronchial tree*** (including the ***bronchi*** and ***bronchioles***) and finally the lungs. Of course, the mouth, which is normally considered a part of the digestive system, also can play an important role in breathing when the nasal passages become clogged. The whole system couldn't function without the ***diaphragm*** — a large sheet of muscle that separates the chest cavity from the abdominal cavity and is part of the musculoskeletal system.

The role of the respiratory system is to get oxygen (constituting about 20 percent of the air we breathe, the rest being mostly nitrogen) into the body, to provide a mechanism for transferring the oxygen over to the circulatory system, and then to rid the body of unwanted carbon dioxide (CO_2) and water. Both CO_2 and water result as waste products from the processes of metabolism, which creates the energy the body needs from the fuels we provide by eating and breathing.

Answers from the Family Doctor (Questions 36-65)

The act of breathing is called *respiration* and the process can be divided in three separate parts: Inhaling air, or breathing in, is called *inspiration*, followed by exhaling, or breathing out, called *expiration*. Then, there is a short rest period before the process begins again. Normally, when we are sitting, or are not active, respiration will occur from 12 to 17 times a minute, each time drawing in about one-half liter (about one-half quart) of air. However, during periods of intense exertion, such as strenuous exercise, the rate can increase to as much as 40 times a minute, and each inhalation can contain nearly five liters (about five quarts) of air.

Let's put the breathing machine into motion and see how all of the parts work together. First, the diaphragm contracts, flattening out as it moves down, out of the *chest cavity*. At the same time, the *intercostal muscles*, which are located between the ribs, also contract. The action of these rib muscles is to move the ribs up and out, which together with the diaphragm's contraction, increases the space within the chest cavity. That reduces the air pressure, so the outside air rushes in to fill the larger space and equalize the pressure.

The air flows through the nose, where it's warmed a bit and moistened. The nostril hairs serve to filter some of the larger particles in the air. The *mucous membranes* that line the nose help moisten and warm the air, in addition to trapping some of the dust and bacteria that may enter with each inspiration. The air then passes to the back of the throat, past the tonsils and adenoids, and continues for a short distance in the *pharynx* (throat) before it turns off past the *larynx* (voice box) and to the *trachea* (windpipe).

The trachea divides into two main bronchi (tubelike structures): one that goes to the left lung and the other to the right. These are the beginnings of the right and left bronchial trees, which — just as other trees in nature — begin to divide, giving off ever smaller branches called bronchioles. The bronchi are lined with a special tissue, coated with mucus and covered by constantly moving hairlike structures called *cilia*. These cilia catch the particles of dust and debris in the air, as well as many of the bacteria, and sweep them upward, out of the bronchi to the throat. There the material is coughed out, sneezed out or just swallowed, but most importantly, it doesn't get to lodge in the delicate tissues of the lungs.

The air continues its journey through ever-dividing bronchioles, which become narrower and narrower, ending up in spongelike sacs composed of groups of *alveoli*, which are lined by a thin layer of cells. There are about 300 million alveoli lining the lungs. If we could spread them out, they would cover a space 50 times greater than our skin, or about 70 square meters (84 square yards). A single alveolus fills and empties about 15,000 times in the course of a single day's breathing. The bronchi, bronchioles, alveoli and surrounding tissues form the organ we call the lung. Part of the surrounding tissue is composed of a framework of strands of fibrous tissue, which serve to support the bronchioles and keep them open.

The left lung differs from the right lung in that it is a bit smaller and consists of only two lobes. The larger right lung has three lobes. The lungs surround the heart and the large blood vessels that carry blood to and from the heart. Behind the heart and between the lungs lies the *esophagus*, the long tube that carries food from the mouth to the stomach. All of these organs are contained within the protective housing formed by the spine at the back and the ribs curving around to attach to the *sternum* (breastbone) in the front. This whole structure is called the chest cavity, or the rib cage if you will.

The lungs are covered by a special tissue called the *pleura*. This is composed of two membranelike layers: one layer that surrounds the lungs, and the other that lines the inside of thc chest cavity. Between the two, there is a small amount of fluid that serves to lubricate the tissues to reduce the friction and allow the lungs to move freely within the chest cavity. When too much fluid is present, due to an infection or inflammation, it is called *pleurisy*.

Within the lung, embedded in the surrounding structure of the supportive tissues, is a most important element in the working of the lungs, the network of millions of very fine *capillaries*, which are the smallest structures of the circulatory system. These capillaries are a single-cell thick here — so narrow that only a single red cell can pass through at a time, and the blood flow is limited to red cells moving along in single file. Each alveolar sac is surrounded by these capillaries. It is here that the first process necessary for the real function of respiration takes place.

Respiration is actually defined as the process by which the body uses oxygen in the *metabolism* of the body, which creates the energy needed and involves the production of CO_2.

The *red cells*, which form about 40 percent of the blood volume, contain *hemoglobin* — a chemical compound that gives the red blood cells their color and has the ability to grab onto the oxygen atoms contained in the air. There are about 25 billion red cells in one teaspoon of blood. When hemoglobin combines with oxygen, it turns a brighter red, which is the color associated with arterial blood. The red cells filled with oxygen-rich hemoglobin pass through the circulatory system and carry their important cargo to all parts of the body. There the constant process of metabolism is taking place, converting food into energy. The metabolic process requires oxygen, and so it is here the hemoglobin releases the oxygen. In exchange, the blood picks up the waste products that are formed by the energy-forming reactions, namely CO_2 and water vapor. The hemoglobin now turns to a darker color, a deep reddish-purplish, giving blood the hue we associate with venous blood. It then returns by way of the circulatory system to the lungs.

Gases are exchanged by a process known as *diffusion*, which is when a gas passes from an area of higher concentration to one of lower concentration. The inspired air is rich in oxygen but very low in CO_2. In contrast, the hemoglobin in the blood returning to the lungs from the body's tissues and organs now carries an increased load of CO_2 and a very reduced amount of oxygen. So in the brief moment when the blood passes through the capillaries surrounding the alveoli — less than a second — the hemoglobin gives up its burden of CO_2 in exchange for a new cargo of oxygen. Thus, though the inspired air contained 20 percent of oxygen and only 0.3 percent of CO_2 on the way in, it leaves with only 16 percent of oxygen and about 4 percent of CO_2. The air we breathe out is also saturated with water vapor. The body will lose about a liter (about a quart) of water a day in the air that is exhaled.

Now it is time for this "used air" to leave the body. The diaphragm relaxes and moves back up into the chest cavity. The intercostal muscles relax, allowing the ribs to move down and back. These two actions reduce the space in the chest cavity, increasing the pressure in the chest cavity and squeezing down on the flexible lung tissue. This forces the air out of the lungs, back through the bronchial tree and trachea to exit the body by way of the nose or mouth.

On the way out, the current of air moves over the vocal cords located in the larynx. Normally the vocal cords remain open and still during breathing. But when they're drawn closer by the muscles that control them, the passing air will cause them to vibrate. That movement creates the sounds we use to speak and sing, and of course, scream and yell. The more the muscles contract, the tighter the cords become and the higher the pitch of the resulting sound will be. But the control of speech and language is the responsibility of the brain. And that subject matter is for another chapter.

Questions and Answers

36. ***I still smoke around the house, though certainly less than before. My wife literally screams at me each time she smells even a bit of smoke, and says that not only am I killing myself, but I'm ruining her health as well. How could this be? Is there any truth to my wife's opinion?***

I believe your wife probably has done some reading that you haven't, for there have been many investigations into the effect of smoke on people who breathe in these secondhand fumes.

A draft report from the Environmental Protection Agency was reviewed by a panel of scientists who concluded that secondhand cigarette smoke caused about 3,800 cases of lung cancer. And it is felt that the risk to children may be even more overwhelming.

There arc many effects from breathing in the smoke from someone else's cigarette (sometimes called passive smoking), and perhaps outlining them for you may help you deal with your wife's ire.

Smoke is an irritant that can affect the eyes, throat and nasal passages, causing tearing and sneezing. From there the smoke is absorbed into the bloodstream through the membranes of the nose and throat. In the bloodstream, the smoke is picked up by red blood cells, reducing their ability to carry oxygen. This causes the heart to work harder as it tries to make up for the deficiency. The chemicals in the smoke can injure cells inside the blood vessels, which speeds the formation of fatty plaques, which are the primary cause of blockage.

In the lungs, the smoke particles cause irritation that provokes the production of excess mucus. Indirectly these same particles may cause damage to the walls of the alveoli (the tiny sacs in the lungs), through which oxygen passes into the bloodstream. This reduces the efficiency of the lungs, requiring more effort to breathe. And all of this occurs in someone who is breathing your smoke secondhand. Can you imagine what is going on inside *your* body?

37. ***They've discovered asbestos in the walls of my plant. They're removing it all, but I would like to know what are the chances that I've suffered a medical problem. Can you tell me what risks I may have run?***

In recent years, the full picture on asbestos has begun to emerge. What was once thought of as a simple insulation and fireproofing agent has turned out to be a highly carcinogenic (cancer-causing) substance, particularly when its fibers break down and particles of the material float free in the atmosphere.

Exposure to asbestos increases the risks of developing asbestosis, which is a chronic lung ailment resulting in shortness of breath and permanent lung damage, as well as dangerous lung infections. A variety of cancers also have been associated with asbestos, including lung cancer, mesothelioma (affecting the membranes lining the chest and abdomen) and cancers of the larynx, stomach, colon, rectum and esophagus.

It's impossible to give you a simple yes or no answer without conducting a thorough physical examination, including a chest X-ray and lung function tests. Specialists trained in evaluating such information would examine the results to develop a prognosis.

Complicating the picture is the fact that asbestos-related diseases take a surprisingly long time to develop — in cases of lung cancer, usually 15 years and often between 30 and 35 years following exposure. In cases of mesothelioma and asbestosis, the delay can be as long as 40 to 45 years.

By all means, check with your doctor, company or union health office immediately. If the asbestos insulation currently being removed was relatively intact and not flaking or decaying, you're probably at lower risk.

If you're a smoker, this is yet another good reason to kick the habit. Exposure to both tobacco and asbestos multiplies the impact each has on the body; smokers heavily exposed to asbestos are 90 times more likely to develop lung cancer than non-exposed non-smokers.

38. ***My friend has black lung and I would like to know how this disease is like — or perhaps different from — emphysema. There is emphysema in my family, and so now I'm trying to learn as much as I can about both of these lung conditions.***

This interesting condition received its name because of the color of the lungs found on post-mortem examination in patients with the disease. Black lung is one of a number of similar conditions grouped together under the classification of Occupational Lung Disease.

Black lung also is known as coal workers' pneumoconiosis (CWP) or anthracosis. In this condition, coal dust is inhaled into the lungs where it becomes trapped, forming "coal macules" around the bronchi of the lungs.

Coal is not one of the dusts that lead to the excessive formation of fibrotic or scarlike tissue in the lungs, and so the structure and function of lung tissue is not greatly disturbed. However, in some cases the accumulation of the dust causes the bronchioles to dilate, giving rise to the name focal dust emphysema. But in contrast to emphysema, this condition doesn't cause obstruction to the airflow and doesn't involve the alveoli (air sacs) of the lung.

A complication of CWP, which occurs in about 1 to 2 percent of miners, is known as progressive massive fibrosis. This condition can cause extensive lung damage and associated symptoms. In many cases, the disease is complicated by emphysema and obstructive lung disease from such causes as smoking.

Another related disease known as silicosis is the result of breathing in particles of silica dust, and is seen in such industries as hard coal mining, lead, copper, gold and silver mining, as well as in foundries, pottery making, and sandstone and granite cutting. Fibrosis or scarring of the lung may be extensive, and breathing problems, coughing and sputum production are considerable.

There are no cures for these diseases, and treatment is directed at improving the flow of air and reducing the amount of secretions that are present in the lung.

39. *I know doctors use telescopes to look into your bowels and stomach. However, my problem lies within my lungs, and my doctor has suggested the same procedure to look into my lungs. Can that be done?*

Those aren't telescopes, they are endoscopes. And yes, there is a special endoscope for looking into the throat and lungs. A bronchial endoscope, or bronchoscope, uses optical fibers to view the lungs, the throat, the voice box and the windpipe. It also can remove foreign objects or take a small sample of tissue for analysis.

You can undergo bronchoscopy either as a hospital patient or as an outpatient. Before the test, you'll be given a medication to relax you and to reduce secretions in your lungs. While you lie on a table, your doctor will spray your nose and throat with a local anesthetic and insert the tube through either your nose or mouth. Breathe slowly and try not to cough. Although your throat will feel full, you will still be able to breathe around the bronchoscope.

The test will provide your physician with a great deal of very important information about your lungs that can be important in establishing the correct therapy for your condition.

40. ***I'm trying to find out everything I can about bronchiectasis. My doctor mentioned that I might have this. He seems to think there isn't much that can be done about it. I would like your opinion.***

Bronchiectasis is a condition that may develop at any age, frequently beginning in childhood, although the symptoms may not become apparent until later in life. The bronchi are part of the system of tubes that carries the air from the mouth and nose to the alveoli, or tiny grapelike clusters of sacs that transmit the oxygen to the bloodstream while retrieving carbon dioxide.

In bronchiectasis, the condition may be congenital (rare) or acquired. The acquired form may result from a variety of causes: damage to the bronchial walls after infection, breathing toxic fumes of various kinds over long periods of time, immunologic reactions, or abnormalities in the arteries that supply the bronchi with needed nutrition. The disease may affect both lungs at the same time and is most common in the lower lobes.

The most common symptom is a chronic and productive cough (which produces sputum) that fails to disappear after a severe pneumonia. Typically the cough is worse in the morning and late afternoon with the rest of the day relatively free of symptoms. Coughing produces large amounts of material, often containing blood (hemoptysis). Other symptoms include shortness of breath, wheezing and other signs of a poorly functioning respiratory system.

Chest X-rays are very valuable in helping to make the diagnosis, and bronchoscopy, which is a tube inserted into the lungs through the mouth to permit the physician to examine the bronchi closely, is frequently advised.

While it may not be possible to restore the lungs to normal, a "nothing more to be done" attitude is unacceptable. There are many treatments that should be used to prevent the condition from worsening.

Antibiotics must be used to fight the frequently occurring flare-ups of infection. Antitussives (cough-suppressing medications) help control the cough symptoms, and medications and physical therapy help promote drainage of the secretions.

41. *Despite the fact that I have no problems with my lungs or breathing, a chest X-ray is always included in my yearly examination. What can the doctor see on this examination that would make it worthwhile?*

While the chest X-ray is a fine examination of the lungs from at least one point of view (the other is a pulmonary function test, which tells us how lungs work rather than how they look), there are many other organs and structures that may be viewed and evaluated from a routine chest film.

The physician can see the ribs, the clavicles (collarbones) and the breastbone (sternum). Thus the idea of checking bone structure health is one possible gain. The heart is outlined in a chest X-ray, and an enlarged heart is easily diagnosed, as well as many other heart abnormalities. Lungs and the tissues that surround both heart and lung can be evaluated, plus the presence of any fluids, growths or infections.

One of the real values of routine examinations is that the physician can compare one year's result to a previous examination and thus detect any important changes that may have occurred.

We all know that medical costs must be controlled. So the cost and usefulness of such an examination must be calculated against the possible savings we can obtain from early diagnosis and treatment of newly developing diseases — which can be the most valuable outcome of all.

42. *My physician has identified my recent breathing problem as asthma. This took me by surprise but set me to wondering if there might be something on my job that could cause this disease to develop at this stage of my life. I'm a 32-year-old male, and there is no history of such ailments in my family. What can you tell me?*

I could probably tell you a lot more if you had indicated your type of employment in your letter. This is another example of just how important a patient's history is in tracking down the cause or origin of a disease.

It's not easy to point out any specific agents that could provoke the bronchial constriction that typifies occupational asthma, as there are more than 100 known causes. However, we can develop a workable search plan by dividing the possible causes into animal, vegetable or mineral (chemical) categories, and you can figure out those that might apply in your case.

The most common animal sources are hair, dander and saliva. These particles, which are carried through the air, cause an immediate response, and it is characteristic of the type of asthma seen in people who work in close contact with animals on a daily basis. Of the vegetable-type sources, flour is the most common. It may be made of any of the cereal grains, including wheat and barley. This is frequently called baker's asthma or miller's asthma. However, wood dust, particularly from the western red cedar, is another vegetable cause that affects millworkers.

One of the most common chemical agents known to cause asthma is toluene diisocyanate (TDI). This chemical is found in many products, such as polyurethane foam, paint products and acrylics. About 5 to 10 percent of people exposed to this powerful chemical will develop asthma. The onset of symptoms may not be immediate but will become apparent hours after the workday exposure is over.

If you work at a large plant, you may be able to get more help from the plant's medical staff, which may have seen cases like yours in the recent past. Once you have a suspect, further testing is necessary to establish the exact cause of your asthma.

43.

While visiting my son in Minnesota, he and I took a brisk walk before dinner. The evening was cold, with snow on the ground. We hadn't made half a mile before I experienced a tightness in my chest, a dry cough and wheezing. I could barely breathe. A trip to the emergency room convinced all of us that it wasn't a heart attack. After I returned home to Florida, I rushed home one evening walking farther and faster than in Minnesota, and nothing happened. There has got to be a logical explanation.

With the data you provide and the fact that you have been cleared of any cardiac problems, my best guess is that you suffered an attack of exercise-induced asthma, which was provoked by the cold climate that seems to be the important element in your case.

It's a common enough condition and can be diagnosed with a pulmonary function test and a better history and examination than is available to me. The asthmalike attack is caused when the bronchioles, or small tubes that carry the air to and from the lungs, contract because of irritation or reaction to substances to which they're sensitive.

In the case of exercising — even a brisk walk in the snow — it's possible that the dry air you were breathing dehydrated the airways and caused them to contract. When you performed the same activity in the warm and moist air of your hometown, the factors that caused the attack previously were absent, so there was no attack.

Because this is but one answer to an interesting medical situation, I strongly advise a thorough physical, with special attention to your past history, and the necessary tests to establish the performance patterns of your lungs.

44. *My breathing difficulty has been diagnosed by my physician as COPD. Could you please tell me what my condition is and how it is treated?*

COPD stands for chronic obstructive pulmonary disease, and many diseases can cause it. Essentially, COPD is difficulty in breathing and shortness of breath due to limited airflow through the lungs. Chronic bronchitis or chronic emphysema can contribute to COPD, as can other diseases like cystic fibrosis. Some COPD patients also suffer from asthma.

The most common contributor to COPD is smoking, which is the leading cause of chronic bronchitis and emphysema. Because of smoking, COPD is a significant health problem in the United States. The number of cases will only increase as more people who have spent a lifetime smoking grow older. Exposure to air pollution is another risk factor in developing COPD, as is severe bronchial infection.

In most COPD patients, the airways of their lungs either have become permanently narrowed, or the tissue has lost its elasticity like a balloon that is stretched out of shape. COPD usually develops slowly, over the course of years. Many patients show the symptoms for years before finally seeing a physician because of increasing shortness of breath.

There is no cure for COPD, and all treatments include eliminating factors or situations that exacerbate the problem. If you still smoke, the most important thing to do is to stop smoking. This will slow the progression of the disease, but your condition will not reverse. Other steps to take are to eliminate dust, animal hair and other irritants from your home environment.

Several types of drugs can be used to treat COPD. These will alleviate symptoms and work to reduce potentially serious complications. Bronchodilators are commonly used to treat COPD, since they open the air passages and make breathing easier. Corticosteroids are used to reduce inflammation. Antibiotics may be necessary to clear infections. It's also important to keep to a minimum the secretions in the bronchial tubes (air passages), and both sufficient fluid intake and medications may be helpful.

You must be careful to try to avoid catching colds or respiratory infections, because your lungs already are weakened. I hope you had your flu shot this season, as you're just the person who can profit from this type of disease prevention.

45. ***My friend is a wonderful woman, but even I, her best friend, don't know what to tell her about her terrible breath. Perhaps if I knew more about this I could help. Can you please tell me what causes bad halitosis?***

Halitosis — severe and persistent bad breath — usually is related to periodontal disease. When dental plaque, decaying teeth, food trapped under dental restoration such as bridgework, oral ulcers or other problems allow the growth of bacteria, they can produce bad-smelling chemicals. Chronic infection of the salivary glands also can cause odor.

Another category of causes of bad breath involves infection or debris in the nose or nasal passages and sinuses. A careful examination, including CT scanning or magnetic resonance imaging, may detect the source of this problem.

Medications or problems such as kidney disease and diabetes can cause bad breath. Another possibility is a diet that includes a lot of sugars, fat or milk products.

If none of these is the cause, it could be a pulmonary infection, such as bronchiectasis, or gastric reflux from either a hiatal hernia or disturbed esophageal motility (digestive movement).

Mints and mouthwashes may improve the situation for short periods of time, but eventually only treating the underlying causes will rid the sufferer of this embarrassment.

46. ***There is a man who lives in the same adult home that I do, whom I see coughing up blood several times a day. I tell him that he must do something about it, but he claims it's nothing and will go away. Do you know what this condition is, and what I should do about it? I feel sorry for him, but am also afraid that it might be catching and dangerous to all of us.***

Your concern is not without good reason, and your efforts to obtain help for this man are important. Coughing up blood is called hemoptysis in medical terminology and can be classified as mild, moderate or severe, depending upon the amount of blood that is coughed up.

It's hard to tell you an exact diagnosis, for there are more than 100 causes of this symptom listed by the American Thoracic Society, and you have not provided me with enough details to even make a guess in this case.

In about 20 to 40 percent of the cases, the underlying disease is either bronchitis, which is caused by an infection, or bronchiectasis, which is a condition of the lungs where the bronchi have become dilated and possibly infected as well. Lung cancer certainly can be at the root of this problem, and we cannot overlook the possibility of tuberculosis. These conditions probably account for more than two-thirds of all the cases of hemoptysis.

While small amounts of blood loss are not too serious and won't endanger this man's life, things can become progressively worse if not attended to. And death can result both from asphyxiation (when the blood blocks off the breathing tubes) as well as from excessive blood loss itself.

Your responsibility to the others living in your home as well as to this individual makes the need for your intervention quite clear. A talk with your health personnel, nurse or physician, or an administrator of the home is in order.

47. *My hiccups sometimes go on for days. Are there any medications that can help me?*

I presume that you've tried physical approaches, such as swallowing granulated sugar or bitters, and deep breathing or rebreathing into a paper bag, for example. Sometimes a doctor will find that inserting a nasogastric tube into your esophagus is enough to "break" the hiccup (or hiccough) reflex.

If these conservative maneuvers haven't produced results, drug therapy may be the next course of action required. Two relatively mild ones are chlorpromazine (brand name Thorazine) and metoclopramide (Reglan). If these don't stop your hiccups, your doctor will want to investigate some more serious causes of hiccups, such as kidney trouble, lung infections, tumors or other sub-diaphragmatic (underneath the diaphragm, the muscle that contracts to produce the hiccup) process. These abdominal causes include disorders of the stomach and esophagus, bowel diseases, pancreatitis and even pregnancy.

Should your tests turn out normal, then your doctor will move on to the anti-convulsant drugs, such as carbamazepine (Tegretol) or phenytoin (Dilantin). A few patients respond to a stronger anti-convulsant drug called valproic acid (Depakene), a heart drug called nifedipine (Procardia), an anti-psychotic called haloperidol (Haldol), or tranquilizers in the benzodiazepine group like diazepam (Valium).

All of these medications can be obtained only with a prescription, and should be taken only under medical supervision. As the long list of medications indicates, hiccups may be difficult to treat successfully.

48. *Can you tell me the causes of hoarseness? Can it ever be anything serious, and how can you tell the serious kind from the ordinary kind?*

Most hoarseness comes from a simple viral infection of the larynx, or voice box. You can tell the common kind because there's no pain and no difficulty in breathing associated with it. If hoarseness has come on suddenly and has lasted only a short period of time, it's probable that it may pass simply by resting your voice and gargling on a regular basis. A post-nasal drip may create morning hoarseness, resulting from the accumulation of mucus on the vocal cords.

My favorite gargle for these conditions is a teaspoonful of salt in a glass of warm water (except when extra salt is prohibited by other medical considerations). Frequent gargling brings extra humidity to the larynx and aids in the rapid resolution of the problem.

However, if hoarseness persists for a long period of time, let's say more than two weeks, and doesn't get better with these simple procedures, then your physician probably will perform an examination called an indirect laryngoscopy. That's the procedure in which he uses a mirror to look down your throat to take a careful look at your vocal cords. This special examination, plus the presence of other symptoms — such as difficulty in breathing, pain in the throat that may be associated with ear pain, fever and cough that can be associated with sputum streaked with blood — all indicate the presence of something more serious than common ordinary hoarseness.

The good news is that in 90 percent of patients who do complain of hoarseness, the diagnosis is the simplest one that has no long-lasting ill effects.

49. ***Is there any truth to the stories that humidifiers in the home can be a good method of curing a common cold? My sister-in-law swears that it's so, but some of my friends chuckle when I bring it up. I get more colds during the winter months than I can count, and I can use all the help I can get.***

I'm afraid your relative is wrong. While the presence of a humidifier in the home may help to reduce some of the annoying effects of a cold, it can neither prevent nor cure the infection. The cold air of winter cannot hold as much moisture as the warmer breezes of summer, and when that cold air passes through the heater or furnace in your home, the amount of moisture it contains drops even lower. This dry air may affect our breathing apparatus, leaving the nose and throat dry and the lips chapped.

When a cold does strike, the mucus dries up as well, blocking the nasal passages and causing distress and difficulty with breathing. Warm, moist air can reverse these conditions and make breathing a bit easier. But that is not curing a cold, it's just making it a bit easier to put up with.

You have a wide choice of methods and materials to get that humidity back up over the 30 percent level, which is judged to be comfortable. Simply boiling water in a pot will help, but steam vaporizers that can be moved about cost less than $25 and are helpful for small areas. The mist they produce is pure, as the boiling has killed any bacteria that were in the water.

Not so with cool-mist vaporizers, which cost about $50 and can provide atmospheric moisture for a moderate-sized room. They must be cleaned carefully, as bacteria can survive in cool water.

Ultrasonic humidifiers also are available at a cost ranging from $50 to $200. They must be maintained properly, including changing filters regularly and using distilled water.

Whatever your choice, read the labels carefully and get as much information as you can about the benefits of the model you choose.

50. *I keep reading the term emphysema in medical magazines but have absolutely no idea what it refers to. Perhaps you can help. What is it? How is it treated?*

Emphysema is a lung condition that is marked by shortness of breath. It's diagnosed when the small air sacs that make up our lungs have become weakened and lose their elasticity.

Normally, these sacs, which are called alveoli, expand with each breath and then return to their normal, small size between breaths. In emphysema, each sac is stretched like an old balloon and doesn't return to a small size. In addition to being stretched, the weakened alveoli do not exchange carbon dioxide for oxygen as they should.

Because the alveoli are not working properly, the respiratory muscles of the chest must work harder. This leads to a barrel-chested appearance in many emphysema sufferers, who also lose weight and tire very easily.

Emphysema has a biochemical cause that is created or worsened by environmental factors. Normally, chemicals called proteases fight off bacteria and viruses in the lung and are regulated by another chemical called alpha-1-antitrypsin. In emphysema, alpha-1-antitrypsin is inactivated or missing and the proteases go wild and start to attack healthy lung tissue. Smoking inactivates alpha-1-antitrypsin, which is why smoking is the leading cause of emphysema. However, some cases of emphysema are related to genetic biochemical defects.

There is no treatment for emphysema nor is there any way to reverse the damage once it has begun. However, stopping smoking will prevent lung damage from progressing.

51. *When I tell my doctor that I seem to be getting little relief for my breathing problem, even though I use my inhaler regularly, he merely tells me to use it properly and increase the dosage. The nurse seems to give me a slightly different story each time I ask for instructions. I know others who do well with this type of medication and wonder if you might offer me the instructions I can't seem to get from my doctor.*

The use of metered dose inhalers has become an important and widely used method of taking medications to manage a group of lung diseases known as obstructive airway diseases.

A variety of medications can be used in these inhalers to open the airways and help restore the normal passage of air to and from the lungs. These inhalers are a convenient and useful method of taking medications, since they measure the dose precisely and are easy to carry around, but many people experience some difficulty in their use. There is even some confusion among professionals as to the correct use of inhalers; when used incorrectly, the dosage of medication they deliver to the lungs may be reduced by as much as 90 percent.

Here are the six steps I recommend:

1. With a properly assembled inhaler, remove the cap and shake the inhaler well before using.
2. Hold the inhaler upright, mouthpiece below the canister that holds the medication, about two finger-breadths in front of the widely opened mouth.
3. Empty your lungs, then start to inhale SLOWLY, and press the canister once, to obtain one dose.
4. Continue your slow inhalation to expand your lungs fully over a five- to 10-second period.
5. Hold your breath for as long as possible, as many as 10 seconds, then exhale.
6. Wait at least one minute between doses.

The angle of the inhaler and the distance from the mouth are important factors in assuring the maximum delivery of medication to the lungs. In cases where patients have difficulty in using the inhaler properly, a "spacer" or holding chamber may be attached to the mouthpiece.

52. ***Assuming that all the cells in the body die and are replaced sooner or later, can one say that after 30 years of smoking, a five- to seven-year period of not smoking will give someone pristine "new" lungs?***

An interesting question but, unfortunately, based upon a wrong assumption. It's true that we replace all our red cells every 100 days, and that many other body cells die and are replaced in the normal process of living. But some of the damage inflicted on the lungs by 30 years of smoking never can be repaired.

Chronic bronchitis, emphysema and chronic obstructive airway disease are all possible outcomes of long-term cigarette smoking. The smoke has an adverse effect on lung defenses and provokes a low-grade inflammation that in turn leads to changes in lung anatomy and function.

But I don't want to take a completely negative approach to your question. It's true that if lung function is measured by certain tests in smoking individuals and then compared to the results of the same test after a period of smoking abstinence, a notable improvement can be measured. Many of the symptoms of coughing and shortness of breath also improve considerably, as the lung cleanses itself and revitalizes after the constant irritation of smoking is removed. However, if the seeds of cancer have been sown during a 30-year experience with tobacco, stopping the habit now cannot eradicate the tumor.

It's nice to think of the human body as being constantly renewed and repaired, but it's mortal and, with time, begins to show the signs of wear and tear that we inflict upon it. Good health habits allow the body to function at its best and offer the best hope for a long life.

53. ***I have a lush growth of hairs inside my nostrils. They irritate me, cause me to sneeze and look just terrible. However, when I do try to cut them back, my wife says they're there for a purpose and that all kinds of calamities will befall me if I don't quit. Please tell me what to do.***

Well, your wife does have a point. The hair that grows inside the nostrils does serve a function. By partially blocking the opening, the hair strains out large particles of dirt and dust, which are prevented from entering the air passages when we're breathing.

The size of individual hairs differs from person to person. While most people have no problems, the hair may be thick and voluminous in others. When it becomes too luxuriant, I see no danger in carefully clipping it back to a more discreet look. All you need is a good mirror, a pair of fine scissors and a steady hand. Nail clippers and other nonscissors cutting tools should be avoided, as accidents can happen and this is a bad place to sustain a cut.

To be honest, I have seen many a fine barber in my day who made this procedure into a real art and solved the problem during a regular haircut visit.

54. ***A letter from an old friend has us confused about the health of a mutual acquaintance. The letter speaks of "pigeon lung," but we can't find any mention of this condition in our home medical advisor. Do you know what our friend is talking about?***

I think so. The disease is also known as bird fancier's lung or pneumonitis of pigeon breeders. It's a type of pneumonia that is seen in individuals who breed or care for pigeons.

The symptoms of fever, chills, cough and difficulty in breathing come on about four to six hours after exposure to the birds. The disease is believed to be caused by an allergy or hypersensitivity to the pigeons.

The disease can be treated with corticosteroids, which are cortisone-like medications, and will disappear by itself in many cases if contact with the birds is avoided for 12 to 24 hours.

If your friend is the owner of these animals, it looks like a short-lived hobby. Prolonged or repeated contact can result in chronic lung disease, which is certainly too high a price to pay for the enjoyment of raising these graceful creatures.

55. ***My mother had severe chest pains recently that turned out to be pleurisy. Can you fill me in on this condition or infection? Is it like a cold that can be cured, or is it more like a condition that stays with you?***

The pleura is a membranelike tissue that covers the lungs and also lines the inside of the chest cavity in which the lungs are found. Between these two sheets of tissue is a space, which is normally closed as the lungs fill and move against the chest wall.

However, in certain circumstances, the pleura becomes inflamed — swollen and congested — and produces a thick, liquid (called a fibrinous exudate) that begins to fill this space. This fluid is sticky and can cause the tissue that covers the lungs to adhere or become fixed to the lining of the chest wall. That forms an adhesion and causes pain when the lung moves to and fro as the patient breathes.

Pleural effusions occur when the pleura is injured, usually as a result of a lung infection or some type of trauma, but it also can be caused by tuberculosis, uremia or even asbestos. The pain of pleurisy usually comes on quite suddenly and can range from a mild discomfort to a stabbing pain. It's made worse by deep breathing and coughing. When the physician examines the chest with a stethoscope, the sound of rubbing can be heard, and this helps with the diagnosis. Chest X-rays may be of some help in confirming the diagnosis, particularly when there is a quantity of liquid present.

The treatment of pleurisy depends upon its cause and may include antibiotics and pain medications. Chest pain can be relieved in some cases by wrapping the entire chest with wide elastic bandages, which provide support to the wall of the chest and reduce the movement the chest makes during breathing.

Pleurisy may take a while to heal, but it usually does with the proper treatment, leaving but a small scar on the pleura to mark where the injury occurred. Thus pleurisy is not a condition that stays with the patient, and your mother can look forward to a normal existence without pain.

56. *My sinuses are a never-ending cause for concern. They just don't quit giving me problems. But I still don't understand the causes and reasons for sinusitis. Please explain.*

Sinusitis is an inflammation of one or more of the paranasal sinuses, which are cavities in the skull connected with the nasal passages. They're arranged in four pairs, with members of each pair on the right and left side of the head.

Doctors are not 100 percent sure of the functions of the sinuses. The sinuses are thought to help the nose circulate air, warming and moistening it as it is inhaled. Therefore, the lungs do not get a shock as cold or dry air is inhaled. The sinuses also play a minor role in voice production, as they're believed to act as resonating chambers.

Sinusitis often occurs during an upper respiratory infection. Sometimes excessive or strong nose blowing may cause the infection to spread from the nose to the sinuses. There are, however, many, many other causes of sinusitis, which is why it's such a tricky, annoying problem.

Some factors that trigger sinus troubles include allergies, infectious diseases such as pneumonia or the measles, air pollution, diving and underwater swimming, sudden extreme changes of temperature, structural defects of the nose, or a complication from a tooth infection.

When you have a sinusitis flare-up, you may feel pressure on the sinus walls, which in turn causes discomfort, pain, fever and difficulty with breathing. This happens because the mucous membranes of the sinus are inflamed and the openings of the sinus cavities become partially or fully blocked. The blockage often causes headaches and may lead to nasal discharge.

Sinus sufferers also complain of dizziness, weakness and general discomfort. People suffering from these symptoms certainly should seek a doctor's help. A physician can use many diagnostic tools to confirm sinusitis, including radiography, ultrasound, multiple X-ray exposures and computed tomography.

Most cases of acute sinusitis will respond to antibiotics. The antibiotics most commonly prescribed are ampicillin, amoxicillin, cefaclor, trimethoprim-sulfamethoxazole and erythromycin. If this treatment is unsuccessful, your doctor should do further testing with X-rays to determine whether your case of sinusitis is infectious, allergic or caused by another factor.

Decongestants also may help the sinusitis patient by increasing drainage. Discomfort can be relieved through inhalation of steam or warm, moist air.

If you've been suffering with sinus problems for a long time, you may be one of those unfortunate people who have chronic sinusitis. This condition occurs when the mucous membranes in the sinuses thicken and normal drainage becomes obstructed. If the previously mentioned treatments don't clear up the problem, surgery may be necessary.

Since the sinuses are close to the ears and brain, it's important to treat sinusitis aggressively to minimize the risk of spreading the infection to those organs.

57. ***My husband claims that when you sneeze, your heart stops. Isn't this an old wives' tale? He will have sneezing episodes for anywhere from three to 15 minutes. What causes this and what damage is he doing to his heart? He claims he has had such episodes for about 20 years.***

Sneezing is an uncontrollable reflex that occurs when something irritates the upper air passages, such as the nose or pharynx (throat). First, a large amount of air is pulled into the lungs and then pushed out by the breathing muscles in a rapid and forceful manner, so that a large volume of air passes through the nose and mouth at great speed. This is designed to clear the passages of the cause of the irritation.

The heart doesn't stop during this action, although the rate may be altered by the changes in the timing and pattern of breathing. Your husband, therefore, is inflicting no damage to his heart, as his 20 years of experience surely prove.

Sneezing is frequently caused by allergens, such as pollen, or the increased mucous flow in the nasal passages provoked by a cold. However, other irritations may be the root of the problem, such as cigarette smoke, an abrupt change in air humidity or temperature, the smell of certain perfumes and even bright light or high-pitched sounds in certain sensitive individuals.

No damage occurs, provided the sneeze is not suppressed but allowed to happen, while the mouth and nose are gently covered to prevent the spread of germ-carrying droplets.

58. *My 86-year-old father is in the hospital with what the doctors call bacterial pneumonia. Could you please explain what this is?*

Let us first define the term pneumonia. Sometimes called pneumonitis, it's an acute infection of lung tissue. When it's confined to just one lobe of the lung, it may be known as lobar pneumonia; when it affects the bronchial tubes, it's called bronchopneumonia. The term bacterial pneumonia tells us that the infection is caused by bacteria rather than viruses or fungi.

Bacterial pneumonia is the most common kind. It can be caused by a wide variety of bacteria, including pneumococcus, streptococcus, staphylococcus, legionella, klebsiella and hemophilus influenza. And it's a most serious condition. About 2 million Americans get pneumonia each year, with about 40,000 to 70,000 deaths reported. It ranks sixth among all categories of disease as a cause of death.

Despite the many tests available to physicians, it's sometimes quite difficult to determine just what germ (bacteria) is causing the illness, and no culprit is discovered in up to half the cases. Pneumonia frequently follows an upper respiratory infection. It may start with shaking, chills and a high fever. Patients find it difficult to breathe, sometimes experience pain when pleurisy develops, develop coughs and also may experience nausea and vomiting. Both chest X-rays and blood tests help make the diagnosis.

Hospitalization is generally necessary to properly treat the condition, especially in older folks, who lack the resistance and strength to fight off the infection. Fortunately, a large number of powerful antibiotics are effective in combating the infection. An antibiotic is chosen for its particular ability to kill the germ that has been identified as the cause of the pneumonia.

Other measures used to treat pneumonia patients and keep them comfortable are bed rest, fluids (including the intravenous route), analgesics for pain, cough medications and oxygen for patients who may not be able to take in enough oxygen for their systems because of the pneumonia.

It may take a while to subdue the infection and an even longer period for recovery, but a total cure is possible in most cases.

59. *A friend of mine, a notorious snorer, has told me his condition is a life-threatening situation he called sleep apnea. Is this an exaggeration? What is sleep apnea; what causes it; and how do you treat it?*

Sleep apnea, a condition that affects up to 4 percent of the adult population, is a sleep disorder in which the sufferer actually stops breathing for several seconds and the heart slows down. This episode may be followed by a jerky body movement, respiration resumes and the heart speeds up considerably.

Subjective symptoms not withstanding, these patients experience no difficulty sleeping through the night, though they usually complain of fatigue and headache upon awakening. Objectively, their sleep partners testify that the symptoms of these disorders are more life-threatening than the patient suspects.

For instance, while sleeping, apnea sufferers often stop breathing for 15 seconds to as long as 60 seconds, and these episodes may be repeated as frequently as four to 30 times an hour. During this time the oxygen content of the blood is reduced, taxing both the heart and lungs. Apnea sufferers then may seem to fight to regain their breath, and then continue with a more quiet sleep. While personal problems, such as divorce, sometimes are blamed for the onset of sleep apnea, it might be the result of the noisy, on-and-off pattern of loud snoring that is so frequently associated with this condition.

Snoring, a sign of temporary and incomplete obstruction of the upper airway, is very common in patients with sleep apnea. Obesity, tonsillitis and pulmonary problems are only a few of the contributory factors a physician will be on the alert for.

An accurate diagnosis, however, can best be obtained by requesting that the patient spend a night or two in a sleep laboratory, where his or her sleep cycle can be electronically monitored through polysomonography.

Once a clear picture has been established, a conservative course of treatment can begin. In obese subjects, unless life-threatening abnormal heart rhythms are present, weight loss is a good first step. Studies have shown that even a small reduction in weight in grossly obese patients greatly improves sleep disorder symptoms. Eliminating depressants, such as alcohol, hypnotic drugs and sedatives, also improves control.

If these initial efforts prove unsatisfactory, the use of respiratory stimulants (such as medroxyprogesterone) or surgery may be necessary. Successful surgical procedures range from removal of obstructive tissue to tracheostomy. However, a recent advance in sleep apnea management — nasal CPAP, or continuous positive airway pressure — is yielding some dramatic results.

Nasal CPAP involves the use of a tight-fitting nasal mask and a small compressor that generates enough constant air pressure to keep the air passages open and prevent obstruction. It takes just a bit of getting used to the increased pressure, but this is rapidly achieved. Admittedly, this "deep sea" equipment is not the most alluring nightwear, but for many patients it's a most acceptable alternative to surgery.

60. *Although not sickly, my 12-year-old son comes down with throat infections very frequently. His doctor is advising that he should have his tonsils and adenoids removed. Just what do these glands do, and is removing them in a youngster considered the right thing to do?*

Although these glands have an important health role in infants, they probably have accomplished all they ever will by the time the child is three years old.

In the first few years of life, these glands are responsible for sampling the incoming air and catching some of the germs and viruses that may be present. An infection then can develop in this tissue, causing the body to develop antibodies to help combat the infection. In this manner, an immunity to similar infections is developed that protects the individual against future infections.

You easily can see the state of your son's tonsils for yourself by looking in his mouth. The tonsils are the glands located just behind a fold of tissue at the back of the mouth, and they may be filled with small pockets (crypts) that are filled with cheeselike material, resulting from infections and abscess formation. They may be causing bad breath but, more important, they are the reason for repeated infections and possibly breathing difficulties as well. You can't see the adenoids without special instruments, as they're located high in the throat behind the nose, but they probably would look similar to the tonsils if you could see them.

There is nothing unusual about removing tonsils in a child the age of your son, and tonsillectomy and adenoidectomy (T & A) is the second most common operation performed on children, numbering about 400,000 operations per year. When the symptoms of frequent and recurrent sore throats, fever and chills, bad breath and nasal congestion or obstruction occur frequently and cannot be permanently relieved with antibiotics, a T & A is considered sound therapy.

61. ***It seems that almost from my adolescence, I have had a pair of weak lungs. Most of my adult life I was plagued with chest colds, and I developed severe shortness of breath later on. I attributed that to my smoking habit. When I retired two years ago, I decided to change my life for the better. I gave up smoking and moved to Florida, and I'm doing much better. However, I'm now under the care of a new, young doctor who strongly recommends that I take a pneumonia vaccine. What do you think of the idea? Do you think it's necessary, and does it work?***

I think it's a great idea, especially for you. You're one of the people this vaccination is most recommended for: someone who's over age 65 (I presume?) with a history of chronic lung problems. While it's true that some clinical trials failed to show dramatic results with the vaccine, it's also true that the vaccination will provide some degree of protection in older and high-risk patients.

In addition, you need only one injection to gain a lifetime immunity, there are very few side effects, and the vaccine is inexpensive and widely available. Your new young doctor is using his head in recommending this to you, as preventing disease is the order of the day. It's better to avoid the complications of diseases and their cost than to have to conquer them once they have developed. And as a friend of mine has remarked, in this case "It certainly can't hurt!"

62. ***The good news is that our high school team won, but the bad news is that no one in the family could talk for days afterward. Gradually our voices returned along with the noise level at the dinner table, but we can't help but wonder just what happened. We know we "strained" our voices, but just what does this mean? Could you please explain?***

To help you understand, let us first look at the mechanism that produces sound and how it works. The voice box (larynx) is located at the upper part of the air passage, between the trachea and the base of the tongue, or about the middle of the neck. When the air passes out of the lungs into the airway, the vocal cords vibrate to produce a sound. Then the mouth, tongue and lips all take part in shaping the sound into speech or song. These actions proceed most smoothly in the normal state.

However, screaming or cheering can slam the edges of the vocal cords together quite forcibly, irritating these sensitive tissues and causing them to swell. Talking without pause for long periods of time or even clearing your throat too frequently also can result in the same condition. So can raising the pitch of your voice to a level higher than you normally use. All of these elements can occur during the excitement of a game, or any event where cheering is part of the fun.

The treatment is quite simple in uncomplicated cases. It consists of several days of resting your voice as completely as possible, drinking plenty of liquids, and using glycerin-based throat lozenges to help lubricate and soothe the throat.

63.

A splitting headache drove me to the doctor's office, where after an examination, the diagnosis of sinusitis was made. A prescription for an antibiotic was given to me, but I sensed that my doctor was very concerned. I was required to return in just three days, but everything seemed to be going fine. Can you tell me what he was worrying about?

It's not difficult to imagine the concerns of a caring physician who is faced with a case of acute sinusitis. He already was visualizing the possible complications and was planning your care to avoid those possibilities. The sinuses are actually hollow spaces within the bones that form parts of the skull. They're normally filled only with air and are lined with delicate mucous membranes.

When an infection strikes, the membranes become swollen and may close the small holes (ostium) that provide drainage for the liquid normally formed by the tissues and allow for the free passage of air in and out of the sinus. As a result, the air in the sinus is absorbed by blood cells in the membranes and the pressure within the sinus drops (vacuum sinusitis), which can be painful.

If this condition persists, the membranes then produce large amounts of fluid that fill the sinus cavity and can serve as perfect breeding grounds for bacteria. As the body attempts to defend against this infection, it pours additional serum and white blood cells into the area. This action soon creates a positive pressure within this closed space, causing pain, often described as "splitting," and tenderness. This can lead to the extension of the infection beyond the sinus, provoking infections in the orbit of the eye (orbital cellulitis), as well as within the skull itself (meningitis and brain abscesses).

However, full doses of appropriate antibiotics — ampicillin or amoxicillin, in most cases — for 10 to 14 days is usually sufficient to prevent serious complications. Drainage of the sinus may be aided by using a vaporizer, which helps to reduce the pressure, relieve the pain and hasten the recovery.

64. *I have symptoms that are bothersome, but fear the diagnosis more. My shortness of breath is worsening and I can't rid myself of this cough. Now I've begun to wheeze and wonder if the time has come to see my doctor. What's your advice?*

I think you have already made up your mind and just need a few words of encouragement from me before making that important appointment with your physician.

Although there are a number of possible diagnoses, the three symptoms you describe — shortness of breath, cough and wheezing — make chronic obstructive pulmonary disease (COPD) the most likely choice. Usually a mixture of chronic bronchitis and emphysema, this frequently seen disease strikes about one in 14 people over the age of 45. It develops gradually, as in your case, and may be detected first by a physician when a bad cold or the flu strikes and a visit to his or her office is needed. COPD tends to run in families, and its No. 1 cause is smoking.

Other factors, such as exposure to dust, chemical fumes or other irritants, can contribute to the development of COPD. The lung passages become inflamed and swollen, producing mucus, which blocks the flow of air to and from the lungs. This produces the symptoms that are bothering you.

While there's no cure, many treatments are available that will reduce the symptoms and make you feel better. The cigarettes must go, and there are a few other lifestyle changes that can dramatically improve your outlook for the future. You also might wish to consider dropping any extra pounds you are carrying and starting an organized activity program.

65. ***Please do not laugh at my question, but since I've been unable to find an answer to it, I thought you might be able to help me. I would like to know why we yawn, and why everyone seems to do it at the same time.***

Actually, that is a very good question, since it may interest many people. There has not been a tremendous amount of medical literature written about the process of yawning, but it certainly is something we all do, at one time or another.

A yawn is not simply opening the mouth wide, but it's usually accompanied by a deep inspiration, filling the lungs fully with air. That circumstance has led to a theory that yawning has something to do with the physical state of the lungs at the time the yawn comes along.

The lung is filled with millions of minute air sacs called alveoli, where oxygen is taken out of the air and transferred into the bloodstream for transportation to all the cells of the body. After we have been sitting for a prolonged period of time, perhaps in a slumped position, some of the air sacs collapse. When enough of them have been affected, the lung cannot function as it should and so we yawn to re-expand all of the lung tissue once again.

If we search for a logical reason for everyone yawning at the same time, it might be because they're all doing the same thing, for example sitting in a room with stale air, watching a show or television, not exerting themselves too much. That is a time when shallow breathing sets in. Therefore, it could be speculated that everyone would need to yawn at the same time. Of course, it also has been written that yawning can be induced by the power of suggestion, and we sort of "catch" it from the next person. Or it could just mean the show was boring, and the yawn was a display of disinterest. Now take a deep breath and take your pick.

3.

The Bones, Joints and Muscles

It is shameful for a man to rest in ignorance of the structure of his own body, especially when the knowledge of it mainly conduces to his welfare, and directs his application of his own powers.

PHILIPP MELANCHTHON
German religious reformer (1497–1560)

When a baby is born, its skeleton is made up of 350 bones. As the child grows through adolescence into adulthood, however, some of the bones fuse, resulting in only 206 bones in the adult skeleton. At that time, the skeleton accounts for about 18 percent of the total body weight.

Bone is composed chiefly of inorganic salts, mostly calcium phosphate and calcium carbonate (52 percent), in addition to organic substances (27 percent) and water (21 percent). Bone is the body's major reserve of minerals, providing calcium when it's required for the chemical actions that are part of all living tissue. And bone is a vital and living tissue, rich in blood vessels. It's constantly undergoing a process of change, responding to the needs of the individual. Under physical stress, bones become stronger, as ***osteoblasts*** (bone-forming cells) lay down rings of mineral salts, mainly calcium and phosphorus, which are the substance of new bone. During periods of inactivity, bones become weaker, losing calcium and strength. This process of constant renewal continues throughout life and provides many skeletons during an individual's lifetime, averaging a new one about every two years in a healthy young adult.

The outer layer of a bone is composed of hard *compact bone*, sometimes known as solid bone, which provides most of the bone's strength. Tiny canals, called *Haversian canals*, run through this bone. The Haversian system carries tiny arteries and veins, lymph vessels and lymph fluid to all parts of the bone. Compact bone is covered by a tough, fibrous membrane called the *periosteum*, which can form new bone and so plays an important role in the repair of fractures.

In the center of a bone, the appearance of the bony tissue is a bit different. Here the structure is more porous and resembles a sponge by comparison with the outer layer, and so the name spongy bone is often applied. Also known as *cancellous bone*, it's formed of rigid beamlike structures called *trabeculae*, which can provide the greatest strength with the least weight.

In the center of many bones, particularly the long bones that form the legs and arms, lies the *bone marrow*. It's in this tissue that blood cells are formed. About 5 billion red cells are manufactured here each day, and it's their color that helps to tint the marrow. In children, the marrow is normally a rich red color. As an individual grows older, this tissue becomes filled with fat cells, turning the color of the marrow in some bones to a yellowish gray.

Although often considered merely the scaffolding upon which all the other organs of the body depend for support, the skeleton actually has three important functions. To be sure, it does provide the framework of the body, and in so doing, supports the body's weight and maintains the shape of the body. But it also serves to protect the internal organs and, along with the muscles, enables the body to move. The basic skeletal structure is called the *axial skeleton*, which is composed of the skull, spine and rib cage. To this "main frame" the *appendicular skeletons* are attached, the upper limbs connecting by means of the *shoulder girdle* (*clavicle* and *scapula*) and the lower limbs attaching to the hip bones, or *pelvic girdle*.

The protective function provided by special skeletal structures is clearly demonstrated by the skull, itself composed of 29 bones. The *cranium*, which encloses and protects the brain within its bony armors, is made up of eight bones, with 14 facial bones, three tiny bones in each middle ear that conduct sound, and the *hyoid* (at the back of the tongue) completing the count.

The spine, which is composed of seven *cervical*, 12 *thoracic* and five *sacral vertebrae*, demonstrates another protective adaptation. The vertebrae form a bony canal that contains and protects the *spinal cord*, which is the main nerve "cable" that runs from the brain to the rest of the body. The thoracic vertebrae connect to 12 pairs of ribs, which curve around to the front of the body resulting in the ***thoracic cage***. There, the 10 upper pairs of ribs connect to the ***manubrium*** (breastbone) by cartilage connections, while the two lowest pairs form the ***floating ribs***. The ***thorax*** contains and protects the two lungs, the heart and the esophagus, which runs from the mouth to the stomach.

It's the function of locomotion that provides the most amazing adaptations seen in the construction of the skeletal system. Wherever bones come together to join, a ***joint*** is formed. It's the structure of the joint that either permits motion or provides strength, which is desirable in a system that provides support for the body. In some cases, where a great range of motion is required, the freedom of movement permitted by joints is quite extensive. These are classified as ***mobile*** joints. This is seen in the ***ball and socket*** joints of the hip and shoulder, which permit movement in all directions. ***Hinge*** joints, as in the knee, allow a wide range of motion, but in only one direction.

To withstand the friction caused by motion, the ends of the bones in these joints are covered with a pad of resilient, smooth cartilage. The joint is surrounded by a tough capsule containing a special membrane (synovial membrane) that secretes a liquid that helps to lubricate the joint. ***Ligaments*** of strong fibrous connective tissue form part of the joint and strengthen it by connecting one bone to another.

Where strength is needed and motion is less important, a joint can be ***slightly mobile***. This can be seen in the joints between the vertebrae. Great strength is required, but a small amount of flexibility also is needed, to permit the body to bend forward (flexion), for example. Here a pad of cartilage lies between the edges of the bones, to provide the limited mobility that is necessary, along with substantial strength. This ***disc*** allows the necessary motion to occur and acts as a shock absorber for the spine as well. These joints also are held together by ligaments, which provide extra strength.

In still other circumstances, strength is the only concern, and movement is not a consideration. Here the bones may be joined together in an ***immobile*** joint. This can be seen in the skull. The edges of the bones are sawtoothlike and irregular, and are bound together by a tough fibrous tissue to form a rigid joint called a ***suture line***. Because of the solid connection created by this method of joint union, there are no additional ligaments needed, and so none are present.

Now that the chassis is in place, it's time to consider the muscles, which provide the force that moves the bones. There are three types of muscle, which share in common the ability to contract. About 35 to 45 percent of the body's weight is composed of muscle tissue. Each muscle is composed of many small *fibrils*, which shorten when stimulated. The more fibrils that are affected, the greater the force of the muscle contraction.

Of the three types of muscle, only *skeletal muscle* can be controlled voluntarily. Both *cardiac muscle* and *smooth muscle* function without conscious control, and their anatomical structure is different from that of skeletal muscle. Cardiac muscle is made of branched cells, which interweave and form thick bands of muscle that spiral around the ventricles of the heart. They operate under the influence of the heart's own pacemaker as well as nerve impulses from the autonomic nervous system. Each time the heart muscles contract, they squeeze the chambers of the heart closed and thus propel blood through the circulatory system.

Smooth muscle is found in the intestines, the blood vessels, the iris of the eye, the bladder, the ureter, the Fallopian tubes and the uterus. In the intestines, smooth muscles produce the wavelike contraction called *peristalsis*, which moves food through the system during the digestive process.

However, it's skeletal muscle (sometimes called *striated* muscle because of its appearance under the microscope) that provides the force for movement. The cells of skeletal muscle, each having several nuclei, are long, some as much as 20 centimeters (8 inches) in length, and are made up of long filaments called *myofibrils*. These fibers are arranged in a parallel manner, running lengthwise through the muscle's cell. The cells group together in bundles, surrounded by connective tissue. The main body of a muscle, where many bundles are assembled together, is often referred to as the belly of the muscle. At each end of a muscle are the *tendons*, which are strong, resilient tissues formed of fibrous connective tissue that connect the muscles to the bones. The origin, or beginning, of the muscle usually is formed by a short, broad tendon, attached to the surface area of bone. When this bone serves as an anchor, other muscles may contract to hold the anchor bone steady and in place. This permits the contraction of the muscle that originates on the anchor bone to draw another bone toward the origin.

The tendon on the other end of a muscle may have a long, tubular, circular shape, which may run like a cable over other structures of the body to "insert" into another bone. The area of this insertion is usually smaller than the origin, and so directs the energy provided by the contracting muscle to a fairly specific area.

When a muscle fiber contracts, it shortens, often to just one-third of its original length. And each time it contracts, it does so as completely as it can. To provide an even flow to the force of the contraction and the movement it induces, groups of muscle cells within the body of the muscle will contract in sequence. Only the number of cells necessary to produce the needed force, or to reduce the muscle length by the required length, will contract during a given movement. The fine control of these contractions is provided through the *central* and *peripheral nervous systems*, and it's under voluntary control.

Since muscles can provide force in only one direction as they contract, they're usually arranged in pairs. After one muscle has drawn a part of the body toward it (*flexion*), the opposing muscle partner can contract to reverse the action (*extension*), while the muscle that created the original motion relaxes. Muscle tone is the product of the ongoing action of two opposing muscles or muscle groups, as they constantly contract and counterbalance each other.

Muscle activity accounts for much of the energy used by the body. It uses oxygen from the blood and glucose stored within the cells for its first efforts, and produces heat as it does so. This is why you get hot as you exercise. It's the action of many muscles working together in absolute coordination that permits the actions needed to achieve locomotion, for example. More than 200 muscles are involved in the "simple" act of walking. Many muscles are at work even when you're sitting down, just to maintain your position and keep your body erect.

Questions and Answers

66. *Have you ever come across the term "boxer's fracture"? Though I suspect I might figure this one out, I would appreciate your explanation?*

A boxer's fracture is simply cracked knuckles, which is a common side effect of fist fighting, and is frequently called this even when caused by other circumstances. There are several options for treating such a fracture. The final decision on how to treat it depends on the severity of the injury, how important the hand's function is to the patient, and how often he expects to be using the hand as a weapon.

For instance, if he uses his hands in his work or hobbies, he may opt for more aggressive treatment. If the patient is a regular fist fighter, then the possibility of reinjury must be considered before advising extensive and delicate surgical repair.

The choices for treatment of boxer's fracture mainly revolve around whether to operate or to treat more conservatively with protective splinting. More time is lost from work when surgery is chosen, because recovery is slower. There's some controversy over whether the functional and cosmetic improvements gained in surgery are worth the delayed recovery that it involves.

The best results in treating boxer's fracture occur when the extent of the injury is fully evaluated, considering how the hand is used in occupational and leisure pursuits and how important cosmetic results are. Based on this information, the patient can decide with the physician on the best course of action.

67. *I returned to my favorite hobby of carpentry, only to develop a painful wrist and a burning feeling in my fingers. My physician has made a diagnosis of "tunnel syndrome," but I need some more explanation.*

Both your history and the description of your complaints make the diagnosis of carpal tunnel syndrome a most likely one. The condition is a common and painful one that affects people in their 50s and 60s most often, and usually is seen in women more often than men.

Carpal tunnel syndrome is caused by pressure on the median nerve that passes through a structure called the carpal tunnel, which is formed by the bones of the wrist (carpal bones) and a tough, fibrous ligament attached to these bones. The median nerve carries impulses to the muscles that control the action of the thumb. It also transports sensations from the thumb, index and middle finger, and half of the ring finger.

After unusual or unaccustomed activity of a repetitive nature, like using a hammer, or the constant strain placed on your tissues by the consistent stress of typing for hours on end, the symptoms of this condition may develop.

Although your history is typical, some testing is necessary to assure the diagnosis and help direct the therapy. A test that measures the speed of nerve impulses in the median nerve (electromyography) can confirm the diagnosis with great accuracy. You will have to give up your hobby for a while, and will probably have to wear a splint to support your wrist for as long as three weeks. Your physician may choose to inject a cortisonelike steroid into the carpal tunnel, or attempt to reduce the inflammation with oral medications, such as non-steroidal anti-inflammatory drugs (NSAIDs). Vitamins (B_6) sometimes help as well.

If these treatments do not help after a six-month period, or the condition worsens, a surgical procedure that cuts the tunnel open may be necessary. The treatment offers almost immediate relief of the pain and is a permanent cure.

68. *A few years ago, when boxer Mike Tyson was diagnosed as having "costochondritis" and refused to fight, a lot of eyebrows were raised. What is it? What are its symptoms?*

Costochondritis is pretty common. Taking the word apart we find "costo," which denotes a rib, "chondr," which means cartilage, and then the familiar "-itis," denoting an inflammation. Together it means an inflammation of the cartilage of the ribs, normally found at the end of the rib where it attaches to the sternum (breastbone).

The history usually is enough to make the diagnosis, upon hearing the story of pain or discomfort in the chest, sometimes sharp, sometimes dull, and aggravated by motion of the trunk. Usually the patient can put one or two fingers on the exact area of the pain. Any pressure applied directly to the area reproduces the pain. Occasionally, a physician can feel a swelling of the cartilage at the exact location of the tenderness.

It's not a very serious condition and is considered in the same category as a strain. In ordinary mortals, there's not too much that need be done, for the condition will usually disappear in a week or two on its own and doesn't interfere much with normal activity. However, when a boxing champion's performance depends upon his being in top shape, and since he was likely to be at risk for more than a few sharp raps to the chest, the point of view is very different.

It's probable in Tyson's case that the pain would have been more than slightly exaggerated. As to the validity of this diagnosis in postponing a bout, I'm going to side with Tyson. I think he played it safe and, as a doctor, I like it that way.

69. *A knee injury has left me confused and crippled. All I can gather from my doctor's explanation is that I need more tests to find out how badly my "cruciate" is damaged, and that it may take surgery to get me back up and running. Would you give me more information to make a good decision?*

Answers from the Family Doctor (Questions 66-95)

From the information you have provided, I can gather that you have sustained an injury to one of the two ligaments that help support the function of the knee: the cruciates (from the Latin meaning "shaped like a cross").

However, it's not clear which ligament you have injured, the anterior or the posterior. That diagnosis is sometimes difficult to make after an examination. When the anterior cruciate ligament is injured, there's an immediate swelling of the knee, pain to the back of the knee and varying degrees of joint instability sufficient to make you cease your activity.

In the case of a posterior injury, which may be caused by a fall on the knee or a blow to the front of the leg, there is pain, but swelling may be slow to develop, and the injury will not make you stop your activity.

Physical examination may lead to a correct diagnosis, but standard X-rays may not show too much. Magnetic resonance imaging (MRI) may be helpful in determining the extent of the injury, or tear to the ligament. But in most cases, when there's much instability, it will take arthroscopy to determine the exact extent of the injury to the ligaments, as well as to the other components of this vulnerable joint. Using a telescopelike instrument, which is inserted into the knee space through a small incision, the surgeon can inspect the ligaments, cartilage, bone and other tissues.

When the ligament is severely torn, reconstructive surgery can be used both to repair the damage and to restore full function and stability to the joint. This may be your physician's plan when he indicates that more tests and surgery is necessary in your case.

70. ***My doctor says I have a pretty rare condition called "Dupuytren's contracture." What is it? Where could it have come from? What can I do now? Please make your answer simple to understand.***

Just under the skin of the palm of your hand lies a sheet of fibrous tissue known as the palmar fascia. For reasons still unclear, but possibly involving repeated mild injuries, this tissue begins to thicken and contract, usually without pain. As it does so, it sticks to the skin, which becomes puckered, and affects the fingers, causing them to curl, contract and lose their ability to straighten out and function properly. It's far more common in men than in women and usually starts after the age of 40. It's also more common in people with chronic disease.

Dupuytren's contracture is pretty easy to diagnose, since the effects of the disease are readily apparent and you can feel the nodules that form in the fascia simply by touch. The disease is a progressive one, but it's not possible to predict either the speed or the extent of damage it will do.

The only sure way of dealing with it is to have the damaged tissue removed surgically, since medications — even injections of cortisonelike substance — don't work. After surgery, whirlpool baths and an exercise program can help rehabilitate your fingers more rapidly.

71. *I'm sure I saw something about this on a TV program recently, but it makes no sense to me: Have you ever heard of using electricity to heal a fracture? If so, please explain.*

Yes, I've heard of the process you saw televised. The usual therapy for a broken bone is to immobilize it (with a cast, generally) until the fractured ends knit or heal together. Most fractures heal within six months. However, there are always a few breaks that either heal more slowly or refuse to heal at all, and for these there's the choice of using electric bone-growth stimulators or undergoing bone graft surgery.

In the 1950s, it was found that bones that were mechanically stressed (by normal exercise) produced small electrical charges. This mechanical stress helps bones to grow stronger, and researchers theorized that an external electrical charge would do the same thing, which is how the stimulators are thought to work. The results from using bone-growth stimulators are roughly comparable to those of bone graft surgery, with success rates of between 75 and 85 percent as compared to between 85 and 95 percent for bone graft surgery.

Because the technique is non-invasive, it's worth a try in those difficult cases where the bones just won't knit.

72. *My fibrositis condition still confuses me and is very difficult to deal with. Perhaps you can offer some new insight. What is the difference between it and fibromyalgia? Are there any treatments that give relief?*

A confusing disease indeed, even its name can cause confusion. Fibrositis and fibromyalgia are the same disease (also known as myofascial pain syndrome). The term fibromyalgia (meaning muscle pain) is now preferred, for there is no inflammatory process (-itis) seen in this syndrome.

It's classified as a rheumatic disorder that can cause pain, tenderness and stiffness in muscles and tendons at specific "trigger points" that are distributed over the back of the neck and shoulders, the sides of the breastbone and the bony points of the elbows and hips. In addition, there are a whole flock of nonrheumatic symptoms to complicate the patient's life: poor sleep, anxiety, fatigue and even irritable bowel symptoms.

While this confusing syndrome makes accurate studies hard to find, it's estimated that as many as 10 million Americans may suffer from the condition. It's most common in women, and occurs between the ages of 35 and 60.

Since there is no cure, I can list the types of treatment that may offer you some relief, over and above the use of analgesics, such as aspirin, or nonsteroidal anti-inflammatory drugs (NSAIDs), such as ibuprofen. Other types of treatment include both ice packs and heat treatment, relaxation techniques, stress management, biofeedback and stretching exercises. Low doses of tricyclic drugs at bedtime may help sleep problems and reduce pain. A tender point may be injected locally with a 1 percent lidocaine solution in combination with a 40 milligram hydrocortisone acetate suspension.

Your prognosis may be favorable by utilizing a comprehensive, supportive program along with your physician's advice.

73. ***During an examination at summer camp, my 7-year-old son was found to have flat feet. We took him to his doctor for some help, but he didn't seem too concerned and did not prescribe any supports for my son's shoes. When my husband was younger, he had the same problem and was required to wear special shoes to correct the problem. What do you think will happen if I follow my doctor's advice? Do I need a second opinion? I would very much appreciate your advice. Thank you.***

It's more than likely that your son will grow out of the situation or have no problems with his flat feet. There's growing evidence that flat feet will improve by themselves over a period of time, and that problems are more common in people with high arches than with flat feet.

In years past, it was common to "correct" flat feet with special shoes or arch supports, and many people who received this treatment still believe that this is the way to go. But the "wait and see" theory is gaining more and more attention from practitioners, who see excellent results.

There are certain clues that help predict that these flat feet will correct themselves. Children with long, slender limbs or hyperextendable joints seem most likely to improve on their own.

Try this simple test for yourself: Have your son stand on tiptoe. If an arch then appears in his feet, your chances are very good that the flat feet will resolve over time.

If you're not sure of your findings, check with your doctor again. He may have used this same test and based his decisions on its results. If all of this does not convince you or calm your fears, you can seek a second opinion, although, in my opinion, you really don't need one at this time.

74. *I have a chronic pain in my heel. I can't tell you what makes it worse, but nothing makes it better. What causes it? What can I do about it? I hope you can figure something out for me. I'm stumped.*

If you haven't already done so, you should see your doctor. About half of the people with heel pain have a spur, which is a tiny projection from the bottom of the heel bone. The spur can be seen in an X-ray. Although it may be less than 6¼ millimeters (one-quarter inch) long, it can cause you a great deal of discomfort.

The other main possibility is an inflammation of one of the tissues that attaches to the bottom of the heel bone. If your problem is caused by inflammation, your doctor can prescribe pills to reduce the swelling or he can give you steroid injections.

In order to recover from the problem, you must relieve the stress on the muscles and other tissue that attach to the heel bone. You can do this by wearing shock-absorbing shoes or heel cushions and arch supports. In rare cases, surgery may be required for people with heel spur pain.

The best way to treat the pain, however, is prevention. You always should wear footwear with shock-absorbing qualities, and replace them with new ones before those shock absorbers are worn out. Also, if you participate in athletic activities, such as running or aerobic dancing, it'll be necessary to ease into those activities gradually to prevent the problem from flaring up.

75. *I had a hip replacement several days ago and am now in my initial period of recuperating, working hard to get back to normal. I have a fine surgeon, who thoroughly explained my operation to me, but as I sit here I can't help but wonder what the future holds in store. Just what can I expect now, and how long will this new hip hold up?*

Answers from the Family Doctor (Questions 66-95)

The news I have for you is certainly optimistic, but let me first state that I'm going to have to make a few generalizations, as I do not know all the specifics of your situation. Younger patients do better than older ones, not too astonishingly. And your body weight is a real factor, as hips do fail more frequently in individuals who weigh more than 81.8 kilograms (180 pounds).

An interesting sidelight is that hip replacements will fail more frequently than knee replacements, probably because hip patients feel almost completely normal after the operation and tend to put more stress on their new joint than they should. But that's the greatest thing about the operation, the relief of pain, which was probably a key indication for having the operation.

You're passing through a period of great importance to the eventual success of the procedure. That's when the correct physical therapy program will get you back on your feet in the gradual but continual manner that attains the best long-term results. The good news is that you can count on 10 to 15 years of service from your new hip, possibly longer, while following the golden rule of all patients with joint replacements: "Use it, but don't abuse it."

You do have to be aware of some special precautions, which consist of proper antibiotic treatment before certain dental and surgical procedures. Be sure to inform any doctor or dentist of the presence of your hip, and obtain the correct prophylactic antibiotic treatment when necessary.

And if the surfaces that bear the weight and provide the ability for movement (articulating surfaces) begin to show wear after a time, it's not always necessary to replace the whole prosthesis, but merely replace these surfaces, which is a bit like getting new brake pads for your car.

76. ***After sitting around for a while and then getting up to walk about, every so often I feel and hear a cracking sound in my hip. I know I'm not imagining this as my wife can hear it, too. It doesn't hurt, but it isn't a pleasant experience. Do you know what causes this and if it's a serious situation?***

Sounds that come from the joints are not too uncommon, especially in people with a bit of arthritis. There are a number of causes, and none of them is too serious.

If the surfaces inside the hip have become worn and damaged by arthritis, there can be a sound created by the rough surfaces grinding against one another. Sometimes there are loose bodies, bits of cartilage or bone, that float around inside the joint space and can cause a sound as they're moved about by the motion of walking.

Most of the time, however, the sounds are made by the tendons and muscles around the joint as they slip over a bump on the bone. Near the hip joint is a sac called a bursa, over which tendons pass. If it's inflamed, it too may be a source of sound. While the sound may be startling at times, it's usually of little consequence and shouldn't cause you any undue concern.

77. ***I was awakened from a deep sleep with a terrible pain in the calf of my leg. It was a long while before the pain went away and I could feel my leg relax again. This has never happened to me before, and I'm very worried. Do you know what this is, what caused it and what I can do to prevent it from ever happening again?***

You've described a leg cramp quite clearly, and these painful episodes may occur either during exercise or sleep. In your case, you probably stretched your foot or toes downward, causing the big muscle in your calf (gastrocnemius) to contract. However, instead of a normal contraction, the muscle went into a spasm, becoming hard and tense, and as you felt, quite painful.

This leg cramp usually lasts for but a few minutes and then lets up on its own. You can help ease the cramp and reduce the pain by massaging the area. Try to point your toes toward your head, which will stretch the muscle again. Getting out of bed and standing on the leg can also help.

The cramps occur most often after a day of unusual activity or exercise, for strenuous exertion can fatigue these muscles. Wearing a high-heeled shoe or one that is higher than you may be accustomed to also can contribute to the formation of a cramp at night. They're more common during pregnancy, in individuals with diabetes or those who suffer from circulatory problems.

Similar cramps also may attack an individual during exercise, but they're provoked by muscle fatigue, excessive sweating and loss of potassium, and dehydration. Drinking plenty of water during periods of exercise can help to prevent cramps.

If your muscle spasms are an occasional happening, there's nothing to worry about. However, recurring episodes should be reported to your physician, who may wish to prescribe a muscle relaxant to be taken before bedtime.

78. ***Aren't the two terms "lumbago" and "sciatica" one and the same? It seems to me I have heard even physicians use both terms to refer to a bad back. Maybe it's just calculated to confuse the patient, but I want to know.***

They're not the same. Lumbago, from the Latin word *lumbus*, or loin, may refer to any pain in the lower back, usually of muscular origin, but applicable to arthritic or bony pain as well.

Sciatica, or sciatic pain, is caused by a compression of the sciatic nerve, which runs from the low back, across the buttocks and the back of the thigh, into the leg, calf and foot. The pressure on the nerve may be caused by bony changes in the vertebrae, or from the bulging of cartilage that occurs with a slipped disc (intervertebral disc).

The treatment in lumbago is to reduce the spasm or pain in the muscles, and in sciatica, to reduce or remove the pressure on the sciatic nerve. Heat and analgesics frequently are used in both cases, which may be the origin of the confusion, for I'm unaware of the use of this term, or any other, just to confuse patients.

79. ***I've developed a most annoying and painful condition that is preventing me from getting around as much as I want to. It's a pain in the ball of my left foot that sometimes feels like I have a stone in my shoe, when there is nothing there. Is there something you can recommend to help me get rid of the pain and start me back on my walking program?***

It's pretty hard to make an exact diagnosis from the information you've provided. There are 26 bones that make up your foot, bound together by ligaments and many tendons that link muscles to the bones and provide the power that enables you to walk.

The area you describe, the ball of the foot, is the area in which five slim bones, the metatarsals, are located. Pain in this location is known as metatarsalgia and can be the result of a number of conditions. When the skin in this area is irritated from bunions or calluses, pain of this nature may result. However, arthritis is often the cause, a condition easily diagnosed with the help of an X-ray.

Sometimes physicians are surprised to find a stress fracture present as the culprit. Many people who must stay on their feet a great deal, or are overweight, or even pregnant are at risk. Sometimes a benign tumor of the nerve that passes through this spot can be the cause of the pain (Morton's neuroma).

While each condition requires its own treatment strategy, there are a few general tips I can offer. Check your shoes for fit, and stay away from tight-fitting shoes or those with high heels. A metatarsal pad, carefully fitted by a podiatrist or physician, may relieve the pressure that is causing the pain. Many over-the-counter pain medications, including nonsteroidal anti-inflammatory medications (NSAIDs), have been found useful. Injections of corticosteroids into the tender area may be used in rare cases, and surgery may be necessary to remove a Morton's neuroma.

Your best course of action is to have a thorough examination and careful evaluation to help choose the best treatment for your condition. Don't delay, it probably won't disappear by itself.

80. ***A friend of mine seems to have become a new person. He used to be one of the most uptight people I knew. Now there's a new relaxed way about him. He told me he does something called Progressive Muscle Relaxation. Please tell me what this is.***

Progressive muscle relaxation is a technique that aids in stress reduction by working through each muscle group in the body to remove stress. It's based on the concept of the mind-body connection — that relaxation of the musculature produces mental relaxation.

The technique involved is actually quite simple, and the effect quite successful. The best way to do progressive muscle relaxation is in a recliner with head and foot rests, but a couch or a pad on the floor with a pillow under your head will serve well, too. The room should be quiet and peaceful, with no phones or other interruptions. Soft background music can be used if you want. Clothing should be loose and comfortable, and no shoes should be worn.

You should begin by lying down and stretching comfortably. Arms and legs should not be crossed. Breathe deeply, then begin by clenching each hand to create tension, then releasing that tension. Concentrate on the difference between the tense and relaxed muscles. Proceed to tense and relax each part of the arms — the forearms, biceps, triceps, neck, shoulder, upper back. Then go on to the facial area. Wrinkle up your forehead, then release the tension. Tense your eyebrows, then release. Proceed to the jaws, lips, tongue, throat area and neck. Now do the same tensing and relaxing procedure going down slowly through your entire body.

Take time several times a week to practice this relaxing technique, and perhaps you, too, will feel like a new person.

81. ***Is there a condition in which the muscle turns into a bone? A friend of mine had an X-ray of his arm, and there was a piece of bone seen that normally isn't there. The doctor says that the only way to treat it is to remove it with an operation, but he wants to wait a while to see how big it's going to get. Is this right? Please help us.***

The condition is one that is known and bears the impressive name of myositis ossificans. It really isn't muscle turning into bone, although that is the meaning of the translation of these words, which come to us from both the Greek (*myo*, meaning "muscle") and the Latin (*ossificans*, meaning "to make bone").

The process begins with an injury, usually a contusion or strain, in which the muscle is torn, and blood collects in a clot called a hematoma. The most common spot for these types of injuries is the thigh, followed by the middle of the arm. The bone formation usually occurs only in severe injuries, or in a clot infection after a respiratory infection.

Slowly the clot is transformed into bone, possibly with bone cells that came from an injury at the same time to the covering of the nearby bone (periosteum). The bony mass keeps enlarging, for as long as six or seven weeks, after which a process of resorption begins. Small masses may disappear completely, but when a large bone mass remains after a longer period of time, the only way to remove it is by using surgical techniques.

Interestingly enough, there's another situation in which such benign bone growth may be seen, called drug user's elbow. Here the process starts with injury to muscles and surrounding tissues caused by the unskilled use of a needle in search of a vein. Instead, the needle rips the other tissues in the area. The brachialis muscle of the upper arm is the muscle most commonly injured.

If the doctor believes that your friend's injury is recent, he's correct in waiting a bit to see what develops before attempting to remove abnormal bone.

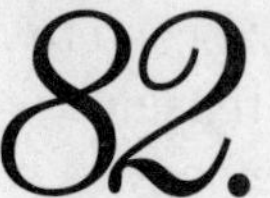

Arthritis of the knee has become more than I can cope with these days, and my family physician has set me to thinking about an operation to give me a

new knee. It sounds like a tremendous operation to me, but I wonder if it's the right thing for me. Could you give me enough information to help me make a wise decision?

It certainly is a tremendous operation, and a most wondrous one as well. Such operations that permit skilled surgeons to replace a joint destroyed by disease are among the most important developments in the care and treatment of arthritis to have come along in the past two decades.

With operations of the hip and knee topping the list, joint replacements, including the shoulder, elbow, finger and wrist, total well more than 500,000 annually. You should weigh many factors, with pain being the primary consideration. If the pain in your knee is so great that it disturbs sleep or makes your everyday activities difficult or impossible, you're probably a good candidate. Other considerations include the ability to carry on your job or occupation, and whether the quality of your life is jeopardized to the point where continuing in the present state is more than you wish to bear.

Meanwhile, your physician has thought about your type of arthritis, whether or not this operation can help, and whether your present medical condition permits this operation. To my mind, the fact that he has asked you to think about it means that he feels you will profit from the experience. If you do choose this type of treatment, you should exercise care in choosing a surgeon skilled in the procedure and an institution where these operations are routine.

Planning the operation may take some time, and you probably will undergo pre-admission testing and evaluation about 10 days before actual admission. You may be asked to donate your blood, which will then be stored and given back to you at the time of surgery. After the operation, look forward to a period of rehabilitation and physical therapy to help get you up and running in style.

83. ***My 12-year-old daughter, who has high hopes of an athletic career in tennis, is suffering from a swollen knee that was diagnosed as Osgood Schlatter Disease. We've looked up the condition in a medical book and are horrified with what we learned. Yet our wonderful doctor keeps telling us not to worry. Can you please explain the causes and proper treatment of this condition?***

The history of this answer to you took an interesting turn, for when checking my sources to refresh my memory, I found that my material spoke in optimistic terms about the outcome of Osgood Schlatter, a disease that strikes the knees of young teen-age boys and girls. I was all set to provide you with the reassurance that your doctor was correct, when my studies took me to our small public library, and I decided to try to duplicate your experience. Naturally the books available were all a bit dated, and when I read the explanations offered, I quickly understood your anxiety.

The description of the cause was "avascular necrosis of the ossification center of the tibial tuberosity," which translates into "the death of the bone-producing center of the tibial bump due to loss of circulation." While that may have been the accepted cause when Drs. R. B. Osgood and C. Schlatter first described the condition in 1903, it's a theory that no longer is generally accepted. Instead, it's believed that the condition — a swelling, very tender and painful area over the bump on the shinbone just below the knee — is most probably due to the strains and stresses that result from active participation in athletic competition.

While once a condition seen primarily in boys, girls are rapidly catching up as their involvement in sports increases. The good news is that Osgood Schlatter is considered a benign disorder, which in mild cases can disappear by itself. Treatment consists of pain medication as needed and restriction of physical activities, particularly those that require frequent deep-knee bending. Knee braces can be used, or even a cast to immobilize the knee if symptoms continue. A two- to four-month period of rest, followed by reconditioning and strengthening exercises, will soon have your young athlete back on her feet and playing her favorite sport.

84. ***Would you please explain the difference between osteoarthritis and rheumatoid arthritis? I'm always confused when these two terms are used. I'm at a point in life when I need some information. Are the treatments the same for both?***

While both conditions affect the joints in the body, they really have two quite different mechanisms. Rheumatoid arthritis is a chronic inflammatory disease that has a course of acute periods alternating with periods of remission. It can range from a barely noticeable disease to one that is crippling and mutilating. Although an infecting agent, such as a virus, has been sought, none has been found, and it's thought that the immune system is involved in the process. It's treated with anti-pain medicines and anti-inflammatory agents as well as medicines that repress the working of the immune system.

Osteoarthritis is a joint disease characterized by degeneration and loss of cartilage, and is sometimes known as degenerative arthritis. It's the most common type, seen increasingly as age advances, and it affects more than 10 percent of the population over the age of 60. Inflammation rarely is seen in this type. Pain is increased when the joint is in motion and relieved by rest. Though both aspirin and non-steroidal anti-inflammatory drugs (NSAIDs) are useful in its treatment, so are other treatments using heat and cold, and physiotherapy.

85. *I have a soft lump on the back of my knee that hurts when I straighten my leg. My doctor told me it was a Baker's Cyst, but I can't find anything about it in my medical books. Is this anything to worry about? Can it turn into cancer? It isn't getting any better, and I've had it for six months.*

It's also called a popliteal cyst, since the back of your knee is the popliteal area. It may be the result of a hernia, or pushing outward, of the fibrous capsule of your knee or of one of the bursa that are located in this area. A bursa is a sac or saclike formation that contains the thick, viscid fluid that helps to "oil" the joint and prevent friction.

Although a Baker's cyst (named not after breadmakers, but after Dr. W. M. Baker, who described it first) may occur at any age, it's seen most frequently in men age 15 to 30. Its cause is unknown, although trauma to the knee is suspected, and it never progresses into a cancer of any type.

Conservative treatment using anti-inflammatory medications or aspirating the fluid out of the cyst and injecting it with corticosteroids may help reduce the symptoms temporarily. However, your only hope for a permanent solution is to have the sac removed surgically.

The surgeon dissects the cyst away from the surrounding tissue and ties off the neck of the sac. When performed properly, this has a permanent effect and prevents the cyst from increasing in size and extending down the leg. The pain also will disappear, and you will regain normal function in your knee and leg.

86. *I'm a longtime sufferer from Paget's disease. I find it difficult to believe that all that can be offered as treatment are some simple pain pills. Can you tell me a bit about this disease, what causes it and what medications can possibly help me?*

Paget's disease of the bone, also called osteitis deformans, is a chronic disease occurring in adults where hyperactive bone is replaced by a softer, bonelike structure in various parts of the skeleton, such as the pelvis, thigh bone and skull.

Bone is in a constant state of remodeling, a process of breakdown and buildup. However, in Paget's the new bone is faulty and cannot perform all the duties of normal bone. The cause is unknown, but about 3 percent of adults over the age of 40 suffer from the condition, with men more commonly affected, in about a 3-to-2 ratio over women.

Many times there are no symptoms, but when they do occur they include pain, stiffness, headaches, some loss of hearing, increasing skull size and a general feeling of weariness and loss of energy. The diagnosis often is made by chance on an X-ray taken for other reasons, which shows the typical pattern of bone growth.

Generally, pain may be controlled by salicylates and nonsteroidal anti-inflammatory drugs (NSAIDs), such as ibuprofen. Two other medications are used to successfully treat and control the condition. Etidronate disodium may be taken in a dose of 5 to 10 milligrams per kilogram (2.2 pounds) of body weight, in a single dose each day for six months. Calcitonin also may be effective.

87. ***What is TMJ? Would you please discuss it and its treatment? It may help — and surprise — you to know that it was my dentist, not my doctor, who made this diagnosis.***

TMJ stands for temporomandibular joint and usually refers to problems with that joint. This joint is the one that allows your jaw to open, shut and slide your chin forward. It's a joint that takes a lot of stress, even under the best of conditions. Its proper alignment and function depend on many factors, including your teeth, the muscles of your face and mouth, and your ways of coping with stress.

The range of problems with TMJ is broad, but any disruption of its function usually results in a misalignment of the teeth and jaw and gradual deterioration of the joint.

The causes of TMJ problems are varied, and I'll discuss a few of them. Mouth or jaw injuries, such as those occurring in auto accidents or sports injuries, often start the TMJ problems. The jaw becomes misaligned due to the injury, and the joint wears unevenly due to the misalignment. The TMJ problems may develop slowly over a period of years after the injury. Personal habits such as chewing pencils or ice, grinding teeth or clenching the jaw from tension also can create a TMJ problem.

What are the symptoms of TMJ? Face or jaw pain, noises such as a clicking when the jaw is opened, or difficulty in opening the jaw are all symptoms. Some people report that the jaw pain travels to the head, neck, ears, shoulders and arms. TMJ should be suspected in anyone who suffers from frequent headaches that have no known cause. The symptoms worsen over the years unless the problem is treated.

Accurate diagnosis of TMJ is important before treatment can be begun. Specialized X-rays, especially a process called video arthrography, are part of the diagnostic work-up. Determining exactly how the different parts of the temporomandibular joint function in relation to one another is crucial to treating the problem with success.

The problem may not be in the joint itself; it may be located in the powerful muscles of the jaw. If this is the case, muscle relaxation is the goal. This may be accomplished by learning to control stress, using physical therapy to exercise the jaw muscles or using local anesthetic pain control. Sometimes muscle relaxants are prescribed to help the jaw muscles relax and heal. In some cases, a special mouthpiece is designed to realign the mouth and ease the pressure on the jaw joint.

If the problem is severe and doesn't respond to less permanent treatment, the alignment of the jaw and mouth must be altered. This can be accomplished in a variety of ways but should be undertaken when other methods fail, because the treatment is permanent and cannot be reversed. Changing the alignment of the teeth and jaw should be attempted only by someone who is well-experienced in successful treatment of TMJ. Sometimes the alignment of teeth is altered by grinding the surfaces, so that the upper and lower teeth meet more harmoniously. In more severe cases, surgery is performed to repair the temporomandibular joint. If the jaw joint is found to be deteriorated beyond repair, an artificial joint can be used to replace it.

In some parts of the country, arthroscopes are being utilized to diagnose and treat some forms of TMJ disorder. This shows great promise, because the physician can see directly into the joint with only a minimal incision and treat the problem without extensive surgery.

88. ***I have a lot of questions about steroids, from hearing all about the things that happened to professional athletes. Are these the same steroids that are used for skin rashes and allergies? Isn't it true that the***

bad side effects probably have been overstated by the press? I can't believe any sane person would take the risks some of the reporters talked about. Please give us the straight "dope!"

Pun noticed and accepted. To begin with, we're talking about another type of steroid than those included in creams and medications for rashes and allergies. Such medicines are called corticosteroids, and resemble the natural hormone cortisone produced by the adrenal gland. They have nothing in common with anabolic steroids, which are more closely related to the male hormone testosterone.

Therefore these drugs have both an anabolic, or building, effect, as well as an androgenic, or masculinizing, effect. Whether they are taken orally or by injection, it's the liver that must handle the chemical actions and changes that occur within the body. After these chemicals are used by the body (metabolized), the leftover fragments of the chemical (metabolites) are excreted by the kidneys and may be found in the urine tests used to check amateur and some professional athletes.

Let's look at some of the side effects, and I will let you be the judge of the press reportage of possible dangers. Among the minor side effects are psychological disturbances, including abnormal aggression, mood swings and even psychiatric problems. Add sleep disturbances, changes in sexual activity and libido, acne, masculine traits in women (chest and lip hair, enlarged clitoris and baldness) for completeness.

Now to the major side effects. They include liver tumors, peliosis hepatitis (a condition of the liver in which many small blood-filled cystic spaces develop in an area where liver tissue has died), hepatitis, leukemia, and an imbalance of the types and amounts of cholesterol in the blood.

Overstatement by the press? Not in my book. This is one time the press is to be complimented in taking the hard stand against the misuse of potent and dangerous drugs. As to the "why" of these actions by athletes, take a look at the tremendous amount of dollars involved in product endorsements and try to calculate the pressures they exert on many young people who are striving to rise above their disadvantaged beginnings. I, for one, am glad this is now in the open, giving us all a chance to re-examine our own attitudes.

89. ***My husband works too hard at a very demanding job. He also has been running three to four times a week for more than an hour at each session. When he began to have a pain in his right foot, he did nothing about it***

until it became so bad he could barely walk. Now the doctor tells him he has a stress fracture, and he must take it easy. Was it the stress on the job, or just running too much that brought on this problem?

While it may be true that your husband is undergoing much mental or emotional stress on the job, in this case it was the physical stress on the bones in his feet that caused this fracture. This is a common problem in runners and is the result of the repetitive shocks to the bone that happen during running, rather than by a sudden forceful blow.

The break may be seen in any bone that receives this type of stress, but it's found most frequently in the lower third of the tibia (shinbone) and in the bones of the foot. It's sometimes a difficult diagnosis to make if there is no local swelling, for the normal X-ray may not reveal the presence of the break until three weeks or more after the injury.

While one of the reasons this occurred may be overuse, your husband's running schedule does not seem to be excessive. But there are times when old and worn running shoes are to blame. If the cushioning is worn out, then the shoe has lost its shape and ability to properly support and cushion the foot.

Rest is the answer, of sufficient duration to give enough time for the bone to heal properly. If your husband tries to push it and begins his exercise routine before all is ready, then the fracture may never heal completely, or it may heal improperly. Many compulsive runners start up when the pain disappears, which can be too soon for the bone that's still in the process of repairing the fracture.

As your husband suffers through this enforced repose, he might do well to consider scheduling other types of relaxation activity to help relieve some of the stress that his occupation may be thrusting upon him. That might help resolve some of his other problems and turn this period into a "lucky break!"

The school nurse thinks my 13-year-old daughter might have scoliosis. Frankly, I can't see what she is talking about. Is there any way I can see for myself?

Scoliosis, a sideways (lateral) curving of the spine, usually appears in pre- and early adolescence. You, as a concerned parent, can do a preliminary screening of your daughter.

Have her stand tall with her back toward you. Frequently, in scoliosis, the head alignment appears to be to one side of the buttocks, one shoulder appears higher, one hip seems more prominent, and an unequal distance is seen between the arms and body. Now ask her to bend from the waist: Normally, in this position, both sides of the upper and lower back should appear symmetrical and the hips level. Any uneven symmetry in the rib cage or lower back is a possible sign of scoliosis.

After these preliminaries, if you at all suspect scoliosis, call your family physician and tell him or her your concerns. An experienced eye always detects this condition a bit more readily. Scoliosis is most easily and effectively treated in the growing years of adolescence, so you will want any necessary therapy to start as promptly as possible.

91. *Is it possible for rheumatism to attack your muscles, not your joints? I live in a retirement community and have been very friendly with an active woman who has suddenly stopped wanting to do things. She says she has "rheumatism," not arthritis. I can't get her to see a doctor, because she says it will pass.*

There are several disorders that leave a person with musculoskeletal stiffness and/or pain that generally spare the joints. Doctors usually refer to them as soft-tissue rheumatism — so your friend's diagnosis of her own condition may be close to accurate. However, it's very important for her to see a doctor, because the risks of permanent damage increase when the ailments are allowed to settle in the body without treatment for a long time.

The most common forms of soft-tissue rheumatism are bursitis and tendinitis. The bursa are soft sacs filled with lubricating fluid, which are located in connecting tissues, usually near the joints, where friction would otherwise occur.

When a bursa is irritated, by either pressure or injury, the little sac may become inflamed and fill with fluid — thus bursitis results. Usually bursitis will clear up when the inflamed area is rested for a while. However, it's important to do conditioning exercises once the attack is brought under control to restore function to the area. Too often, bursitis sufferers will abstain from using the affected area again, and reflex sympathetic dystrophy will set in — that is, the muscles will degenerate and lose strength.

Tendinitis is an inflammation of the tendons, which are whitish, fibrous bands of tissue that connect muscle to bone.

Treatment for both tendinitis and bursitis may include nonsteroidal anti-inflammatory drugs (NSAIDs) or injections of steroids into the affected area. If the swelling is severe, the doctor may insert a needle to draw off excessive fluid and bring down the swelling. The worst cases of recurrent bursitis may be helped with surgery. If the inflammation keeps coming back to the same bursa, it may be wise to have that bursa removed.

There are several other disorders that come under the broad category of rheumatism. Try to encourage your friend to see a doctor, so that she can begin effective treatment to clear up her problems.

92. *What can be causing my shoulder pain? The pain is always there, but dull. I know this is not much information to go on, but I just can't describe it much better.*

The shoulder joint is the most versatile joint in the body, possessing an enormous range of motion. It allows us to perform strenuous tasks, such as lifting and throwing, as well as simple manual tasks, like writing or sewing. Because of the shoulder's anatomical complexity, however, a trade-off is made. The shoulder's extraordinary range of motion, a great advantage for many activities, is counterbalanced by an instability that makes it subject to injury.

To diagnose the cause of shoulder pain, a great many factors must be considered, including bones, muscles, tendons, ligaments, vessels and nerves. Since countless causes can be involved, the first step in diagnosing the problem is to determine the exact location of the pain. The more acute the problem, the more likely the patient can pinpoint it. How the pain started is important to determine as well. Knowing if there was an injury or if the pain came on gradually is a key point in a diagnostic evaluation. If certain movements cause pain or are impossible to perform, they should be noted, as should any movements that relieve the pain. Swelling, burning, tingling or numbness in the arm will influence the diagnosis as well.

Knowing the type of activity a person engages in is also a key factor when diagnosing a shoulder ailment. For example, sedentary activities, such as writing, typing or sewing, force shoulder muscles to contract. Prolonged engagement in such tasks can cause shoulder spasms. Exercising to stretch the muscles can prevent the problem and should be performed, because if the joint is not allowed to move freely it can "freeze" and cause the formation of fibrotic adhesions.

On the other hand, strenuous activities, such as swimming or overhead work, cause certain tendons to stretch and compress. Such violent, repetitive action may traumatize the tendon and its sheath, producing pain. Other possible causes of shoulder pain can include chronic inflammation of a shoulder joint that may develop if a shoulder injury doesn't heal properly or if the joint is strenuously worked and abused. Even years after an injury, simple activities, such as rolling on the shoulder during sleep, may cause pain, tenderness and spasms. Arthritis, tension, fibrositis and bone calcification are still further possible causes of chronic shoulder pain.

If you're suffering from undiagnosed shoulder pain, I suggest that you see a physician in hopes of determining the cause. Simple, five-minute examinations have been designed to quickly pinpoint possible causes, and it's certainly worth your while to investigate them. Relief can be achieved readily in many cases.

93. ***My 37-year-old son has been diagnosed as having a type of arthritis in which his spinal column may fuse and become one bone. We're desperate for information that can help him prevent this terrible disease from progressing and robbing him of his youth. Please help.***

Without a doubt you're referring to a rheumatic disorder known as ankylosing spondylitis (AS), or sometimes referred to as Marie-Strumpell disease. It's a disease that is three times more common in men than in women, and strikes between the ages of 20 and 40.

The most common complaint of patients with AS is stiffness, particularly in the morning, which is gradually relieved by activity. Although the stiffness may occur in any joint — knees, ankles, shoulders and hips — it's the back that is the eventual target, with back pain of varying intensity occurring, frequently at night.

The term "ankylosis" means stiffening, while "spondyl" refers to the vertebrae and "-itis" denotes inflammation. The disease process is one of inflammation, with the tissues around the joints of the body, particularly the spine, becoming inflamed and swollen. This creates the pain, and the patient attempts to reduce the discomfort by keeping the joint immobile, which of course leads to more stiffening. As the joint attempts to heal, new bone is formed which may eventually join one vertebra to another. But it is the extremely rare case where the whole backbone becomes a single fused bone.

Much can be done to help your son. To start, the joint pain and stiffness, as well as muscle spasm, may be relieved by using nonsteroidal anti-inflammatory drugs (NSAIDs). In addition, a program of daily exercise to maintain both correct posture and flexibility is vital.

The good news is that even in patients who are not correctly diagnosed or treated, the condition may not disrupt their lifestyle, or cause a deformity. However, continued care and attention to therapy frequently can reduce this condition to occasional episodes of backaches and spasm, without deformity or compromised posture.

94. *Aren't the words "strain" and "sprain" used for the same physical condition? It seems that the doctors always give me the same advice no matter which one of these two terms is used as the diagnosis.*

No, actually strain and sprain are two separate situations, although I'm sure that many of us have used these words as if they were interchangeable. A strain results from overstretching or overexertion of a muscle. When you try to use a muscle once it has been strained, you'll know it, because it hurts and you often can actually put your hand over the area of injury by feeling for the aching muscle.

A sprain, however, is a joint injury and occurs when some of the fibers in the ligaments that form that joint are torn or ruptured. The ligament as a whole still remains intact, but the injury provokes pain in that area. A typical injury of this type is an ankle sprain. Because this joint bears most of the body weight and is subject to accidental twisting during walking, running and athletics, almost everyone has had to deal with this frequent sprain.

Obviously, whether it's a muscle that has been injured or a joint, your doctor is going to recommend rest, applications of heat to the area, and possibly some type of analgesic or painkiller. Nonsteroidal anti-inflammatory drugs (NSAIDs) like ibuprofen also are useful to reduce the inflammation and swelling that may be present. You would be wise to take that advice and not to overuse either the joint or the muscle until all signs of pain or tenderness have disappeared.

95. *Would you please define a leg tendon and a leg ligament. I have often read about football players undergoing surgery for a torn ligament. However, surgery of the tendon, to my knowledge, has not occurred.*

Although both structures are made up of fibrous tissue, the difference between the two becomes more apparent when we look at their shapes and their functions in the body.

Ligaments are bands of fibrous tissue that connect bones or cartilage, and serve to support and strengthen the joints. Tendons are cordlike structures that connect muscles to bones and transmit the power of the muscular contraction to the bone to produce movement. You can observe this easily by watching the action of the Achilles' tendon at the back of the ankle. You can wiggle your foot by contracting the muscles in the calf of the leg. This force is transmitted along the large tendon to the heel bone (calcaneus) and then your foot moves.

The jarring contact that occurs in football puts great strain on the ligaments, particularly those that surround and reinforce the knee joint. When the feet are planted in the turf and held in place by the cleats on the shoes, then a tackler comes flying in about knee high, even the tough fibrous ligaments can give way and tear as the lower leg is pushed into a position that nature never intended. Modern orthopedic surgery can repair these tears and put the player back on the field, after time for healing and reconditioning.

While the action of the tendons gives them more flexibility, and they are located in positions better protected against injury, they too can be torn if there is sufficient trauma. In such cases, they can be repaired by orthopedic surgical techniques, which can restore their function to normal in most cases.

The same information applies to tendons and ligaments found in other locations throughout the body.

4.

The Skin, Hair and Nails

Skin for skin, yea, all that
a man hath will he give for his life.

JOB 2:4

Stop and think for a moment. If someone asked you to list all the organs in the body, how likely is it that you would forget to include the skin? Most people do. Yet the skin is an organ, and a most important one at that. If you spread out the skin of a normal, average adult male, it would cover about 1.62 square meters (18 square feet), weigh over 12.5 kilograms (27.5 pounds) and account for about 15 percent of the total body weight. That makes it the largest organ, and deserving of a bit of respect.

The skin is the waterproof envelope that retains all body fluids and protects all the other organs from dirt, bacteria, the sun's damaging rays and the invasion of other harmful substances. It's flexible, permits full movement, helps keep our internal temperatures within the narrow margin that permits normal function and life, and contains an impressive array of sensor cells that provide the brain with constant news about our surroundings by conveying information about touch, pressure, heat, cold and pain.

The skin is the first thing that others about us see, yielding information about our age, race, color and sex. Since appearances are so important, the skin provides motivation for a multibillion-dollar industry devoted to products that make us "look better." A close examination of the skin's clarity, texture, temperature and color also can provide important information about our state of health. Not bad for the organ you forgot to list.

Answers from the Family Doctor (Questions 96-125)

The skin is made up of three layers. From the outside in, they are the *epidermis*, the *dermis* and the *subcutaneous layer*.

The epidermis begins with a layer of live cells called the *Malpighian layer*. It sits on the underlying dermal layer that is rich in capillaries and nerves. While in the Malpighian layer, the cells continually reproduce, push their way outward and gradually undergo several changes. As they leave the nourishing arteries that flow in the dermal layer below, they die and become compressed, so by the time they reach the surface, they form a hard, horny layer that protects the underlying tissues. It takes about a month for the cells to make the trip from the living layer in which they were formed to the outer layer of the epidermis. These dead cells contain a substance called *keratin*, which provides the strength and toughness to the outer cell layer. These cells are continually worn off and replaced by more cells growing up from below. It's these dead cells that provide most of the substance that forms the "ring around the tub" after a bath.

Within some cells of the Malpighian layer is another important substance. It's a pigment called *melanin*, and it's responsible for the color of the skin. There's very little melanin present in the cells of light-skinned individuals, but repeated exposure to the sun's rays may cause more melanin to be produced, resulting in a tan. Melanin is produced by cells called *melanocytes* (pigment cells). All races of people have the same number of these cells present in their skin. However, genetic (inherited) differences influence the amount and speed of melanin granule production within the cells. It's these differences that are a major factor in the variations of skin color in individuals.

The epidermis is a very thin layer, only about 0.2 millimeters (eight-thousandths of an inch) deep, but it becomes thicker where the skin is exposed to hard wear. The soles of the feet or calluses that develop on the hands and fingers are examples of thick epidermal layers.

The dermis gives the skin its elasticity and is composed of connective tissue and elastic fibers. This layer is rich in specialized nerve endings that can sense pressure, pain, heat and cold. This is where the *eccrine glands* (sweat) are located, equipped with ducts that bring the sweat to the surface of the skin. These glands are located throughout the skin, but are particularly numerous in the hairless regions, the soles of the feet and the palms of the hands. As sweat evaporates, it carries heat away and helps cool the body. However, the glands also may secrete fluid under the influence of the parasympathetic nervous system: the "cold sweat" of fear or emotion. In some parts of the body, the sweat glands become modified and produce a thicker fluid. These *apocrine glands* are located in the axillary (armpit) and pubic regions. When bacteria living on the surface of the skin break down apocrine gland secretions, body odor may be the unwanted result.

Sebaceous glands are located close to the roots of hairs, which also grow in the dermal layer. They produce a fatty substance, ***sebum***, that oils the hair and lubricates the skin. When these glands produce an overabundance of secretions, an "oily" skin results, often with large pores visible. An oily skin is seen in many individuals who develop acne, but this type of skin resists wrinkling. By contrast, when the sebaceous glands do not secrete much sebum, the skin becomes "dry," with a greater tendency to develop wrinkles, but in which acne rarely, if ever, is seen. A balanced skin is neither oily nor dry, while combination skin has patches of oily skin and other areas that are dry or balanced.

Many capillaries run through the dermis. They, too, help to maintain the correct body temperature. When we become overheated, because of physical activity or fever, the blood vessels dilate (expand) and permit more blood to flow through the skin. This causes our skin to appear red or flushed. Since the temperature outside our body is usually lower than our inner temperature, blood becomes a bit cooler as it passes through the network of capillaries in the skin. The heat is lost through a process of radiation, rather than evaporation, which is the heat loss process that makes sweating an effective cooling mechanism.

Another mechanism also can turn the skin red and create a warmth from within. This is the skin's response to challenges from the immune system. Special cells located in the dermis level can produce chemicals, such as histamine, bradykinin and various prostaglandins, when activated by allergens. These chemicals cause the capillaries to dilate, which produces the red hue, heat, swelling (as liquids exit from the capillaries into the surrounding tissues) and pain (from local nerve stimulation). All of these signals — redness, warmth, swelling and pain — are signs of inflammation, which is the result of an allergy or infection.

When the body temperature begins to drop, the blood vessels in the skin constrict (become narrower), which reduces the flow of blood to the skin. Smooth muscles (erector muscles) that are attached to the base of the hairs may contract and cause the hairs to stand up or, in areas where the hairs are less noticeable, cause goose bumps to appear. This really works to the advantage of fur-bearing animals (fur is just a form of dense hair), for as the hairs become more erect, the coat becomes thicker. This way the fur can trap more air between the hairs and increase the depth of the insulation that helps keep the body warm.

Unfortunately (from the point of view of retaining heat), humans possess little of this fur covering, except between the sixth and eighth months of fetal development, when the fetus is covered by fine hairs called *lanugo*. Normally this hair is shed before birth. As adults, we grow hair everywhere on our bodies except the palms of the hands, soles of the feet, lips, eyelids, nipples and parts of the external genitalia, but it is usually too short and too fine to notice. Hair is dead tissue that grows from a layer of cells in the hair root. The new cells push the older ones upward at the rate of about 13 millimeters (one-half inch) a month on the scalp. Most hair can grow to a length of about 70 centimeters (27 inches) before it falls out. Normally about 50 hairs fall out of the scalp each day. The hair follicle rests for about three months, then begins a new hair. The cycle of hair growth can be divided into three phases: *anagen*, when hair growth takes place; *catagen*, when growth stops and the hair is shed; and *telogen*, when a new hair begins to regrow.

The hair as seen in cross section under a microscope contains three concentric layers. The outermost layer is called the *cuticle* and is composed of thin overlapping cells in a pattern that looks like shingles on a roof. The middle layer, called the *cortex*, has many elongated cells, while the center layer, the *medulla*, has rectangular cells. The rounder the hair follicle is in cross section, the straighter the hair is, while a flat follicle produces curly hair, and an oval follicle produces wavy hair.

Hair color is produced by the same substance, melanin, that influences the color of the skin. There are two types of melanin in the hair: dark brown and red. The combination of the two is responsible for all shades that hair can exhibit. When the melanocytes die, the hair turns white (or gray, if you will).

Hair growth is controlled to a large extent by testosterone (male hormone) and is influenced by our inherited makeup. Hair growth is different in men than in women and is therefore considered a secondary sexual characteristic. While facial hair is rare in women, women do keep the hair growing on top of their heads at an age when many men must satisfy their need for hair by growing a beard. Balding tendencies run in families, with some people maintaining a luxuriant growth even through the aging years.

Below the dermis lies the subcutaneous layer of the skin, which is essentially a layer of *adipose tissue* (fat cells). This layer also functions to preserve heat, as the layer of fat provides another insulating blanket for the body. Different parts of the body are endowed with layers of different thickness, with the depth around the thigh, for example, being much greater than around the ankle. Women tend to have more subcutaneous fat proportionally than men.

The skin thickness is not the same throughout the body, measuring a mere millimeter (one-twenty-fifth of an inch) on the eyelids, to about 3 millimeters (one-eighth of an inch) on the palms of the hands and soles of the feet, with an average of about 2 millimeters (one-twelfth of an inch) elsewhere on the body.

The nails also are formed of dead cells and contain keratin, which is the same protein that gives toughness both to the outer layer of the skin and the hair. The same substance can be found in the horns of animals, which is another special adaptation of skin. The nails grow from special tissue located under the cuticles, called *nail beds*. The half-moon seen at the base of a nail results from the fact that the nail is not firmly attached to the skin below at that point. Fingernails grow at an average rate of 0.1 millimeter (.004 inch) per day, or 3 to 6 millimeters (one-eighth to one-quarter inch) per month. It takes about 5½ months to replace a fingernail from bottom to top. Toenails grow about one-third as fast as fingernails, and both grow more slowly with age, during cold seasons and at night. However, their growth is more rapid in women during pregnancy and the premenstrual period.

To conclude this discussion about skin, hair and nails, please remember that any changes in blemishes, freckles, moles or other skin markings might be the first signal of serious skin or systemic disease and should be examined by your physician as soon as possible.

Questions and Answers

96. ***I'm sure that I read somewhere that you never should open an abscess with a needle, for fear of starting an infection. My husband insists that all such things must be opened as soon as they're "ripe," to prevent the spread of the poisons through the body. Would you please clear this up?***

Your husband gets the nod on this one, provided he restricts his activity to abscesses. Blisters are another thing, however. Your beliefs probably stem from the warning not to open blisters caused by friction or prolonged activity. The tissue beneath the liquid pad formed by the blister has been damaged by the trauma. The fluid inside the blister, which protects the area from further damage, is sterile and should not be drained. The blister should be covered with a thick bandage to add another layer of protection to the injury.

Abscesses are another story. They're collections of pus beneath the skin, formed by white blood cells assembled to fight an invading bacterial infection. Abscesses begin as cellulitis, which is an inflammation within the solid tissue, and are noted by the redness, heat, swelling and tenderness that accompany the inflammation. As the tissue dies, a space is created that becomes filled with tissue fluids, white cells, bacteria and parts of the destroyed cells, forming pus and creating the abscess.

Abscesses can grow, destroying adjacent tissue and eroding blood vessels. When the bacteria get into the bloodstream (septicemia), the infection may spread to all parts of the body. Incising an abscess allows the contents to be drained away, reducing the chances of spreading infection and allowing the body's own power to repair itself to begin healing the wound. However, such surgical procedures are best left to the expert hands of your physician — they are not something to try at home with a needle.

97. ***My 15-year-old son has a whole lot of pimples popping out on his chest. If I didn't know better, I would think it could be acne, but I believe acne only crops out on the face. What could this rash be?***

Acne can cause pimples on the chest and back as well as the face. Teen-age boys suffer especially from acne pimples in that location. But there are other skin conditions or infections — and some medications — that can cause skin outbreaks on the chest.

The best way to find out what your son has is to see your doctor. All skin eruptions are best diagnosed when examined directly. Acne pimples are primarily blackheads (comedones, in medical terminology). If this outbreak is composed of small whiteheads (pustules) or reddened bumps (papules), the condition may be folliculitis (an infection of the hair follicles), or perhaps it's just a case of prickly heat. However, neither of these usually occurs on the chest.

The problem may be a skin infection, and your doctor can check for this by seeing if there are bacteria in the pustules. It sounds like this problem is causing a bit of anxiety, which only can be relieved with the personal diagnosis a physician can supply.

98. ***What do you make of a diagnosis of "tropical dermatitis" for someone who hates the sun and who certainly hasn't been in the tropics? This is the diagnosis from my doctor. I'm a high school freshman and need some answers.***

Dermatitis is an inflammation of the skin. Since I know of no condition actually called tropical dermatitis, I think I can safely assume from your brief history that what you have is atopic dermatitis. As many as 5 percent of the people in the United States are believed to have this skin condition, which causes an itchy rash.

Researchers don't know exactly what causes atopic dermatitis, but they know it's inherited and is related to an allergy. Diagnosis of atopic dermatitis can be made by checking your family's history and by having your doctor examine your skin. This same condition is sometimes referred to as eczema.

Treatment is usually topical, using medications that you apply to the skin. Cortisone-derivative creams or ointments, or antibiotics, may be prescribed. In some mild cases, cold compresses may do the trick.

You can help yourself by avoiding contact with things that commonly cause itching, such as certain soaps, detergents, some perfumes, dust, furs, wools and synthetic or scratchy fabrics. Bathing too frequently can worsen the condition by drying the skin. Above all, don't scratch. It will aggravate the rash, can cause bleeding and may damage the skin. Scratching can lead to a secondary bacterial infection that will only complicate matters.

This is not a serious condition when treated properly — it's just a nuisance. One positive thing is that this disease often burns itself out, so that many people who have suffered through childhood, the teen years and young adulthood with atopic dermatitis often are free of it by age 30. I hope this is the case for you.

99. ***While fighting an ongoing battle with bedsores in our aged and ailing mother, who is being cared for at home, we're constantly on the alert for a possible magical cure that can help her. What can you add to our understanding of this terrible condition, and do you have any secret potion to aid us?***

I wish that I had the remedy that could rid all sufferers of their bedsores (or decubitus ulcers, in medical jargon). Over the centuries there probably have been thousands of treatments suggested or tried to relieve bedridden patients of these gaping sores.

During the era of Hippocrates, a warm water wash followed by a vinegar sponging, a surgical trimming of all dead tissue, and then a poultice of verdigris (copper acetate), flower copper (copper oxide), molybdaina (lead oxide), alum, myrrh, frankincense, gall nuts, vine flowers and wool grease was used. This is not a concoction I would recommend today. But even in our modern times, we use remedies without scientific data to prove their effectiveness, such as aloe vera, gold leaf, insulin, sugar, vitamins and even iodine.

Three major factors contribute to the development of skin ulcers: pressure, time and friction. Pressure on the small capillaries that nourish the skin tissues compresses them, reducing the nourishing flow of blood to the cells, which leads to their death. The longer the patient remains in one position and the longer the blood flow is reduced, the more damage occurs to the cells. When the patient is pulled across wrinkled bed sheets, or the skin moves over the bony prominences of the body, friction results, which may cause blisters or abrasions that can lead to the formation of pressure or bed sores.

A sound program of treatment takes all these factors into consideration. The treatment consists of frequently turning or carefully changing the patient's position, and keeping the wound free of infection and clean of dead, or necrotic, tissue to aid natural wound healing. A wide variety of topical agents, including silver sulfadiazine or povidone-iodine, are applied directly to the skin. Newer, moisture-retaining materials reduce the number of dressing changes needed and reduce the loss of newly developed epithelial cells, which are the body's attempt to heal the wound. Maintaining good nutrition is a must. Surgery may be needed to clean or close a wound or place skin grafts in position.

The care of these patients is indeed difficult. You might consider studying the nursing literature, where many excellent articles about decubitus care can be found.

100. ***I have a bad case of blackheads, mostly on my face. Though I know you're not supposed to, I "pop" them from time to time, because I can't stand the dirty look it gives me. But what should I do? I wash as carefully as I can, several times a day.***

Blackheads are not a sign of dirt, nor of oily skin, which is commonly assumed. So your soap and water treatments are to no avail. Blackheads form in the pores of the skin, which are the surface openings of skin follicles. The follicle produces a waxy substance called sebum, which makes its way along the narrow channel to the surface of the skin. Along the way it picks up dead skin cells, which are shed by the lining of the follicle. This can form a sticky clump that can clog the opening of the pore. Oxygen in the air turns this mass black (a process called oxidation) and forms the blackhead you see.

Any over-the-counter medication containing benzyl peroxide may be sufficient to control a mild case of these unsightly blemishes. Ask your pharmacist to suggest one for you.

In more serious cases, a prescription medication (Retin-A) can be used. The treatment may take a few months to become totally effective, so it will require more patience on your part. Retin-A can cause dry skin and some peeling, so it's important that you use this medication under the supervision of your physician. Follow the instructions carefully, as doubling up on doses or applying the cream more frequently than indicated will not speed up your recovery, but it will increase your chances of having unwanted side effects.

101. ***Please help settle a discussion between two sisters. It's about the proper care of blisters on the feet. I still abide by the precautions my mother taught me, and break the blister with a carefully sterilized needle and then put a bandage on. My sister claims this is old-fashioned and that modern antibiotic ointments are the proper solution. Which treatment is correct?***

Frankly, I'm not impressed by either method, and certainly vote against the old sewing needle procedure. A blister is formed as a natural protection for the injured tissue beneath the blister. The correct manner of dealing with these annoyances is to keep them intact, clean and dry.

Removing the protection of the skin by puncturing the blister is an open invitation to infection. Try an ice pack first to reduce any swelling or inflammation. Then prepare a bandage or dressing with a hole in the middle to preserve the blister, but protect the area against further rubbing or friction. You may find "ready to use" moleskin bandages of this type at your pharmacy.

If the blister does break open, wash the area carefully with soap and water and dry completely. Then you may apply an ointment or cream containing an antibiotic or antiseptic, keeping the broken skin in place as it is the best covering of all. A sterile bandage to cover the sore area completes the treatment. Of course, you must now check your shoes to find the cause of the blister. Then remedy that situation or face the possibility of more blisters the next time out.

102. *I'm a bit awkward and so constantly knock myself against tables and chairs, with the result that I usually have a bruise somewhere on my arms or legs. While the bruises may be sore for a while, they're not too burdensome. I often have wondered whether there is a correct method for dealing with them. I usually just put a hot washcloth over the spot and hope it helps. What should I be doing?*

You should try to be more careful in getting about, and change your method of treatment. Whenever there's a possibility of swelling or bruising, the correct measure is to apply cold to the area. A bruise is an area where an injury is causing bleeding to occur just below the skin. A cold application helps contract the blood vessels and reduce the amount of bleeding.

Heat does just the opposite and can make things a good deal worse. Incidentally, don't try to treat the pain or swelling with aspirin, as that may reduce the ability of the blood to coagulate and increase the amount of bleeding in the area.

103. *I'm basically a thin person but have cellulite on my hips and thighs. Is there anything special I can do to get rid of this? Can you explain what cellulite is?*

Cellulite is really no different from regular fat. It's a word used to describe the bumpy orange-peel appearance of fat that most frequently appears on women's hips, thighs and buttocks.

Researchers have compared biopsies of fat taken from people with cellulite deposits to fat taken from people free of cellulite. They found that the fat is essentially the same. The ripplelike appearance is thought to be the result of the connective tissue that envelops each fat cell and separates the cells into compartments. These compartments bulge as more fat is stored in them due to weight gain.

Although some men are afflicted with cellulite, more women develop the problem because their outer layer of skin is thinner and fat distribution in females is more concentrated in some areas.

If you're thin but have patches of cellulite in the typical areas, then it will be tough, if not almost impossible, to get rid of it. Fat does not accumulate evenly over the entire body but has a higher concentration in some anatomical areas.

Unfortunately, there's no such thing as "spot reduction." I advise you against believing advertisements that promise such results. In reality, exercise along with a low-calorie diet will help take fat off all areas of your body, and may be of some help. Exercising the areas where you have cellulite will tone the underlying muscles, but it won't necessarily remove fat from that area of the body.

104. *A lot of your readers suffer from corns and calluses. I'm sure they all would like to know where they come from, what they are and what to do about them.*

This is an important health question that affects many people. According to a recent survey, about 155 people out of every 1,000 have some type of corn or callus, although fewer than four of those people will require medical attention.

The causes of both of these skin changes include friction and pressure. The skin responds by becoming thicker and tougher as a protective mechanism. The horny outer layer of the skin, called the stratum corneum, becomes thicker in the area of increased pressure or rubbing (for example, from a tight shoe).

A corn has a hard core a bit like an upside-down pyramid, with the base at the surface of the skin and the point pushing inward as a result of pressure from the surface. When this point presses against the nerve endings in the nearby tissue, a stabbing pain may result. Although a callus is formed from similar tissue, it has no hard central core, which is why it differs from the corn.

The treatment of both begins by attacking the cause: preventing the friction and relieving the pressure on the area. That means checking shoes, particularly athletic gear, for a correct fit. It may require stretching the shoe a bit in areas where corns and calluses now exist. Try using thick socks to absorb some of the pressure, or use corn and callus pads directly on the feet to reduce the pressure to the irritated areas.

Home treatment may consist of soaking the corn or callus in hot water, and then trimming the surface very carefully with a sharp knife or razor. Specially medicated plasters containing chemicals that can dissolve the tissue (keratolytics) are frequently very helpful. When these simple home remedies fail to correct the problem, it's time to seek professional help, where more aggressive treatment techniques can be used to rid you of these annoying and painful conditions.

105. ***My wife showed me a blister or two that had formed on her arm. They're not large or tender, and look like any ordinary blister. I wanted to puncture them with a needle sterilized in a match flame, but she wouldn't let me, saying that they could be the sign of something serious. I don't need unnecessary medical bills. Is she being overcautious or should I just perform my minor surgery?***

Unless you can find a rational explanation for the formation of these blisters, your wife may be justified in her concern. Blisters (doctors call them bullae) may result from many ordinary circumstances, such as a burn or the irritation of a tight-fitting shoe. When you know the cause to be a simple one, the blisters are best left alone without your surgical assistance, for they break and heal in their own good time as the tender skin beneath re-forms.

However, there are a number of other reasons why such lesions develop that require more attention, and the examination and advice of your physician may be truly necessary.

Certain drugs can cause eruptions of blisters, including medications used for arthritis, infections (antibiotics) and hypertension. Of course, not everyone develops these liquid-filled bumps when taking the drugs, but it may happen in those who are particularly sensitive to medications. Exposure to excessive heat, cold or harsh chemical products may be the reason. Poison ivy, oak and sumac also produce similar lesions. In addition, there are several diseases that may be the cause of the problem, known as bullous disorders.

Your best action is to take stock now and determine whether any such explanations can account for the presence of the blisters. Are they changing or spreading? Are any other symptoms developing, such as fever and fatigue? Have other skin problems or rashes developed? If they have resolved by now, as I suspect they might, there never was any cause for alarm. If not, put your needle away. It's time for your wife to see her physician.

106. ***I'm 22, have been a diabetic for five years, and I don't really follow my diet. Lately I've been thinking about getting a tattoo, but I was told that diabetics shouldn't get tattoos because we have a slow healing process. I'm willing to take the risk.***

It looks as though you have already made up your mind. If you're expecting to get me to approve this foolishness, you had better think it through again. I don't want to put all the blame on you, for certainly society and my profession are a bit at fault for not getting through to you, but I can't help but wonder what is going on inside your head. All the educational information available about diabetes and the dangers of its complications seems to have missed you.

Perhaps at 22 you feel immortal, but the chronic perils of your untreated disease will soon chop away at your years and shorten your time with us here on Earth. Not only do you risk poor healing, but the dangers of infection in an uncontrolled diabetic are frightening.

Once the protection against infection provided by the skin has been pierced by that little needle, a local infection can extend to cellulitis and blood poisoning and can even permanently affect your kidneys as well. We're not talking here about an infection that is easy to treat with antibiotics, but one with serious complications that lead to permanent damage and death.

Don't tell me that your tattoo artist is careful about keeping his instruments clean. If he takes you on as a client (that is if you admit your problem to him), he's submitting you to a risk no sensible person would be willing to undergo.

107. ***During a recent skiing vacation, one of the instructors kept harping on the prevention of "frostnip." We thought it was a cute term for frostbite, but after returning home we began to wonder if it represented some other problem. Have you ever come across this term, or do you know what it refers to?***

A true frostbite, improperly treated or ignored, may take a large chunk of tissue as its price. A frostnip is a little bite, if you will, and refers to a superficial or less damaging frostbite.

Frostnip affects only the surface cells of the body. With proper care, no tissue is lost. Though the affected tissue may look white and waxen and feel cold, it's still soft and springy to the touch. The frozen part should be warmed promptly, but never rubbed with snow, or even massaged vigorously, as this friction can break the skin and open the path to infection. Warm water or the body heat obtained from an unaffected hand may be used to gradually return the tissue to normal.

Of course, prevention is the best method of treating any cold injury, with proper clothing as the first line of defense. A bit of reading on this subject before your next outing seems advisable.

108. ***Whenever there's an extra chill in the air or whenever I'm startled or emotional, my skin breaks out in a crop of "goose bumps." I know it's not harmful, but I can't help wondering what it means. Please tell me what causes these peculiar bumps?***

It's all part of some leftover reactions we inherited from our primitive ancestors. Thinking about our pets, whose hair stands on end when they're frightened, will help you understand your own situation.

Each hair is supplied with a tiny muscle called the arrectoris pili (which means it causes the hair to stand erect). In some areas of our skin, this muscle, which is part of the hair follicle, is still present although the skin is hairless.

When we're frightened or aroused — in fact, affected by anything that stimulates the production of adrenaline in our system — these muscles contract. If there is hair present, it "stands up." In hairless skin, it produces goose bumps or goose flesh, if you will. It's an interesting reaction, but it can give your thoughts away if you become emotional in front of someone who is a careful observer.

109. ***I have a difficult time keeping my hands clean because of my job, and I have real trouble with hangnails. It may seem like a simple problem, but let me tell you, it's no joke for the person who has the pain. Where do these things come from, and what is the solution?***

No problem is too simple to be answered, especially when it is such a common situation that affects many readers.

The hangnail is really not a nail at all, but a small spit of skin that occurs around the nail. It is the result of trauma to the fingers, dryness and the use of degreasing agents for cleaning the hands, including soap. Most of the pain develops when the hangnail becomes infected and inflamed. Then the familiar redness and soreness develop, often leading to sharp, constant pain.

The infection is provoked by tearing the hangnail away, instead of the recommended technique of cleanly cutting away the excess skin with scissors or clippers. Sometimes the source of infection is the mouth, as many people habitually try to trim the hangnail with their teeth. Any tearing of the skin in the presence of bacteria opens the door to a painful infection.

Prevention is the best course, by regularly using a hand cream or moisture cream to keep the skin soft and prevent drying. When a low-grade infection sets in, an ointment containing an antibiotic is useful in controlling the problem. If the infection becomes more severe, it's time for a doctor visit and a prescription for oral antibiotics.

110. *I frequently break out with large red blotches all over my body that seem to come and go. I've never been able to get a doctor's appointment while I still had something to show him. My boyfriend says they're hives and nothing to worry about, but I'm still anxious. Can you tell me what the condition is and what I can do about it?*

It's always difficult to make an accurate diagnosis about a skin condition without actually seeing the lesion or rash, but since your doctor seems to be in the same boat, let me try.

Your boyfriend's assessment of the situation may be correct. Hives are itchy red blotches that suddenly appear anywhere on the body, and then tend to fade out with a new crop arriving within minutes. They may be as small as a pea or as large as a dinner plate, with all sizes in between occurring at the same time. The appearance of the skin changes constantly for the duration of the "hives attack," which may last anywhere from a few minutes to a few days. Swelling may accompany the rash.

Hives are the result of an allergy or exposure to some type of skin irritant. The allergy may be to food, food additives (such as food coloring or preservatives), medications (either prescribed or over-the-counter), or substances that have been inhaled (dander, dust or pollen). Hives also may result from an infection or insect bite. Some people even develop hives when their skin is exposed to heat or cold extremes.

First aid for ordinary hives requires you to stop any vigorous physical exertion and apply cool compresses to the skin. This will help reduce the itch, which becomes worse when you're warm. Antihistamines also are useful in combating the hives. But the most important thing you can do is to try to discover just what sets them off. Keeping a diary of daily activities can help.

If the hives or swelling become worse or are accompanied by wheezing, dizziness or shortness of breath, an emergency visit to your hospital or physician is a must, because these are signs of a severe reaction. Short of that, hives are more of a nuisance than a severe disease, so you need not be overly concerned.

111. ***I'm having a problem with the nail on my left big toe. It keeps cutting into the flesh, causing me much pain. Now I notice that the same thing is starting on the right toe. Is this a sign of any medical condition and what should I do to take care of it?***

You're describing a condition known as an ingrown toenail, which occurs when the side edges of the nail grow into the flesh of the toe. This can create a painful problem, which can progress into an inflammation or even an infection with abscess formation.

Assuming that you have no particular deformity of either toe, the problem most likely is caused by cutting the nail incorrectly. The nails always should be trimmed straight across rather than rounding them to fit the shape of the toe. This allows a natural growth pattern that permits the nail edges to grow over the surrounding tissue, preventing them from digging into the flesh.

You may be able to correct the situation by trimming away the portion of the nail that is cutting into the skin and soaking the foot in warm water. It may require that you wedge a small ball of cotton or gauze under the edge of the nail to help push back the flesh until the nail grows over the area.

If these simple measures do not remedy the situation, a visit to your physician is necessary, because the nail must be cut back to relieve the pressure and pain. Any infection will need an antibiotic.

112. ***For about a year on and off, I get a rash that itches and makes my skin real tender around my waist, between my busts, around my bra and back. I've changed the soap I wash clothes with, I take a shower without soap, and I rub the rash with calamine baby lotion, but nothing makes it go away. Is there anything that can help me?***

I'll certainly try to help, although dealing with skin problems without actually seeing the rash is not the easiest thing to do. My first thought is that your condition might be a type of dermatitis known as intertrigo, based on your description of where the rash appears and the failure of the types of remedies you've attempted.

This rash develops in the folds of the skin where the surfaces rub together and the openings of the skin pores are covered. Such a condition leads to the breaking down of the cells that lie on the surface of the skin (a process called maceration) and an irritation that provokes redness, tenderness and itching. To further complicate matters, an infection by bacteria or a fungus may occur. This skin problem is most common in obese individuals who live in a hot climate, which provokes constant perspiration.

There are several steps you can take to rid yourself of this annoyance. First, use an antiseptic soap during your shower to help combat any possible infection. You must dry yourself thoroughly, taking care to blot away all the moisture that remains deep in skin folds. The careful use of a hair dryer on its lowest heat setting can be helpful, but never set it too hot or use it too close to the skin, which can cause burning.

If the infection persists, delaying the healing of the skin, you may have to resort to a prescription cream that contains an appropriate antibiotic or anti-fungal agent. With any luck, the problem should clear up in just a few days. The secret to preventing its recurrence is keeping the skin as dry as possible in the areas of irritation.

113. ***I'm annoyed by a constantly itchy skin, which sometimes drives me to distraction. I'm a clean person and am sure there are no critters causing my problem. But there must be some advice you can offer to reduce my torment and make life livable.***

I'm sure you are a meticulous person, but since there are many causes of a persistent itch, it still may be worthwhile for you to have a checkup to try to determine some physical cause.

Doctors label an itch like this pruritus. They know it may be caused not only by "critters," but by allergies, parasites and both skin and internal diseases. However, a dry skin is the most common reason. And there are a few tips I can offer that can help reduce the problem, no matter the cause.

If dry skin is the main problem, maintaining a healthy level of moisture in your home will help, particularly if you live in warm, dry climates or in a heated apartment in winter. A humidifier will be of great comfort. Reduce your bathing habits, as frequent showering with harsh soap can aggravate the condition, as can the use of water that is too hot. A lukewarm shower followed by the application of a moisturizing body lotion is indicated.

Stay away from tight-fitting clothes. Cotton fabrics may be kinder to your skin than wool or synthetics. Dry your skin with pats of the towel instead of vigorous rubbing. Although it may seem impossible to fight the urge to scratch, realize that you can injure your already delicate skin if you do scratch hard, especially with jagged or roughened fingernails.

The last but sometimes most effective measure is to change your laundry detergent to a mild soap, which is less likely to cause irritation, and be sure that all laundered clothes are rinsed well. These are all effective actions you may try for yourself, but a physician's diagnosis and available medical treatments may result in completely ridding yourself of this raging itch.

114. *The topic of dieting came up recently in a discussion with friends. It was suggested that the easiest way to lose weight was by having the fat removed by suction. What can you tell me about it, and how safe is it?*

The physique-conscious American is constantly experimenting to find fast and simple means of improving body image. One plastic surgery technique that has been developed is the removal of fat cells by the use of a suction instrument.

The process has been given many names, such as liposuction, lipolysis, lipodissection and lipoplasty, but they all involve the same technique. The surgeon makes a small cut in the area of excess body fat, inserts a tube into the region and applies suction to remove fatty tissue. People whose skin is elastic enough to shrink back to its pre-stretched size will have the best results.

The most common complications include bruising, skin discoloration and loss of sensation in the area of fat removal. These complications should resolve themselves in a few weeks, but skin dents may be permanent. Approximately 15 to 30 percent of the material that is removed is blood. Sometimes a transfusion is necessary if a liter (about a quart) or more of fat is removed.

Remember that this is cosmetic surgery used for the removal of localized deposits of fat — not a treatment for obesity. Before undertaking this procedure, you should consult with your doctor and have all the details of the risks and benefits carefully explained.

115. *My doctor pays careful attention to my fingernails as part of my regular visit. I'm always curious as to what he's searching for in such an insignificant part of my body, but I've never dared ask. Can you enlighten me?*

Your nails are not as unimportant as you seem to think. They can offer the careful and attentive physician vital information on otherwise hidden details of your personal health. Like the rings of a tree, the nail contains a record of a person's immediate health history. Conditions ranging from nutritional and vascular disorders to the presence of endocrine or infectious diseases can be detected from the evidence at hand (so to speak).

Thickened, ridged nails, for example, can be a sign of vascular inefficiency or renal failure that accompany aging. Discolored, yellow nails can indicate a number of conditions, including syphilis and cancer. A darker colored band running horizontally through a nail may be evidence of congestive heart failure. These and many other specific nail conditions may tip off your doctor to a health-threatening condition that might otherwise pass unnoticed.

116. ***School has just started and I already have a note from the school nurse that there's a case of head lice in my daughter's class. It seems that this happens just about every year at this time. What's a mother to do? I don't want my daughter to bring those things into our house, but I can't keep her home from school either.***

Every fall, school health officials and parents are on the alert for the lice invasion. Your best protection and best hope for prevention is an understanding of the problem.

Since head lice neither jump nor fly, they get from one head to another when youngsters swap headgear of any kind. That means hats, earmuffs and the headsets on their ever-present Walkmans or radios. Sharing combs and brushes probably tops the list of actions that help the lice get from one head to another. Warn your daughter about all such activity. Another path opens when headgear is all piled together in school closets, lockers or where children share storage space for personal belongings.

To prevent lice from spreading in your home, inspect your daughter's head on a weekly basis through the end of lice season, which lasts through November. Look for those tiny, oval-shaped, silver-colored nits (the eggs of the head louse), which are as big as the head of a needle. A magnifying glass will make your task easier.

If you find any lice or nits, then you'll need the help of a special shampoo that contains a medication designed to kill the lice. Several are available over the counter, and your pharmacist can help you select an effective preparation. It's very important to follow the directions on the label. In some cases, a single application will do the job.

You'll have to comb the nits out of your child's hair, because many schools will not allow him or her back until he or she is nit-free (yes, it's called nit-picking). You'll need to use a special comb that comes with many of the shampoos. You'll also need to clean your daughter's environment, clothing, sheets, pillowcases and the like. Items that can be washed should be cleaned in very hot water and left in a dryer set on high for at least 20 minutes. Blankets and stuffed animals should be sealed in a plastic bag for 14 days. This will kill the "buggers," which need to be in contact with human hosts to survive.

117. ***I guess I let it go for too long, and now I have a terrible-looking horn where my big toenail used to be. Could it be the result of a devil's curse? What can the doctor do to help me?***

If you have the condition I think you do, it wasn't a curse that caused it, but your own neglect. You must have realized that toenails don't normally grow this way and should be trimmed on a regular basis.

The condition has a fancy medical name, onychogryphosis, which comes from two words — "onyx," which means nail, and "gryphosis," which means hooked or curved. Sometimes the horn grows so large that it looks like a ram's horn, and can be referred to as ram's horn nail.

At any rate, it has got to go. There are two possible choices of treatment that your physician may offer you. The choice will depend upon the size of the growth and the condition of your feet. It may be possible to cut the nail back to size, using the appropriate surgical instruments. This would cause no pain, but you would have to promise to keep your nails trimmed.

If the nail is really deformed, the physician will have to remove the nail completely and destroy the tissue from which your toenail grows. Just cutting the nail away won't help as a new nail will grow back in four to 10 months, probably more disfigured than before. The operation can be performed with an injection of local anesthetic to prevent pain. See your doctor soon. Things won't get better by themselves.

118. ***My hearing is not what it used to be, and I'm sometimes too embarrassed to ask a question to clear things up. However, I would swear my daughter told me over the phone that my grandson had suffered a "parrot nick" that required a doctor's care. But they don't have a parrot. Is this something serious? I'm totally confused.***

You had me confused, too, so much so that I was going to bypass your question. While on the phone with a friend, I mentioned your letter and when I heard him say parrot nick over the telephone, it suddenly became clear. Your daughter must have said paronychia, which is the name of an infection that is located in the tissue around the fingernail.

Paronychia can start with a break in the skin caused by a hangnail or even a simple bang. Infecting bacteria begin to multiply and a pocket of pus is formed. This painful problem should be treated with an appropriate antibiotic.

While hot soaks or compresses to the area can help, frequently the pocket must be opened with the point of a scalpel to allow the purulent material to drain. Generally that's all it takes. Then your grandson may soon be back to his usual activities without any need for you to worry further.

By the way, a simple solution to your telephone hearing problem is to get a phone with a sound amplifier. There are rather inexpensive models available. You would be amazed at how much they help. I was!

119. ***When our son was born, we thought we had a Gorbachev in the family because there was a big red mark across his forehead. Our doctor diagnosed this as a port wine stain. We also found out that our child is normal in all other ways. Our question is when and how should this blemish be treated? Do you know of any new treatments that can help?***

Port wine stains, or nevus flammeus in medical terminology, occur quite frequently. As many as three out of every 100 children may be born with similar marks. When such "blemishes" (as you put it) are seen on certain parts of the face, it may be part of a condition known as Sturge-Weber syndrome. This syndrome sometimes causes problems in the neurological system of these children, but that occurs in only about 8 percent of all cases. It seems apparent that your son is not one of these.

The fact is that these skin lesions do not fade over time, as some others do, and must be treated. In the past, a variety of techniques were used, including freezing with liquid carbon dioxide, plastic surgery and skin grafts, tattoos and even just an opaque cosmetic cream that matches the patient's skin color to cover the mark. Argon laser therapy, which is considered the best technique generally available, often left scars in place of the red spot.

A new technology, using a new laser, now is receiving high praise from those who have seen its results. Although it may take several treatments to totally erase a port wine stain, there's little risk of scarring when the skin is properly protected.

Early treatment is recommended, since a baby's skin is thinner. Though there are only a few centers offering this technique, it's not that expensive. Charges per visit are in the $200 range, and much of the cost should be covered by insurance. You should consult with your own physician, but my advice is to start treatment as soon as you can.

120. ***Would you please provide some information about the treatment of poison ivy? What I really want to know is if the fluid in these enormous blisters, which are all over my arms and legs, can cause the poison ivy reaction in my children. My mother says it will. What do you say?***

I know that the fluid in the blisters looks pretty bad, but it doesn't contain anything that will cause similar blisters on your children's skin. The chemical that causes the reaction in sensitive individuals is the oil given off by the poison ivy plant. It's called urushiol, and about half the people in the United States are sensitive to it.

The best treatment is prevention. You can do that by avoiding contact with the three plants that cause these reactions: poison ivy, poison sumac and poison oak. However, once the rash and its terrible itch (pruritus) have started, it's too late for that.

The first step in the basic treatment of this contact dermatitis is to be sure that all the oil has been washed away, by using soap and warm water. That will prevent additional spread of the reaction to other parts of the body. All clothes that may have traces of the oil on them should be speedily thrown in the wash.

Mild cases, which cause only a little discomfort, may be treated with calamine lotion to control the itch. However, when the rash is extensive and the itch more than you can bear, it's time to visit the doctor and get some prescription medications. Both antihistamines and corticosteroids can be used to obtain some immediate relief, but it might take as long as two weeks using smaller and smaller doses of oral cortisonelike medication each day before you will really be out of the woods (Ha-ha!). Sorry, I couldn't resist.

121. ***My 47-year-old son has a severe case of psoriasis on his head, which his doctor says he can't help. My son has tried nearly everything anyone suggests, and it's getting worse. Do you know of anything that can help us?***

It's apparent your son has a difficult problem, but there's effective treatment for scalp psoriasis. About 1 to 2 percent of Americans suffer from this chronic and distressing skin condition, and about half of them have some problems with the scalp. Psoriasis can strike at any age, but most often starts in young adulthood. The lesions in the scalp may extend a few centimeters beyond the hairline, but they rarely affect areas that are bald. However, the condition itself may cause hair loss and hair thinning.

Treatment is always complicated and may take some time before the proper combination of medications can be discovered, since there are many preparations to consider. So my first advice is patience. The treatment will include some type of medication to be applied locally. It's important to remove the heaped-up scales first, which may be done by applying mineral oil to the scalp and combing out the scales with a fine-tooth baby comb.

Next your son must find a medicated shampoo to help. Coal tar shampoos can be useful, particularly when used regularly. The shampoo should be kept on the scalp for at least five minutes to be effective. He also can use coal tar mixed in petroleum jelly to be massaged into the scalp and left in place several hours before shampooing out. It's messy but useful in moderate to severe cases.

Other products may contain keratolytics (chemicals such as salicylic acid) used to "dissolve" the scales. Some coal tar shampoos may contain this medication as well. When dealing with a truly difficult case, a physician may employ anthralin, which is most effective, but be careful to avoid contact with the eyes and normal skin.

If local treatment fails (and I have left out a few), your son can turn to oral medications, which include hydroxyurea, methotrexate, etretinate and isotretinoin. The use of psoralen and ultraviolet A (PUVA) may be used for balding patients without much hair. These oral medications are most frequently used when the patient has extensive lesions involving other areas of the skin in addition to the scalp. Applications of corticosteroid preparations to the skin are most helpful, but this cortisonelike material is not recommended as an oral medication for psoriasis.

You may not understand all of these medications, but I have included their names to show you that all is not lost. There's much help still available for your son.

122. *A recent operation has left me with an ugly scar, which my family doctor calls a "keloid." I would like to get rid of it, if possible. What can be done to remedy this situation and what type of doctor can help me?*

Let's take the last part of your question first. To begin, you may need to consult a dermatologist (often called a skin doctor), one who is experienced in the use of X-ray and laser therapy. In some cases, particularly keloid scars about the face, the skills of a plastic surgeon may be required. Your family doctor is the first person to consult, as he or she can help you locate the proper specialist.

Unfortunately, all treatments of keloids, which are really overgrowths of scar tissue that tend to be shiny, smooth and often domed-shape, up to this time have been less than perfect. But don't be disheartened; the treatments can, and do, help correct the unsightly condition.

Among the newer treatments are the removal of the scar with a special type of laser surgery, plus daily applications to the area of a high-potency, steroid-containing medicine, injections of corticosteroids into the scar itself, and/or low doses of X-ray to the keloid. The entire series of treatments takes about four to eight weeks, and additional treatments may be required for as long as two years.

123. *While everyone now is warning against the dangers of a suntan, I still don't understand what causes a tan. If the body produces this naturally, isn't it a good thing? Perhaps you can explain just what causes a sunburn as well.*

Obviously a sunburn with its painful consequences is something to avoid, and it rapidly can change a fun weekend into something far less enjoyable. Actually there are four effects upon the skin from exposure to the ultraviolet (UV) radiation in the sun's rays, all of which attempt to reduce the injurious effects. They are erythema, short-term tan, common tan and delayed thickening of the skin.

Erythema is the name given to the red flush that occurs in the skin after exposure to the sun's rays (as well as a variety of other causes). A substance called prostaglandin is released by the tissues, which causes the capillaries in the skin to dilate (open), fill with more blood and give the red coloring to the skin. This is an attempt to protect the skin and reduce the damage from the sun's rays. It comes on from two to 12 hours after exposure, and its severity is related to the amount of exposure.

A short-term tan is caused by ultraviolet A (UVA) rays. It's created by the oxidation of the melanin (pigment) in the skin and fades away in a day or two.

The common tan takes several days to develop. It's caused by the production of more pigment in the skin as a response to the sun's ultraviolet B (UVB) rays — pigment that acts as protection for the skin the next time it is exposed to the sun.

Over a period of time, perhaps several months, the upper layers (epidermis) of the skin thicken. These thick skin layers also can absorb the UVB rays and reduce the amount of harmful radiation that reaches the lower (basal) layer of the skin.

A word about protection: Of the 1 million new cancer cases that are diagnosed each year, about 30 percent occur in the skin and are thought to be provoked by chronic exposure to UV radiation. A person with a history of more than six serious sunburns in a lifetime is 2.4 times more likely to develop a melanoma, which is a lethal cancer that spreads rapidly through the body. If exposure to the sun can't be controlled, be sure to apply sunscreen with a sun protection factor (SPF) of at least 15 to cut down your exposure to these potentially harmful rays.

124. *I know my condition is called vitiligo, but I know little else about it. I'm under treatment that is long, but I can't see any results yet. Can you offer me some explanations and information?*

Your disease is not all that rare. It affects about 1 percent of the population and touches patients of all sexes, ages and backgrounds. At least half the patients report a family history of vitiligo or other problems with skin pigmentation.

Vitiligo is a disorder of the coloring or pigmentation of skin, in which the cells that produce color (melanocytes) are destroyed for reasons that remain unknown. This results in patches of skin that are lighter than the surrounding areas and can occur anywhere on the body, predominantly on the backs of hands and wrists, the face, neck and around body openings.

Repigmentation may occur without treatment, but when it doesn't, treatment is directed at stimulating the production of cells that produce the color. A medication called psoralen is used in conjunction with ultraviolet light.

It's a long process as you have discovered and can require more than 100 treatments in some cases. About 75 percent of treated patients will have a satisfactory result, although total recoloring never is achieved. Cosmetics or newly developed tanning solutions that do not wipe off on clothing may be used to help cover the remaining areas.

125. ***My kid seems to get common warts by the bushel. I don't know where they come from or what to do about them. Can you offer any words of wisdom to an anxious and worried mother?***

I understand your emotions, but I can tell you that by keeping your cool, you can deal with the problem in many effective ways. The common wart (also known as verruca) may be caused by any one of more than 35 types of human papilloma virus, which may help you understand how they seem to come back time after time.

Warts of this nature are more frequently seen in older children and are uncommon in older people. It seems that in many people a reaction by the immune system can clear up the unattractive lesion without any specific care, and then provide them with a relative degree of immunity for the rest of their lives.

Almost everyone has had a wart at one time or another. Many warts just disappear spontaneously. They also may be treated by a doctor with a flexible collodion solution (resembling artificial skin) containing salicylic acid and lactic acid. If this is not successful, a physician may use liquid nitrogen to freeze the wart or electrocautery to burn it away, usually with little scarring.

5.

The Brain, Nervous System and Organs of Special Sense

Brains, well prepared,
are the monuments
where human knowledge
is most surely engraved.

JEAN-JACQUES ROUSSEAU
French philosopher (1712–78)

If the muscles and bones provide the engines that move the body, and the heart is the pump that pushes the blood through the maze of arteries and veins, then the nervous system can be said to provide the communication network that controls all the body's activities. It is the most complex of all the body's systems, not only regulating and coordinating basic functions of the body, such as breathing and blood circulation, but influencing thoughts, memory, learning and emotions as well. Through the organs of special sense and the nerve receptors that perceive the sensations of touch, pain, heat and cold, the brain receives information about the condition of the outer world. Simultaneously, it takes in additional status reports from all the organs within the body, correlating, sifting and then transmitting the nerve impulses that control and coordinate body actions. Much of this happens without conscious thought and, amazingly enough, with few errors.

It is easy to compare the brain to a computer. Yet the human brain preceded the development of the modern computer and still provides activity that greatly exceeds the capacity of even the most modern and most powerful computer in existence today. However, like the computer, in which all the actions depend upon the simple proposition of "on" or "off" — all the functions of the human nervous system result from the activity of its basic unit, the *neuron*.

A neuron has three parts: the *dendrites*, the *cell body* and the *axon*. The dendrites are branchlike structures that exchange impulses with other cells and provide thousands of terminal "knobs" that are capable of receiving and sending nerve messages. The electrical impulses go to the cell body and from there are carried along the axon to the next cell. In the brain, the cell bodies make up the *gray matter*, while the axons constitute the *white matter*. The axon is the longest part of the cell and in whales may measure as much as nine meters (30 feet). In humans, the longest axon runs from the spinal cord to the toes, about 1.28 meters (4¼ feet). Many axons are covered by an insulating fatty substance, *myelin*, which keeps electrical impulses from short-circuiting to other axons in the same bundle, acting just like insulation does around an electrical wire. A bundle of axons makes up a *nerve*. The speed of conduction of the electrical impulse along the nerve may reach up to about 100 meters a second (200 miles per hour). The thickest nerve fibers carry the impulses most swiftly, while the impulses in a thin fiber may creep along at a mere one meter per second (three-and-three-tenths feet per second).

Neither the dendrites nor the axons are directly connected to the other nerves, but are separated by a gap called a *synapse*. When the electrical pulse reaches the synapse, a chemical reaction takes place, which releases either *noradrenaline* or *acetylcholine*. Called *neurotransmitters*, these chemicals pass a single stimulus on to the next nerve and then are destroyed by the action of *enzymes*, which readies the synapse for the next electrical message. The whole process takes but a fraction of a second.

There are probably more than 100 billion neurons in the brain, which along with cells that support the structure weighs about 1.36 kilograms (3 pounds). The brain and spinal cord together make up the *central nervous system*.

Most pictures of the brain show only the outer surface, the *cortex* or *cerebrum*, which is divided into two halves called the left and right hemispheres. This is the largest portion of the brain. It's responsible for all conscious thought and feeling, voluntary movements, learning and intelligence. The entire brain is enclosed by the three *meninges* (membranes). The outer membrane is made of tough tissue and is called the *dura mater*. The innermost membrane is extremely thin and is known as the *pia mater*. Between the two lies the *arachnoid mater*, which contains many channels that permit circulation of the *cerebrospinal fluid* that flows around the surface of the brain, through the ventricles (spaces within the brain) to the central canal that runs down the center of the spinal cord. It is this fluid, obtained during a lumbar puncture (spinal tap), which can be analyzed to help diagnose conditions affecting the central nervous system.

The two hemispheres are connected to each other by nerve fibers running through the *corpus callosum*. For the most part, the left side of the brain controls muscle actions on the right side of the body, while the right side of the brain runs the left side of the body.

The surface area of the cortex is increased more than thirtyfold by creases that create the *sulci* (furrows or ditches) and the *gyri* (convolutions or rounded elevations) that characterize the appearance of this part of the brain. The cortex on each side is divided into four *lobes*: the *frontal* (the front), *occipital* (the back), *parietal* (upper side portion) and *temporal* (lower side portion). The frontal lobe permits you to control movement, and the parietal lobe assesses sensation and body position. The occipital area transforms the impulses it receives into vision, while the temporal area is concerned with hearing.

Although the actions of all the areas of the cortex have not been identified, certain specific portions of the cerebrum are known to control speech, reading and writing, while the functions of personality, memory and recognition are probably not localized but rather spread throughout the brain.

At the back of the skull, below and partially covered by the cerebrum, lies a smaller structure of the brain called the *cerebellum*. It is an area of the brain over which there is no conscious control. It helps maintain balance and coordination, and permits muscular movement to proceed in a smooth flowing manner.

In front of the cerebellum and beneath the cerebrum lies the *brain stem*. The brain stem is composed of the *midbrain*, the *pons* and the *medulla oblongata*, which forms its lowest part. Atop the brain stem lie the *hypothalamus* and the *thalamus*. The hypothalamus regulates important functions such as sleep, appetite and sex. The thalamus serves to integrate the transmission of many of the body's sensations. The pons connects the brain stem with the balancing control of the cerebrum. The medulla controls some of the involuntary activities such as breathing and blood pressure, blood circulation and digestion. Nerves that carry the impulses to these areas are part of the *autonomic system*, for they help control functions that are carried on automatically. The brain stem is also the area that gives rise to the *cranial nerves*, which control the muscles of the face, tongue, eyes, ears and throat.

Below the brain stem and connecting the brain to the rest of the body is the *spinal cord*, which runs from the brain to the end of the spinal column through a protective canal of bone formed by the vertebrae. As the spinal cord passes through various levels of the body, it gives forth the nerves of the *peripheral nervous system*. These pass through spaces between the vertebrae and connect to muscle cells and special sensor cells in the skin that are able to detect heat and cold, pressure and position. These nerves are part of the peripheral nervous system.

There are two types of nerves in the peripheral nervous system. Impulses from the sensory cells in the skin and the organs of special sense are brought to the central nervous system by *afferent* or sensory nerves. The axon endings of sensory nerves are called receptors, for they are stimulated either mechanically (by touch) or chemically (such as smell). The stimulus provokes an electrical impulse that runs up the axon to the cell body, from the outside to the inside, as it were. The cell body then transmits the impulse out the dendrites and can excite the endings of literally hundreds of other neurons in the brain in turn. The response may be sent back to the surface by way of *efferent* nerves. The efferent or motor nerves carry impulses from the central nervous system to the muscles. When a group of afferent axons is grouped or bundled together in a single nerve, the nerve itself is classified as a *sensory* nerve. If all the axons belong to the motor type, the nerve is known as a *motor* nerve. Some nerves are made up of both sensory and motor axon bundles and are classified as *mixed* nerves.

While the sense of touch is provided by special nerve endings located in the skin, the other four senses — sight, hearing, taste and smell — have special organs to analyze the environment and provide the nerve impulses to the brain. The eyes, ears, tongue and nose are all highly tailored to the functions they must perform. They are remarkable examples of how the body has been able to adapt and provide sensors of unique ability.

The human eye is literally a series of lenses that focus light from a distant or close object into a precise image that falls on the retina, which is special tissue that transforms the light impulses into electrical impulses. The eyeball is about 2 centimeters (four-fifths of an inch) in diameter, nearly spherical, and is formed of tough fibrous tissue, except in the front. The transparent *cornea*, which forms the front, outermost portion of the eye, is the first lens to act upon the light rays, which then pass through the *aqueous fluid* in the anterior chamber of the eye, then the lens of the eye, and finally the *vitreous humor*, a jellylike transparent substance that fills the portion of the eye behind the lens.

All of these areas act upon the light beams just as optical lenses would. The lens of the eye can change its form, at least until we reach the age of 45 or so. That's when the lens' ability to change form and accommodate light rays coming from objects near to the face or from farther away begins to diminish. When this tissue loses some of its flexibility due to age (*presbyopia*), reading glasses may be necessary to make up for this lack. When the lens becomes cloudy, due to a number of possible conditions, a *cataract* has formed, which prevents some of the light rays from ever reaching the retina, causing vision to become dim. If this becomes too pronounced, the defective natural lenses can be removed surgically and replaced with artificial substitutes. The retina is composed of two types of light sensitive cells, the *rods* and the *cones*. There are about 130 million cells in a normal retina, with the rods outnumbering the cones by about 18 to 1. The rods are more sensitive to light than the cones, which are responsible for color vision. The electrical impulses generated by these cells pass by way of the optic nerve to the cerebral cortex in the occipital area of the brain where they are interpreted in the consciousness as three-dimensional vision.

The ear, too, is a wondrously complex organ, with each part serving to enhance our ability to perceive sound. The shell-like formation extending outward from the head is known as the *pinna*. It is formed of cartilage and shaped to help capture sound waves and pass them through the external auditory meatus, which ends at the *tympanic membrane* (eardrum) — about 2½ centimeters (one inch) away from the external opening. Sound waves cause this membrane to vibrate, which in turn sets three tiny bones (*ossicles*) located in the middle ear to vibrating. These are the smallest bones in the body and are named for their shapes: the *malleus* (hammer), *incus* (anvil) and *stapes* (stirrup). The stirrup connects to another membrane in an opening (*foramen ovale*) leading to the inner ear. It transmits the sound waves, as vibrations, to the liquid that fills the inner ear (*perilymph*). The liquid transmits the vibrations to the *cilia* (hairlike structures that activate the neurons of the auditory nerve that carries the impulses to the brain). The entire mechanism can detect sounds from 20 to 20,000 cycles per second, ranging from below 10 decibels (sound of a whispered voice) to the more than 110 decibels produced by a jet airliner taking off. Our ability to hear diminishes with age (*presbycusis*), which is a condition that can often be helped with a hearing aid.

Answers from the Family Doctor (Questions 126-155)

The tongue is the organ of taste. It can detect chemicals dissolved in the saliva and distinguish between four basic flavors. Each of the taste buds that performs this function is sensitive to only one taste, and they are grouped in different areas on the tongue. About 9,000 *papillae* (taste buds) are distributed over the entire tongue, but they, too, grow fewer with the passing years. The buds are located at the base of the bumps you see on the tongue. Those buds most sensitive to bitter taste are located on the back of the tongue. The middle of the tongue is the location of buds that respond to salty tastes and the buds for sweet and sour are distributed at the front and sides. All flavors are made up of a mixture of these basic tastes.

High in the nasal passage is an area of special tissue that contains the receptors that detect odors and smells. The receptor cells have tiny hairs covered with a sticky mucous secretion that helps to trap the minute chemical particles that contain the scent. The sniffing action is used to pull more of the scent-bearing chemicals higher into the nose, where they can come in contact with the receptor cells. The human sense of smell is poor compared to that of animals. Some individuals have trained their sense receptors, which are capable of detecting more than 10,000 different odors, but it's the brain that interprets the impulses as recognizable scents. A cold reduces your ability to smell by blocking the path to the sensitive area, which may in turn affect the sense of taste. This accounts for the loss of appetite that may occur with certain illnesses.

Though we know a great deal about this wondrous neurological system, much is yet to be discovered, particularly about the chemical actions that are the basis for all the activities of the brain and nervous system.

Questions and Answers

126. ***You could do many people a great service by providing information about a problem that many of us must deal with each day: Please tell us what is new concerning Alzheimer's disease.***

There is some good news to report. Progress has been made in diagnosing and managing patients who suffer from Alzheimer's disease, a condition of unknown cause in which the brain cells die prematurely and progressively. That produces memory loss and generalized intellectual deterioration.

The course of the disease is highly variable, and it can last anywhere from two to 20 years from the time it begins until the patient dies. Nearly 10 percent of people over age 65 have Alzheimer's disease and another 10 percent of people in that age group are caregivers to loved ones with the disease.

Areas of progress against the ravages of Alzheimer's disease include advances in diagnosis, communicating information about the disease to the patient and family, and helping the family manage the diseased patient following diagnosis.

The condition is diagnosed much more frequently today than previously for two reasons: One, as life expectancy improves, many more people are reaching advanced old age and are facing an increased probability of suffering Alzheimer's disease. Two, doctors have more techniques for making the diagnosis and now are aware that 50 to 65 percent of all cases of dementia are due to Alzheimer's.

We have learned also that communicating the condition to the patient and family needs to be tailored to the individual's condition. Most patients may be told that they have a memory problem, will need to rely on others to assist them, will need continuing medical care, and that research is progressing on some solutions to the problem. Family members usually are told in private exactly what to expect as the disease worsens. Because the news can be so upsetting, the family may need two or more visits with the physician to fully comprehend what is happening.

Managing Alzheimer's disease is where the most progress has been made recently. Many resources now are available to patients and caregivers. The number of services is great. For patients, services include ongoing medical care, treating various symptoms such as anxiety, depression and agitation. For families, they include continuing communication with the physician, peer support and counseling groups, community day-care services, in-home or institutional respiratory care services and legal and financial assistance.

While research advances are being made on possible new medical treatments, unfortunately none is yet available that arrests or cures Alzheimer's disease. We still do not know what causes the disease nor how we might prevent it, but scientists are working intensely on it.

127. ***Our daughter came home with a note from the school nurse informing us that she may be suffering from amblyopia. She suggested we take our daughter to an eye doctor. What can you tell us about this condition?***

Amblyopia is the most common preventable form of vision loss. It's marked by reduced vision in one eye without an apparent physical condition as its cause. Often, the brain is unable to combine the information it is receiving from both eyes and simply disregards one of the two visual signals — leading to the condition known as "lazy eye."

Amblyopia is diagnosed in children through standard eye tests, and in infants by alternately covering each of the eyes. If the infant is upset when one eye is covered but not the other, there is a strong likelihood of vision loss in the uncovered eye. If treated early with corrective lenses or vision therapy, the lazy eye can learn to be equally effective, thus preventing a lifetime of impaired sight.

128. ***We visited Mother recently after she had a mild stroke. She is doing well now but still can't seem to speak, although she tries and can make sounds. It's just that they don't make any sense. The doctor calls this "aphasia." I would like to know what that means, and what we as a family can do to help.***

Aphasia is the loss of language ability after a brain injury or stroke. There are several different kinds of aphasia and they affect different parts of the language process.

Some people with aphasia may be unable to say the words they want to say. Other people may not know the words they want, although the words are familiar ones. For instance, they may not be able to say the name of a family member, although they know and recognize the family member.

Some aphasia sufferers are unable to communicate in sentences, speaking instead in a sort of gibberish. Others who have aphasia suffer difficulties in understanding what is said to them. Instead of hearing coherent sentences, they hear a string of unrelated syllables. Aphasia also can affect the ability to make sense of the words on a printed page.

There are few things more frustrating than to be unable to communicate with those around us. Patience and support from others are the best allies of a person who has aphasia. Remember that though your mother has aphasia, she probably can understand much more than she can communicate. Be careful to include her in all your conversations, even if she cannot seem to communicate or participate. Prompt treatment by a specialist in speech, language and hearing is very important to helping the person who has aphasia.

129. ***My teen-ager refuses to work at his desk where there is a good study lamp. Instead he reads in the worst light, and I'm afraid he is going to permanently damage his sight. Is that true or is it just another old wives' tale?***

Eyes do not get damaged from use. Excessive close work may tire the eyes, but has not been proved to harm the eyes. Proper lighting is more comfortable. Too much light, especially when it produces glare, can be even more uncomfortable. It's a good idea to encourage rest breaks to avoid fatigue and the headaches of so-called eyestrain. If your youngster rubs his eyes, squints, holds the book in an unusual position or tilts his head in an awkward position, it might mean that he is not seeing properly.

An eye doctor can determine whether the child needs glasses or has some other condition that needs attention. However, when there seems to be a perfect environment for study available that is not being used properly, it indicates that it's time you had a sit-down discussion with your son to find out just why he isn't using his desk. Some of the answers may surprise you, and the remedy for the situation may be simpler than you think.

130. ***Recently I developed a nerve weakness in the left side of my face. My ENT (ear, nose, throat) doctor told me I had an inflammation of the seventh cranial nerve caused from a viral infection and prescribed a week's supply of steroids. My internist said it was Bell's palsy and that it would take time for it to get back to normal. No medication was prescribed. Would you please explain Bell's palsy to me?***

To a great extent, both doctors are correct even if it seems at first glance that they have some difference of opinion. Inflammation of the seventh cranial nerve (the facial nerve) also is known as Bell's palsy, after Sir Charles Bell, who is credited with describing the condition in 1892.

There may be many causes of irritation to the nerve, some of them a bit controversial, including upper respiratory infection, exposure to a cold draft, emotional upset, and even pregnancy and menstrual periods.

Though the exact cause may not be known, the results are pretty well understood. The cause, perhaps a viral infection, creates an autoimmune reaction in the nerve. As a result, the nerve swells inside the tiny bony canal that it runs through, becomes compressed and suffers from lack of oxygen and nutrition. As the nerve begins to fail, the muscles it serves begin to droop and display a typical Bell's palsy appearance.

Some physicians believe that the early use of steroids can prevent the condition from becoming permanent. Since the eyelids do not function normally, special eye care is in order. Dark glasses are recommended for daytime hours or brightly lit areas, and artificial tears should be used regularly to prevent the sensitive tissues that cover the eyeball from drying out.

Though the treatment must be based upon your individual case, the statistics for complete recovery are quite good. In many cases, no special treatment other than for the eye is used.

131. ***I have a condition that makes my eyelids all red and crusty. They itch and burn something fierce. Would you please tell me what you think it is, and can this condition be treated?***

It sounds like blepharitis, which is an inflammation of the edge of the eyelid, usually caused by bacteria. There's often a feeling of something in the eye, such as a speck of dust might provoke. Symptoms include: red, puffy eyelid, sore eye, crusting of skin at base of eyelashes, recurring redness of eye or eyelid, frequent sties, burning of eyes, and the eyelids sticking together in morning.

Many people with "dry eyes" have this chronic inflammation of the lid margins. A visit to the physician is important because untreated blepharitis can result in serious complications that eventually might endanger your vision.

Proper treatment controls blepharitis. Use warm compresses, wash the eyelid carefully with a cotton-tip applicator moistened with warm water and apply prescribed antibiotic ointment as directed. The warm compresses must be applied for a minimum of five minutes to loosen the crusted skin and dirt, which then must be washed away. Avoid getting particles of crust in the eye and be careful not to strike the eye with the applicator. When you apply the ointment, some of it may get in the eye, but it's usually all right. Here's one time when following your doctor's advice exactly will most certainly pay off.

132. ***I know that X-rays are useful for making many diagnoses, but I have been told that they're of little use in diagnosing bleeding in the brain. But then how does the doctor figure out where the bleeding is? What can be done for it if this turns out to be the problem?***

Almost every kind of bleeding within the brain tissue is called intracerebral hemorrhage. When the blood remains pooled in a well-localized superficial location, it may be termed a hematoma.

Before the development of some incredible technology, particularly the CT scan (computed tomography), physicians relied on the different clinical patterns and symptoms that occurred as a result of the bleeding to determine the location. However, these symptoms also might be caused by the mass effect of the hematoma — swelling (edema) of the brain from the irritation, the shifting of the brain, as well as the extension of the bleeding to the ventricles (cavities within the brain).

Performing a spinal tap (withdrawing fluid from the spinal column) also could reveal the presence of blood, which is a sure sign of bleeding somewhere in the central nervous system. Now the CT scan can localize small areas of bleeding with excellent precision.

The single greatest cause of brain hemorrhage is hypertension. The incidence of hypertension in such patients ranges from 25 to 94 percent. The medical treatment therefore might be directed at lowering the blood pressure to reduce the possibility of bleeding and its amount. Once the size of the hemorrhage has reached its maximum, in about one to two hours, reducing the blood pressure will do little to reduce the size of the hemorrhage. When edema strikes the brain tissue and the pressure within the skull rises, additional techniques, including the use of corticosteroids, may be used.

Finally, surgical techniques must be considered in many cases. They can be used to remove the accumulated blood (hematoma), find the area of bleeding and stop the hemorrhage, and finally drain both blood and fluid away to lower the intracranial pressures. The decision to employ surgery also will depend upon other medical factors and the patient's age and state of health.

133. ***Can you please tell me what conditions make a person "brain dead"? I believe that this is the situation that's necessary for the organs to be donated, and my family needs some information to make a most important decision.***

In actual practice, brain dead means that the heartbeat and respiration can be maintained artificially, giving the appearance of life, long after the brain itself has stopped working and is "dead."

While determination of death traditionally has been based on the stopping of breathing and the heartbeat, the development of techniques to support failing lung and heart functions — even when the brain appears dead — has made these signs insufficient to determine the death of an individual and most inadequate under certain circumstances. So recent criteria for the determination of death have been based on an assessment of the brain.

To be declared brain dead, a patient must meet certain clinical conditions, including having no spinal cord reflex movements; no eye opening or other movement — either spontaneously or in response to painful stimuli to the face or trunk; plus other more technical conditions. The fact is that determining whether a patient is really brain dead is not an easy task and sometimes nearly impossible.

To further complicate matters, certain conditions can mimic the appearance of brain death, but in reality are something entirely different. Examples include cases of extreme intoxication and drug overdose.

Yet despite the difficulty, early recognition and declaration of brain death are important. Continued treatment of patients who are brain dead can subject their families to uncertainty and false hopes. Some people feel that treating a brain-dead patient is an indignity to the patient's body. Others say that medical resources should not be expended on treating patients who are already dead. Still others contend that as long as a patient's heart is beating and breath is continuing, that person is alive and deserves any and all treatments available to the medical profession.

In an era in which organs may be salvaged from patients already brain dead, the hopes of many individuals whose lives depend upon such donors are dashed, as the number of organs remains insufficient to meet the need. Though some statistics indicate that approximately 20,000 cases per year might possibly yield donor organs, only about 2,000 to 3,000 actually do.

Other unresolved issues are involved in the declaration of brain death. Some are scientific issues that require formal investigations. Others concern social values and public policy and require debate by ethicists and lawyers.

Additionally, there are questions concerning who should declare a patient to be brain dead — should it be neurologists, neurosurgeons, anesthesiologists or physicians serving in intensive care units and emergency departments? In many institutions, it takes a panel of physicians, with all these areas of expertise, to make the final determination. If you're facing an important decision of this nature, consultations with your own physician and the chairman of this committee may be of great assistance.

134. ***I'm always nervous when it comes to my health, more so these days as I await the day for my cataract surgery. My doctor has been very accommodating and has explained about the insertion of a new lens. I would like the truth about my chances for a good result. Would you please oblige me with your explanation?***

You probably have no reason to be nervous about the operation, because cataract surgery is currently the most common major surgical procedure performed on people over 65 years old who are on Medicare. Most of the operations are very successful, and a very high percentage of those who have lens implantation report a big improvement in their vision.

I found one study that reported the results of cataract surgery with lens replacement on patients between the ages of 70 and 95. Before the operation, 91 percent of the participants rated their own vision as fair or poor. Four months after the surgery, 66 percent of the cataract patients rated their vision as excellent or good.

On a more scientific level, the doctors also noted a significant improvement in the participants' vision. Using a more precise means of measuring vision, the doctors found that visual acuity after surgery improved from about 20/100 before the operation to 20/40 four months afterward.

With this recovered vision, your daily chores will be accomplished more easily and you can return to the joys of reading, which you mentioned as being so important to your mental stimulation. Good luck.

135. ***My baby was born with crossed eyes. Now he is close to 1 year old, but his eyes are not straight yet. Am I safe in waiting another six months to see if they finally will become straight?***

A loud "NO!" should be heard by all parents. Waiting for this to happen can mean serious vision loss to the child.

I'm not talking about the normal infant eye that frequently may seem to move about and be uncoordinated. The tracking system sets the baby's eyes straight by four to six months of age. But after that time, if the baby's eyes turn in, out, up or down, it's vital to see an eye specialist for diagnosis. If you take a wait-and-see outlook, the baby might miss a crucial part of visual development.

Recent findings show that good early vision is essential to normal visual development. Once this visual development is missed, it cannot be regained. Strabismus, as the turned eye condition is called, can cause double vision. The child shuts off vision in one eye, so that the vision seen with the remaining eye is clear. The unused eye and the brain don't get the proper stimulation and development. After a while, the weaker eye goes blind or is severely visually impaired.

If you notice a turned-in eye and bring the child to be checked by an eye doctor, tests can help find the proper means of correcting the condition. The goals are to achieve good vision in each eye, enable the eyes to move together and appear straight, and to develop binocular vision, in which both eyes see one image. The child may be fitted with glasses or contact lenses. The strong eye may be patched, so that the other eye will be forced to develop.

An orthoptist (a person trained in the use of exercises for this condition) may be called in to work with the child under the doctor's supervision. In some cases, surgery may be necessary to straighten the eye, so it can look and see better. Many surgeons feel the best results are achieved when surgery is performed within the first two years of life. It's a relatively simple mechanical operation, which can provide the type of vision that will allow your child to develop normally. It should not be delayed.

136. ***Could you please discuss the meaning of the word "Demilonization," as it refers to nerve disease? Naturally we have a specific person in mind, but if we can just understand this last piece of information, we're sure we can put the whole story into place. Thank you.***

Sometimes it's the last piece of a puzzle that makes the picture clear. Demyelination is a process we see in nerve disease, in which the myelin (an insulating sheath that covers many nerve fibers) either is injured or degenerates because of a lack of oxygen, toxic agents or metabolic disorders.

Myelin is made of layers made of lipoprotein (fat and protein combination) and promotes the transmission of the electrical nervous impulses along the axon of the nerve. When the myelin degenerates, the axon dies, so the impulses no longer can prompt muscles to work or to carry the sensations to the brain. Some types of metabolic congenital disorder, such as Tay-Sachs, Niemann-Pick and Gaucher's disease, affect the developing myelin sheath, which causes widespread neurological symptoms.

Demyelination occurs in the central nervous system as a basic cause of several diseases, known as primary demyelinating diseases. Multiple sclerosis is perhaps the most common of these diseases. In many cases of these disorders, the myelin can regenerate and repair itself, with the return of nerve function or remission. Unfortunately, degeneration can recur, with the pattern of disease exacerbation and remission being common.

137. ***Despite my words of caution, my daughter is forever cleaning the wax out my grandson's ears. It's almost a fetish with her. Can pushing this type of cleanliness to extremes cause any harm?***

Believe it or not, earwax is a bodily fluid that performs an important function. It helps keep the ear canal moist and traps dirt as it enters the ear. When the wax moves to the outside part of the ear canal, then we can clean it and remove the dirt it has trapped. While it's very important to keep ears washed, using cotton swabs to remove normal earwax actually can cause the wax to build up on the eardrum and lead to excessive amounts within the ear. This sometimes can lead to a decrease in hearing.

When excessive wax buildup occurs repeatedly, using over-the-counter nonprescription eardrops will help keep the wax soft, which enables it to work its way out of the canal in a normal fashion. Should any problems with ears arise, then it's time to consult the physician for an examination.

Remember: Using any object to poke about in the ear can puncture the eardrum or irritate the ear canal and cause serious problems.

138. ***When my hands began to shake, I thought it was just a matter of nerves and gave up my smoking. Then, when it got worse, I began to think I had Parkinson's disease. Finally I visited my doctor who diagnosed this as "essential tremor." I would like to know how he could tell the difference and if there are any treatments that could help me now?***

While all tremors may look alike to a casual observer, a careful examination by a physician usually is enough to distinguish among the many possible diagnoses. The most common tremor disorder is essential tremor, which is about 10 times more common than Parkinson's disease. The trembling begins when the patient attempts to move, in contrast to the movement caused by Parkinson's, which occurs when the patient is at rest.

In Parkinson's, the tremor is most common in the hands and legs but never strikes at the head or causes a quivering tone in the voice, which does occur in essential tremor. In essential tremor, there may be a family history of a similar condition; in Parkinson's, there is usually no family history of the disease.

One of the interesting aspects of diagnosing the tremor is to determine how small amounts of alcohol affect it. Alcohol can dramatically reduce the tremors in the essential variety, but has no effect on the shakes caused by Parkinson's. Alcohol also is used as one of the treatments for the tremor and may be very useful when a glass of wine or other alcoholic beverage is taken just before a meal. The calming effect makes eating quite a bit easier for those whose hands are affected by the tremors.

Essential tremor progresses quite slowly, with long periods of time during which there is no worsening of the symptoms. And it doesn't shorten life expectancy, although severe tremors can make ordinary activities in life difficult to accomplish.

Medications are available that are very effective. These are beta-blockers, including propranolol, and primidone. They are prescription medications and require guidance from your physician to adjust the doses to your individual needs.

139. ***I have a problem with my vision. Whenever I look at a bright surface or up at the sky, I see dots and threadlike shapes swimming around. What are they? Are they dangerous?***

The shapes you're seeing are called floaters. They're clumps of gel that form in the vitreous humor, the clear, jellylike fluid that fills the eye. These dots and lines (they also can take the form of circles or cobwebs) are usually harmless and a natural part of aging. Floaters are especially common in nearsighted people or after a cataract operation. The floaters often go away by themselves.

When floaters crop up suddenly for no reason or become dramatically worse, it's a good idea to see an eye doctor. Floaters also can signal a torn retina or, less commonly, inflammation or crystallike deposits within the eye. All of these vision-threatening conditions arrive quite painlessly.

By the way, the flashes of light some people see are much like floaters in that they're usually harmless. But if they're accompanied by numerous floaters or a blacking out of part of your field of vision, again, see a professional.

If floaters ever have gotten in your line of vision while you were reading, you've probably tried moving your eyes back and forth to get the floaters out of the way and had little success. Next time, try looking up and down instead. This will create currents that carry the floater to a less sensitive part of the eye. Then you can return to your reading without this annoyance. But don't experiment for too long a period of time without seeking professional evaluation of your problem.

140. *Because of a new young man in my daughter's life, I'm seeking some very important information from you. Can you tell me about Huntington's disease? Where does it come from, and what are its symptoms and effects?*

It's sometimes called Huntington's chorea, or more precisely, progressive hereditary chorea. It's an inherited disease that is carried by a single dominant gene. This means that if it's present in the genetic makeup of an individual, it always will cause the disease.

The tragedy of Huntington's is that the disease doesn't begin to manifest itself until middle age (35 to 50 years old) when many sufferers already have married and had children. The odds are that one out of two children of Huntington's sufferers also will have the disease, which strikes men and women equally.

Huntington's begins in an insidious fashion, striking at the mind and body. The patient's personality changes, as he or she becomes irrational or apathetic. A manic-depressive or schizophrenia-like illness may develop before the beginning of the muscle problems. Patients cannot walk, may have difficulty in swallowing and eventually cannot care for themselves as the choreic (spastic, involuntary, irregular) movements of the muscles become worse. The disease continues to the inevitable end, as there are no cures or treatments, and medications can only partially reduce the symptoms.

The recent discovery of a genetic marker for Huntington's permits physicians to offer considered counsel. Members of families in which the gene is present are generally advised to avoid childbearing but should seek genetic counseling to aid them in the decision, which they alone can make.

141. ***One of my friends thought her loss of vision was due to a developing cataract, but a visit to her doctor revealed that the condition is one called "macular degeneration." She now is seeking to find out all about this condition that she can. I would like to help her, so please discuss this.***

Macular degeneration is a visual disability marked by a progressive loss of central vision. It gets its name from the part of the eye that is affected — the macula — which is the small part of the retina responsible for sharp central vision. It sends images in the direct line of focus to the brain. Thus the macula functions differently from the rest of the retina, which is responsible for peripheral and night vision.

In macular degeneration, the afflicted individual becomes unable to clearly distinguish objects and colors. He or she loses the ability to see clearly at long distances or to do close-up work.

This impairment involves a breakdown in the membrane that separates the macula from underlying blood vessels that nourish it. As a result, the macula becomes physically displaced with an unrestorable loss of central vision. Severe eye injury, heredity, myopia (nearsightedness) and certain diseases such as diabetes are believed to be contributing factors, especially when young people are affected. But macular degeneration generally is associated with the aging process, which alters the membrane slowly over time.

Unfortunately, there are no perfect cures or treatments for most cases that exist. However, degeneration caused by infection or disease may be treatable if diagnosed early. In addition, laser treatment used to close off damaged blood vessels in the macular area has proven effective in some cases. The use of magnifiers and high-intensity reading lamps provide many patients with an increased ability to read.

142. *Since we now face the need to deal with multiple sclerosis, we're filled with the need for more information to help us cope with the situation. I'm sure you could help us.*

Information is our most precious ally when facing an unknown situation or problem, and we will start with this answer for you. According to the National Multiple Sclerosis Society, more than 250,000 Americans currently suffer with multiple sclerosis (MS).

One of the tragedies of this affliction is that it strikes at the young, with most patients being diagnosed between the ages of 15 and 40, although it can strike people as young as 2 or as old as 60. Women are the victims twice as frequently as men and come down with the disease at an earlier age.

We know some important facts about MS. It's not an infectious disease, so is not contagious, but it probably is due to an abnormality in the body's immune mechanisms. There's an inherited predisposition to the disease though, and we see it more commonly in children of MS sufferers. Finally, the disease is not fatal and patients may lead long, constructive lives.

MS is a disease of the central nervous system, where it attacks the white matter, known as myelin, which sheathes or wraps the nerve fibers like a type of insulation. When the myelin is destroyed, plaques or scars develop. The nerve signals that normally pass along the nerve fibers are stopped. This creates the symptoms of weakness in the muscles, changes in feeling, numbness or tingling, double vision, dizziness or lightheadedness, and many other disturbing symptoms. Which ones occur depends upon the area of damage in the nervous system.

The symptoms may come and go (remission) only to return again. While there's no specific treatment, many currently are used with some effect and more are being developed. Cortisonelike substances are frequently used during acute attacks. You may obtain much more information as well as reports on all the latest developments in treatment from the National Multiple Sclerosis Society, 205 E. 42nd St., New York, N.Y. 10017.

143. ***Our grandson has just recovered from a serious fight with an infection called "meningitis." It seemed to come from nowhere, with scarcely a symptom before he was deathly ill. Would you please tell us where this infection could have come from, and what types of treatments are available to cure it? Although everything is now all right, the family is still curious to find out as much as possible about the disease.***

I can understand your curiosity and am happy to provide you with some information. Meningitis is a painful swelling of the connective tissues that enclose the brain and spinal cord, due to bacterial or viral infections. Its symptoms include an intense headache, fever, loss of appetite, intolerance to light and sound, neck and back stiffness, and rigidity of the hamstring muscles in the back of the legs. In severe cases, there are convulsions, vomiting and delirium, and it even can lead to death.

About 80 percent of all cases caused by bacteria can be the result of infections by one of three common bacteria: Neisseria meningitidis (meningococcus), Streptococcus pneumoniae and Hemophilus influenzae. These bacteria abound in the environment. Such factors as age, head trauma and diseases that reduce the effectiveness of the body's immune system may influence which bacteria become the infecting agent.

The infection is spread through small droplets of liquid in the air, which come from the respiratory system of an infected person, and by close contact. It's often spread by people who either display no immediate symptoms or have only a sore throat. Transmission can occur through the route afforded by intimate kissing, a practice that should be avoided whenever an infection is suspected.

Pneumococcus meningitis is most common in adults and originates from infections in the sinuses, ears and respiratory tract. H. influenzae, the most prevalent form of meningitis in children, tends to affect children 6 months to 3 years old and accounts for 50 percent of all meningitis cases. Middle-ear infections are the primary culprit and deafness may occur within 36 hours after symptoms begin.

A positive diagnosis of these forms of bacterial meningitis usually is made by studying samples of the patient's blood, spinal fluid, or both. Treatment with antibiotics usually is quite effective. Since the disease is so serious, antibiotics are prescribed when the diagnosis is probable, without waiting for the identification of the specific type of bacteria.

Though the symptoms may be the same, viral meningitis is much harder to manage. Bacteria are simple one-cell organisms that reproduce by cell division and can be affected by a number of available antibiotics. Viruses — which can multiply only inside the cells within the body — are infecting organisms that do not respond to treatment with the same antibiotics that are so successful against bacteria. Diagnosis can be tricky, depending on the results of throat and stool cultures, as well as certain cell changes in the spinal fluid, which occur only during a viral infection.

When the disease is caused by a virus such as the kind responsible for mumps, mononucleosis or infectious hepatitis, the severity of the disease can range from no symptoms at all to most severe. However, even these desperately ill patients may recover completely.

144. ***I have a very severe problem because I get so sick whenever I travel. The distress is so great that I'm limited in my choice of vacations and can't even visit friends just a short distance away. What causes this terrible motion sickness and what can I do to control it?***

Although not usually a serious medical problem, motion sickness is the most common complaint voiced by travelers. Its symptoms — dizziness with nausea, vomiting or pale, clammy skin — are caused by an overstimulation of the balance organs in the middle ear. The sense organs (sight, hearing and touch in particular) send messages to the brain whenever our balance is disturbed, either inside or from outside movements. If these messages come too fast or are mixed (your eyes see no motion but your body feels it), the brain gets overwhelmed and sickness results.

To minimize motion sickness, try to avoid lengthy exposure to continuous undulating and rolling motion. Ride with your eyes fixed on a distant, stationary object when possible, so your eyes will see the same motion that your body and inner ears feel. Do not read when traveling and do not sit facing backward. Also avoid heavy, spicy foods that might upset your stomach. If you're planning a trip by plane, schedule a daytime flight and book a window seat, so you have a distant horizon to gaze out upon.

When these simple remedies fail, try some medications recommended by your physician or pharmacist to alleviate the troublesome results of motion sickness. Follow directions carefully, for most of these medications should be taken before the journey actually begins.

145. ***We're concerned with the problems of hearing loss that seem to afflict some of us. In listening to all the "war stories," it would seem that loud noises may have been a cause for some of the damage. Is this true?***

Yes, it is. Excessive noise is the leading preventable cause of hearing loss in this country. Many veterans of past wars, particularly those who were in close contact with heavy artillery, are well aware of this fact.

Excessive noise can be either continuous, such as a jackhammer or industrial machinery, or acute, such as a gunshot or explosion. Continuous loud noise causes degeneration in the tiny hair cells of the cochlea of the ear. These cells pick up sound vibrations and cannot be replaced or repaired. The longer you're exposed to excessive noise, the more hair cells are destroyed and the more hearing is lost. This damage usually results in hearing impairment and only rarely in profound deafness.

Acute loud noises can rupture your tympanic membrane (the eardrum) and other membranes in the inner ear. A ruptured eardrum can heal and hearing can be restored, but inner ear damage cannot.

In the early stages of noise-induced hearing loss, you may experience ringing in the ears, sound muffling, ear discomfort or a temporary hearing impairment for a few hours after experiencing the noise.

The Department of Labor says that more than 5 million American workers are subjected to hazardous noise levels. A good rule of thumb is that if you must shout to be heard over the background noise at work, your hearing is in danger. Use hearing protection such as earplugs or special earmuffs. Even rock musicians are wearing ear protection now during concerts. I wish more of our young people would get the hint and be more careful about the levels of sound they use when listening to music.

146. ***I know there can be many forms of infections to the ears. My youngster recently had a form called "otitis media." What is otitis media and how did he get it?***

Otitis media is any inflammation of the middle ear. Bacterial infection of the upper respiratory tract is the most common cause of otitis media, which is frequently associated with obstruction of the eustachian tube (the canal between the middle ear and the area above the soft palate). The eustachian tube is responsible for maintaining proper pressure in the middle ear. Obstruction of the tube can result in negative middle ear pressure and/or effusion (escape of fluid).

Allergic rhinitis has been implicated in otitis media as well. Frequent re-exposure to an allergen can cause inflammation that leads to eustachian tube obstruction for extended periods of time. Whether viruses are the culprit is difficult to establish, because they're extremely difficult to culture.

The condition occurs most frequently in children ages 1 to 4 years old. The incidence decreases gradually through ages 6 and 7, and it drops abruptly after age 10. However, it can occur at any age.

In cases where the otitis media is accompanied by fluid forming in the middle ear, antihistamine-decongestant therapy may be effective, but various studies about this yield differing results. Because bacteria are found in most cases, antibiotics are the mainstay of therapy.

In patients who don't respond readily to antihistamine-decongestant therapy or antibiotics, other treatment options include corticosteroids, cromolyn or the insertion of a tympanostomy tube (a small tube inserted through the tympanic membrane (eardrum) that separates the middle ear from the outer ear canal) to permit drainage of the middle ear.

147. ***I suffer from pain in different ways, and the hurt feels different at various times. What causes pain? Is it possible that there are different nerves involved?***

Pain is caused by overstimulation of nerves that may or may not conduct the stimulus to the central nervous system — the brain and spinal cord.

Depending on the type of stimulus, pain impulses can travel through two different types of nerves that are quite different in structure and entirely independent. For example, a pinprick sensation (also called fast pain or first pain) travels through small nerve fibers with a myelin sheath or covering (like an insulated cable). Deep pain (also called muscle pain or second pain) occurs when you have a muscle cramp or more severe muscle damage. This type of pain travels slower and is conducted by larger nerve fibers that lack the myelin sheath found on smaller nerve fibers. Thus there are two types of pain receptors, and the two types of fibers are specific for such pain.

The different types of pain may be demonstrated by inflating a blood pressure cuff (or tourniquet) around a limb to restrict its blood flow, then inducing pain, first by a pinprick (first pain) then by pinching a fold of skin (second pain). If the lack of blood flow is maintained by the cuff, the pinprick sensation will disappear but the pinching or muscle cramp-type pain will remain and even increase.

There are two different reflex actions — a rapid withdrawal after pinprick, and muscle contraction and immobility after pinching. It would be impossible for the same circuit to produce reflex responses that are almost opposite in nature (immediate withdrawal and fairly rapid loss of pain versus a dull, cramplike pain that persists). Therefore it is obvious the central circuits from two different types of fibers must be different.

This information helps physicians prescribe the most effective analgesic for the particular type of pain that is causing the misery.

148. *What is a pinched nerve and how can it be treated?*

Nerves, much like electric cables or wires, transmit messages or impulses from one section of our body to another. As a nerve runs along its path, it must pass through holes in bones, between bones and between, under or through muscles, ligaments and tendons. Usually there is ample room for the nerve to pass, but when the passageway is reduced, the surrounding tissue can press upon the nerve or "pinch" it.

Let's use sciatica as an example. Sciatica is a condition in which pain radiates along the course of the sciatic nerve, often into the buttocks and back of the leg. In osteoarthritis, such pain may be caused by the nerve being compressed by new bone growths as the nerve passes through the space between the vertebrae.

Each case of pinched nerve must be evaluated to discover its specific cause and to direct the treatment toward removing it. And that may be a difficult task.

149. *I have a problem that has been with me for some time now. I get a feeling that the whole world is spinning, usually when I'm getting out of bed in the morning. That's the worst time, although I also can feel this*

way when I get out of a chair or a car that I have been riding in for some time. I have no other symptoms, but I am afraid of what the doctor may tell me. Could I have your opinion first, please? I'm a young woman of 71 years.

Your description of your condition is very helpful. However, without the physical examination that your physician would be able to conduct, my opinion really is nothing more than an educated guess, so here it is.

You're describing a true vertigo, which is a sensation that everything is moving about you, rather than an episode of dizziness, which would lead me to another conclusion.

Your problem has occurred repeatedly, over a period of time, yet nothing else has happened (no other complaints or additional symptoms), so it doesn't sound like a condition that is getting worse or progressing.

I believe you suffer from benign positional vertigo. It's common in women of your age or in people who have suffered a head injury. It will occur only when you change position and shouldn't last for more than a minute or two, if you remain still. What is lacking for my evaluation is to observe your eye movements while all of this is going on.

Your physician may be able to provoke the sensation using a technique called the Hallpike maneuver (named after Charles Skinner Hallpike, a British physician who discussed aural and nystagmic conditions more than 40 years ago). By rapidly moving you backward while you're sitting on the examination table, so that your head extends past the end of the table and hangs downward at a 45-degree angle, and then turning your head to the left, your symptoms may be provoked and the movement of your eyes observed. If nystagmus (a rapid involuntary movement of the eyeballs) occurs, in this case in a circular pattern, it's most probable that my diagnosis is correct, and that you have nothing to fear.

A series of head and eye exercises prescribed by a doctor may be all you need to reduce your problem considerably. Without the anxiety it has caused, you will probably feel much better indeed.

150. ***My son was hurt recently in an auto accident. Although at first we did not think his injury was severe, he has continued to have constant pain in his left arm. The physician has called his condition "reflex sympathetic dystrophy." Can you tell me what this means and what can be done to relieve the pain?***

Normally, pain impulses are carried by the sensory nerves in the body, and the nerves of the sympathetic nervous system control such activities as sweating, blood circulation and temperature regulation. However, when the sympathetic nervous system begins to malfunction after an accident, it can affect the area of injury in a variety of unusual ways.

It may change the perception of pain, the manner in which the skin senses cold and touch, the temperature and color of the skin, and the sweating function of the skin. When these symptoms can be related to the injury, rather than to other nerve problems (such as those that result from diabetes, nerve tumors or conditions that cause pressure on the nerve — carpal tunnel syndrome, for example), the diagnosis may be reflex sympathetic dystrophy. There is a burning pain, which is sometimes described as throbbing in nature, and it may affect an entire arm or leg in the region of the injury.

As the condition progresses, there are changes in the consistency of the skin, loss of body hair in the area, muscle wasting and edema (swelling). The nails become brittle and the joints may atrophy.

Corticosteroids may be used in the early stages of the condition, but if the symptoms last more than six months the chance of recovery is remote. Ordinary short-acting painkillers do little to relieve the constant pain. The physician may resort to injecting a local anesthetic or nerve-blocking agent to determine if the pain can be stopped in that fashion. Repeated blocks may be used, but if the help lasts for only a short time, surgical procedures may be necessary, using a permanent sympathectomy, or complete block of the affected nerves, to achieve the needed pain relief. Once the condition is chronic, many patients require anti-depressants, anti-convulsants and narcotic pain medications to control their symptoms.

151. ***I would appreciate some information about a condition that has my mother in much pain. It's called shingles. What is shingles? Is there anything that can be done for it?***

Shingles is a painful condition that primarily affects skin and nerves. The most visible symptom is a blistering rash. Shingles also is called herpes zoster, since it is caused by one of the herpes family of viruses, varicella-zoster, which is also the virus that causes chickenpox. Shingles is, in reality, not a disease that is "caught," but a reactivation of the virus that has been dormant in the nervous system since a childhood bout of chickenpox.

The virus reactivation apparently is due to some physical stress to the affected area, such as surgery, trauma or infection. Before the rash appears, you may have a mild fever and feel tired, or there may be stinging, burning or pain in the affected area. The fever subsides when the first red patch breaks out. Small to large blisters develop within a day or two and last up to two weeks. In most cases, the blisters fill with pus within a few days, scab over and heal by themselves. The rash can be painful or itchy, which can be relieved by using compresses wet with Burow's solution (Domeboro Powder dissolved in water).

Your physician may prescribe one or two anti-viral drugs: Zovirax (acyclovir generically), which is taken orally or intravenously, or Vira-A (vidarabine), used as an ointment or intravenous injection. An uncomplicated case of shingles may not need these medications, however, and your physician may choose to prescribe only pain relievers.

Uncomplicated shingles usually heals well without scarring. Unless the blisters are popped or punctured, an infection is unlikely. Shingles is not contagious in the usual sense, but you should be careful to avoid adults who are ill or have an impaired immune system, or children who have not had chickenpox, since these people are susceptible to varicella-zoster. People who have damage to their immune system are more likely to get shingles that last longer and extend over a much wider area of skin.

Usually shingles occurs on the back or trunk, but it can occur on the face and around the eye. This is a more serious situation, since ophthalmic shingles can damage the eye or lead to a brain infection called herpes zoster encephalitis.

Another complication is pain that lasts after the rash disappears. This is known as post-herpetic neuralgia, which is more common in elderly shingles sufferers. Several medications can be used for this, but not everything works on every patient.

152. *My daughter faints frequently. I've tried to read all I can get my hands on about possible causes of her trouble, but I have become confused about two words that I keep seeing. Can you explain how to tell "syncope" from "seizure" and what they mean?*

Syncope, the medical term for fainting, may be preceded by such symptoms as yawning, a feeling of warmth, flushing or sweating, blurry vision, dizziness or nausea. This leads up to a gradual loss of consciousness and a "soft," limp fall. Although the person may look pale or grayish and may have low blood pressure and a slow heartbeat, he or she will resume consciousness without confusion and will remember the event.

A seizure comes on with no warning signs, although some people experience an aura or premonition beforehand. Loss of consciousness is sudden, causing a "hard" or abrupt fall. The person's color will be normal, but he or she is likely to twitch or move oddly while unconscious. Patients who have seizures often are confused when they regain consciousness and do not remember the event.

Seizures are associated with brain and nerve disorders, such as head injuries and epilepsy. Syncope can be caused by a wide variety of things, some serious and some not. It's always a good idea to consult a doctor about any kind of fainting or seizure, especially if it happens repeatedly.

153. ***I always have prided myself on my cooking and the compliments I receive from guests who sample my dishes. Lately, however, I seem to have lost the touch, because my senses of smell and taste do not seem as sharp as they once were. I visited a doctor who could find nothing wrong with me. Do you have any explanations to explain my predicament?***

I have an explanation, but regrettably no solution. Those wonderful senses of taste and smell become less sensitive and sharp as we grow older, so much so that almost half of people over the age of 65 have some problem with their ability to smell. According to some reports, more than 200,000 Americans will visit their doctors this year alone to complain of a diminished ability to smell and taste.

It's a good time to review any medications you're taking, which may be the cause of the impairment, and for a thorough check for a number of disorders and diseases that may affect these senses. If nothing is discovered, then you may have to learn to cope with the situation, as it probably will progress slowly.

About 75 percent of people over 80 cannot detect certain odors and, at the present time, there are no medications to treat a disorder of impaired taste or smell. The complaint is so widespread that it has interested a number of scientists who are conducting research into new ways of stimulating these important senses.

154. ***A persistent buzzing in my ear has become a constant torment. It started about five years ago (I am now 64) and has become steadily worse. I'm sure there must be something to help drive it away. Can you help?***

Nearly 36 million Americans experience tinnitus, which is the name for ringing or other sounds in the ears, such as buzzing, humming or clicking noises.

The causes of tinnitus can vary. The nerve endings in your ears may be damaged as a result of age or exposure to loud noises. Other ear problems, like infections (which can cause a hearing loss), could be to blame for your problem. Tinnitus also can be caused by such disorders as allergies, high or low blood pressure or diabetes, or as a side effect of certain drugs (aspirin, for instance).

Your doctor can run tests to try to determine the cause. Unless tinnitus is the result of a specific illness or condition, however, treatment may be impossible. You might try different devices that mask the sounds you're hearing by using white noise, which is a soft, rushing kind of sound like the sound of the surf. Certain hearing aids called maskers also can provide some relief by using the same principle to mask out the sounds in your head.

Though provoking at times, this unwanted sound is not life-threatening. A good mental attitude can help you avoid unnecessary and unprofitable anxiety. You also can help yourself by staying in good shape, avoiding stimulants such as caffeine and tobacco, getting enough rest and, in the knowledge that there is little you can do about it, ignoring the buzz that is tormenting you.

155. ***I read a newspaper article recently that used a term to describe the condition of a person in coma. They called it a "persistent vegetative state." Does this mean the person was "brain dead"? Doesn't it refer to being in a state like a "vegetable"? If those definitions are correct, then I can't understand why they were treating the patient as it was reported in the article. Can you explain?***

This term deals with one of the most sensitive issues in medicine today. Contrary to your understanding, a person in a persistent vegetative state is not in a coma, nor are they brain dead or a "vegetable." The condition results from severe and irreversible injury to a complex and vital area of the brain that is responsible for maintaining alertness.

Most neuroscientists believe the patient is in an awake state, but is unable either to sense or respond to external stimuli. Initially the patient suffers a coma, but returns to a persistent vegetative state within four weeks after the start of the coma. The patient no longer displays apparent thinking functions and is totally unable to accomplish the activities of daily living.

No patient who has been in this state for more than one-and-one-half years has ever been reported to improve neurologically, although there is one report of a patient improving after one year. It's clear that more study is needed, along with a clearer understanding of the condition.

6.

The Kidneys and Urinary System

What is man, when you come
to think upon him, but a minutely set,
ingenious machine for turning
with infinite artfulness,
the red wine of Shiraz into urine?

ISAK DINESEN (1885–1962)
Seven Gothic Tales

The excretory, or urinary, system is composed of two ***kidneys***, a pair of ***ureters*** (tubes) — one for each kidney — that go from the kidneys to the ***bladder***, the bladder itself, and the ***urethra*** (tube), which leads from the bladder to the outside of the body.

The main operating organs of the urinary system are the kidneys, for they produce the urine that flows through the rest of the urinary system. It is the kidneys' filtering and excretory abilities that manage the fluid balance of the body and provide the means by which the toxic products that are formed by the body's metabolic actions are removed from the blood.

From 20 to 30 percent of the body's total supply of blood is passed through the kidneys every minute. The entire supply of blood in the body thus passes through the kidneys about 20 times per hour. To put the enormous activity of the kidneys into another perspective, about 1,600 liters (1,700 quarts) of blood pass through the kidneys each day, and they produce 180 liters of a fluid called *glomerular filtrate*, but only about 1½ liters of urine (roughly equivalent to a quart and a half).

Each kidney is about the size of a child's fist — about 12 centimeters (4⅔ inches) long, 3 centimeters (1⅕ inches) thick and 7 centimeters (2¾ inches) wide. The kidneys, which are reddish brown in color, are attached firmly to the back wall of the abdomen, one on each side of the spinal column, slightly above the waist or just below the level of the lowest ribs. They are bean-shaped and look exactly like (you guessed it) a kidney bean. Each kidney weighs about 150 grams (5⅓ ounces), and each is covered by thick layers of fat.

On the inner side, or concave curve, of the kidney is a ***hilus*** (slit) through which pass the renal artery and vein, which carry blood to and from the kidney, and the nerves that serve the organ. Here, too, is the *renal pelvis*, which is a funnellike structure that collects the urine from the kidney and directs it into the ureter.

If a kidney is sliced through its length into two equal halves, another interesting observation can be made. The cut surface shows two distinct areas: an outer, darker band called the *cortex* and an inner section known as the *medulla*. The medulla is divided into sections known as *pyramids* (from their shape). The apex of each pyramid, called the *papilla*, extends into the renal pelvis. In each of these two areas — the cortex and the medulla — lie different parts of the basic unit of the kidney — the *nephron* — and a different process in the production of urine goes on in each area.

There are about one million nephrons (or tubules) in each kidney. At the beginning of each nephron is *Bowman's capsule* (a goblet-shaped, double-walled structure), which continues as a long, winding tube with three different sections. All together a nephron would measure about 3 to 6 centimeters (1⅕ to 2⅖ inches) if it were stretched to its full length.

Inside the inner cup of Bowman's capsule is found a tuft of minute capillaries, about 40 or 50 in number, that carry blood from the renal artery. This tuft is known as the *glomerulus*. These vessels twist and turn on themselves and form a structure that resembles a tangled knot of vessels.

Bowman's capsule and the glomerulus are located in the cortex of the kidney. As these blood vessels leave the glomerulus, they form a meshlike network of capillaries that surrounds the tubules that form the rest of the nephron and participate in the exchanges of liquids and salts that result in the formation of the final product, urine.

Because the venules, or blood-carrying capillaries, that carry the blood away from the glomerulus have a smaller bore than the ones leading to it, the pressure inside the glomerulus is high. This forces about 20 percent of the blood plasma that enters the tuft of capillaries through the capillary walls into the space between the walls of Bowman's capsule. This liquid is made up of water, urea, mineral salts, glucose and smaller molecules. Under normal conditions, the walls hold back the larger molecules and all the red and white blood cells, which continue to flow in the bloodstream.

The liquid that collects in Bowman's capsule is called the glomerular filtrate or sometimes primary urine, but this liquid still has many changes to go through before it becomes the actual urine that leaves the body. If all this liquid were voided as urine, it wouldn't take long for the body to become seriously dehydrated from losing too much liquid — perhaps less than an hour in most cases.

An average adult takes in about 2½ liters (about 2½ quarts) of liquid a day, in the form of both beverages and the water in food. About one-half liter of water is lost as water vapor contained in the air we exhale in breathing, another one-half liter as perspiration and about 1½ liters as urine. This amount of urine represents only one one-hundredth of the amount of glomerular filtrate produced by the filtration process of the glomeruli each day. Where did the rest of the fluid go? We will discover the answer as we follow the glomerular filtrate along the long path of the nephron to the point where it flows into the ureter.

The first step of the journey is from Bowman's capsule into the first section of the nephron, the *proximal* portion of the tubule, which also lies within the cortex of the kidney. Here, additional unwanted waste products are secreted into the filtrate, while substances that are still useful to the body, glucose for example, are reabsorbed into the circulatory system.

The filtrate flows on into the U-shaped *Loop of Henle* (located in the medulla of the kidney), which is the second section of the nephron, and then back up the nephron's third section — the *distal* portion of the tubule. Here much of the water in the filtrate is taken back into the circulatory system, leaving only a concentrated version of the filtrate that is now composed of urea, a few salts, creatinine, uric acid and other minor waste products and water.

Though a great deal of the water in the filtrate is recovered, there is still a great deal included in the urine, which is about 95 percent water even after this process. This urine flows into the collecting ducts that pass through the medulla of the kidney into the papilla and then spill out into the renal pelvis.

The action of the nephron tubules is under the control of various hormones, which act in response to the actual state of hydration of the body tissues. *Vasopressin*, the anti-diuretic hormone, is produced by the pituitary gland. A description of its action can serve as an example to explain the function of most of the hormones that control urine production.

When the day is hot and there is excess loss of fluids through perspiration, the tissues of our body tend to dehydrate, particularly when there is no additional consumption of liquids to make up for the loss. The pituitary senses this and produces vasopressin. This increases the amount of water reabsorbed in the nephrons (as it reduces the amount of *diuresis*, or water loss) and permits a more concentrated urine to be secreted. This concentrated urine is darker in color than normal and has a stronger odor. We drink deeply, quenching thirst and perhaps overcompensating for the previous water loss. The pituitary stops producing vasopressin, and more water is now permitted to pass out of the body. The urine becomes dilute, a very pale yellow to almost colorless liquid with little if any odor.

The urine now passes from the renal pelvis into the ureters. The ureters are hollow tubes of circular and longitudinal smooth muscle, and are about 25 centimeters (10 inches) long, the length varying from individual to individual and depending upon body height. The muscles contract rhythmically and propel the constant trickle of urine from the kidneys down to the bladder, where it can be stored until sufficient amounts have collected to warrant voiding.

The bladder is a hollow ball of strong, interwoven muscles located in the pelvis, between the rectum behind and the pubic bones in front. In women, the bladder is positioned in front of the uterus. It is held in place by the strong ligaments and muscles that form the floor of the pelvis. When these muscles become weak in women due, in some cases, to age, the bladder can drop down into the vagina, which causes a condition known as a *cystocele*.

The bladder can hold as much as 400 to 500 cubic centimeters (about three-quarters of a pint) of liquid. When it is full, the urge to urinate becomes strong. In order for the process of *micturition* (urination) to occur, a *sphincter* (circular muscle) at the exit of the bladder must relax, while the muscles of the bladder contract to force the urine out of the bladder into the urethra and then out of the body. Until a child is about 2 years old, this process is a reflex, with the stretched muscles of the bladder being the only stimulus necessary for voiding to occur. After that age, the process becomes voluntary, unless impaired by neurological disease.

The urethra, or tube that leads the urine out of the body, is composed of fibroelastic tissue. It is about 20 centimeters (8 inches) long in men, but a mere 4 centimeters (1⅗ inches) long in women. This difference in length puts women at much greater risk for bladder infections than men, for bacteria easily can pass up the urethra to the bladder where the urine provides a hospitable culture medium for their growth.

Many diseases of the urinary system, including the kidney, produce few symptoms and often can pass undetected for long periods of time. However, a simple routine test, called the ***urinalysis***, can provide the clues that lead to early diagnosis. While normally there are no blood cells in the urine, white blood cells may be an indication of an infection, and red blood cells announce the fact that bleeding is occurring somewhere along the urinary tract. If the nephrons are damaged, they may permit protein to seep into the urine. Urine is normally sterile, with no organisms growing in the liquid. The presence of bacteria can be established by culturing the urine. This test permits the identification of a particular strain of bacteria and aids in choosing the proper antibiotic to eradicate the infection.

When the basic urinalysis reveals abnormalities, many other examinations and laboratory tests may be used to narrow the number of possibilities and provide the clinician with the information needed to establish the correct diagnosis and formulate the required therapy.

Questions and Answers

156. ***In reading a home medical book I learned that my problem of pain when urinating was caused by diabetes. However, when I bought the strips to test for sugar, they never turned positive. Does this mean the strips are bad or that I don't have diabetes? I still have the pain.***

Pain or burning on urination (dysuria) is not a specific sign of diabetes mellitus, but rather a clue that there is irritation or inflammation of the bladder or of the tube (urethra) that drains the bladder.

The most common cause of this irritation is an infection. Infections of this type are most commonly seen in women because of the closeness between the rectum and the opening for the urethra, and the short length of this passage. This makes it much easier for bacteria to cross over into the urinary passage and cause the infection.

Depending on the type of bacteria, suitable antibiotics can be chosen that can correct the problem readily. Your confusion between diabetes and painful urination is a common one based upon the fact that urinary infections are more common in people with diabetes. The sugar in the urine makes a better growing environment for the bacteria.

You would be well-advised to check with your physician to determine the exact cause of your pain. Only an exact diagnosis can be used to choose the proper method to treat your problem, which may have a cause other than infection.

157. ***We're most concerned about our newborn grandson and a condition called "Hypospadias." Our daughter is so distressed that she will not discuss this with us. We hope you will tell us something about the condition, and if our grandson can ever be a normal person.***

I can understand your distress as well as that of your daughter, but the news is not all that bad. Hypospadias is a congenital defect that occurs rather commonly in male babies. It affects about one in 300 live-born male infants.

The defect affects the urethra, which is the tube that leads from the bladder through the penis and carries the urine out of the body. In cases of hypospadias, the development of this tube is incomplete. The urethra does not extend the full length of the penis and ends in an opening that is located somewhere along the underside of the shaft of the penis. Usually there are no other abnormalities of the urinary system associated with this condition, which is discovered easily during the baby's first examination.

Although in the past surgical correction was performed only on the most severe cases, new improvements both in pediatric surgical techniques as well as anesthesia permit surgeons to correct almost all cases of hypospadias. The operation usually is performed before the child is old enough to retain any memories of the experience, yet mature enough to safely undergo the procedure. Most surgery therefore is performed when the child is between 6 months and 9 months of age. The children do not seem to experience a great deal of discomfort. With the new techniques, a fully functioning penis is constructed that has a completely normal appearance. Complications of the surgery are rare, and the surgery may be performed on either an outpatient basis or with a single night's stay at the hospital.

You and your family all need one another now for moral and emotional support. This will provide you with the patience necessary to await the best moment to schedule the operation, after which much of your personal anguish and anxiety can be put behind you.

158. *From all the discussions at the office, I believe that urinary infection has to be pretty common among women. Could you please discuss this condition?*

Cystitis, or inflammation of the urinary bladder, is a very common condition with one out of every five women experiencing an attack of it during her lifetime. It is caused by urinary tract infections or sexually transmitted disease. Cystitis is marked by burning in the bladder, pain in the urethra and difficult or painful urination. Because of its high occurrence, new diagnostic procedures are evolving constantly, and recommended treatments often vary.

In any case, however, a clinical history and physical examination are particularly important in diagnosing cystitis. A pelvic examination is necessary to rule out the possibility of other diseases, such as vaginitis, being the cause of the symptoms. It's most important to determine if a woman has a history of recurrent urinary tract infections or if she is at high risk for sexually transmitted diseases, because these factors will influence the choice of treatment.

To gain an accurate diagnosis for cystitis, a urine sample taken from a midstream specimen is examined for bacteria and for red and white blood cells. Bacterial cultures are useful in determining the organism causing the lower tract infection and choosing the most effective antibiotic treatment. Escherichia coli (E. coli) is the most common bacteria identified as the culprit. However, if a sexual disease is suspected, chlamydia and gonorrhea should be tested for and treated accordingly.

In an uncomplicated first-time case, where no sexual disease is suspected, cystitis treatment is fairly simple. Single-dose or short course antimicrobial therapy usually cures the infection. If this therapy fails, however, a longer course of treatment is recommended. A three- to five-day regime should be successful, but if symptoms persist, the patient may need to continue taking the drug for 10 to 14 days or even longer in some cases.

Even after extended treatment, some patients experience recurrent bouts of the infection. This can be due to a number of things, such as persistent infection with the original organism, reinfection with the same or different organism, poor antibiotic absorption, or resistance to the prescribed drug.

For high-risk patients, there are a number of precautions and daily practices that may help prevent infection. Drinking plenty of liquids and urinating frequently improve bladder washout. Using prophylactics, avoiding intercourse with a full bladder and urinating after intercourse are also helpful for patients experiencing postcoital cystitis. Soapy bubble baths, which can cause urethral irritation, should be avoided.

Cystitis is a very common disease in women and, for most, is easily treated. However, if a patient experiences recurrent infection, additional testing and more intense treatment are in order. In addition, another painful bladder condition, "interstitial cystitis," may be the underlying disease.

Even when there are no complications, the patient should continue daily precautionary practices, because cystitis, a severe case or not, can cause a great deal of discomfort. Prevention is always the best medicine.

159. ***I have just recovered from a bout of kidney stones, which fortunately passed without my having surgery. We never did get a look at the stone, but I'm now quite curious as to its nature and whether I may have to go through this thing again.***

It's really too bad that you didn't manage to recover the stone as it passed. The first step in deciding upon future treatments and your risks of another episode of renal colic would have been to chemically analyze the stone.

Statistically, the most common composition of renal or kidney stones is calcium oxalate, which occurs in 65 percent of the cases. The next most frequent is struvite (composed of magnesium ammonium phosphate) in 15 percent of the cases. Other types of stones include calcium phosphate (5 percent), calcium and uric acid (4 percent), uric acid (4 percent) and cystine (about 2 percent).

Calcium stones are frequent in individuals whose urinary content of calcium is high, with an output of greater than 300 milligrams per day. Struvite stones are seen in patients with urinary tract infections caused by bacteria that can affect urea, a chemical normally found in urine. Uric acid stones are the most common of the noncalcium stones and are seen in conditions such as gout that produce high levels of uric acid in the urine.

Your chances of recurrence are close to one in 10 each year, and 75 percent of all patients will have at least one recurrence during their lifetime. You have a high risk of repeat episodes if you're a middle-aged Caucasian male, if there is a family history of renal stones or gout, or if you have chronic bowel disease or certain kidney disease.

The good news is that you may never need surgery to rid yourself of these painful pebbles. Between 80 and 85 percent of all stones pass by themselves. The development of techniques that use high-power shock waves to disintegrate stones in the body has reduced the use of open surgical procedures to less than 5 percent.

Your best course is to have a complete, relatively inexpensive metabolic evaluation to try to determine the cause of your stones in the absence of a specimen. Such an evaluation will provide the information necessary to plan strategies that prevent recurrence. In the meantime, keep your fluid intake high, so that production of urine exceeds two liters (about two quarts) a day. This will keep the concentration of stone-forming materials low and help prevent another painful incident.

160. ***It seems as though every type of disease has something to do with the food we eat. Certainly I have read that this is true about heart disease. But my problem is a continuing bladder infection, which is certainly a most unpleasant situation. Are there any foods that affect this condition, and what might they be? I will go to almost any lengths to reduce the stinging and burning sensations I'm experiencing.***

The first important step in controlling and ridding yourself of this annoying but common condition in women is to visit your physician for a proper diagnosis and prescriptions for the effective medications that can wipe out the infection. But there are a number of tips about foods that may help to reduce the discomfort to more bearable levels and are fairly easy to follow.

There are two basic types of foods that provoke the pain and discomfort. The first type to avoid are foods that cause the stomach to produce additional acids and then cause the discharge of histamines (the same body chemical released during allergic reactions). They include coffee, spicy foods and almost all fruits except for watermelon, honeydew melon, berries and pears. Such foods increase the burning sensation already present in an irritated and inflamed bladder.

The second group are foods that contain amino acids, which stimulate the sensory nerve fibers in the bladder and provoke a burning sensation. These amino acids are present in chocolate, aged cheeses, alcoholic beverages and pickled foods, among others.

The secret of success of these dietary restrictions is that they reduce the acid content of the urine, thus reducing the irritation. Some doctors also advise drinking a full glass of water with a quarter teaspoon of baking soda once a day to help neutralize these acids.

You also can reduce acidic concentration by drinking lots of water, as much as eight glasses a day, to help dilute the concentration of bacteria in the urine. And that is a great health hint for most Americans — even for those without bladder irritation — who usually do not consume enough of this health-protecting liquid each day.

161. ***I'm cursed by a problem that I know many women have. I lose my water at the most disturbing and embarrassing times. I have read all I can find about this condition, but I'm looking to you for anything new that might help. There must be something I can do to stop or at least reduce the times I find I must withdraw from a public room and seek the privacy of my own room.***

Urinary incontinence is indeed a most distressing situation. It affects an estimated 10 million Americans, with twice as many women as men facing the problem. Almost half of all people living in nursing homes suffer urinary incontinence. For many sufferers, the only hope is treatment with medications or surgery, both of which may have side effects and risks.

The first step toward any rational treatment is a complete clinical evaluation by your physician, who may discover the exact nature of your problem. Urgency and urge incontinence are characterized by a sudden need to void of such a nature as to occur before reaching the toilet. Incontinence also can occur during periods of exertion, stooping to lift an object or coughing (stress incontinence).

Both situations may be helped by bladder training, which is based on principles of behavior modification. It consists of education and strict scheduling of urination. Patients are instructed to void at specific times even when they feel no desire, and to try to suppress the urge when the need is experienced before scheduled times.

The goal of such a program is to reach intervals of from 2½ to 3 hours between voidings, which is enough time to allow scheduling normal social activities. Such training programs may reduce the number of incontinent episodes by more than half. The results of the training have been shown to be effective six months after the training is completed.

For more information on this subject, you may write for the Age Page on urinary incontinence, which is obtainable from the National Institute on Aging (NIA) Information Center, P.O. Box 8057, Gaithersburg, Md. 20898-8057.

162. ***I'm seeking information about a disease called "nephrotic syndrome." Where does it come from, and what will the future hold for the person who has this illness? The physician's answers to our questions have been most confusing.***

To begin, I must define the word syndrome for you. A syndrome is not actually a disease or an illness, but rather a term applied to a group of symptoms or signs that often appear together. For the purposes of this discussion, a symptom is something the patient experiences or feels subjectively, something unusual or abnormal that can be reported to the physician. Pain, for example, is a symptom suffered by the patient but undetectable during the physician's examination. A sign may be observed by the doctor. It is an objective finding. Fever is a sign, for it can be measured by using a thermometer and easily can be compared with a normal temperature.

The nephrotic syndrome is composed of the following signs and symptoms: swelling around the eyes, feet and abdomen; large amounts of protein found in tests of the urine; increased weight from fluid retained in the body (all of these are signs); and loss of appetite (a symptom).

The nephrotic syndrome may be observed in a number of different diseases. They include diabetes, multiple myeloma and glomerulonephritis as well as systemic lupus erythematosus. Nephrotic syndrome can result from an infection, exposure to certain drugs and toxins, malignancy or even an inherited disorder.

The common element in all of these is damage to the glomerulus, a basic structural element of the kidney. The damage affects the ability of the glomerulus to retain proteins, so they spill out and are found in urinary tests.

Because there are so many possibilities, I can't answer your question completely. When infection is the cause, antibiotics can cure the situation. When the reason for the syndrome is the use of a drug, the syndrome may disappear after the offending drug is stopped. The treatment thus depends upon the cause, and the outcome depends upon the success of the treatment.

Now that you understand the terminology, perhaps your own physician's explanation may make more sense to you.

163. ***I was told that I might get more information about my kidney infection by writing to a kidney association. I can't seem to find that resource and wonder if you could help me out. The discomfort is getting to me, and the treatment is slow to work.***

A urinary tract infection (UTI) can be a painful problem for anyone. It may affect a person of any age or any sex. While women are more susceptible to these infections, the symptoms (pain and burning sensation on urination, an urgent need to urinate frequently, cloudy, bloody or foul-smelling urine) can occur without warning and strike any adult or child. Knowing about the symptoms and signs, causes and cures can be of real value to you, particularly if you're a frequent sufferer.

All that information and more is contained in a valuable publication from the National Kidney Foundation. It's called quite simply "Urinary Tract Infection." You may obtain your free copy by sending a stamped, self-addressed, business-size envelope along with your request to Urinary Tract Infection, Dept. AB, National Kidney Foundation Inc., 30 E. 33rd St., New York, N.Y. 10016.

The National Kidney Foundation Inc. is the major voluntary health agency seeking the total answer — prevention, treatment and cure — to diseases of the kidney and urinary tract. Affiliate services may vary depending upon community resources.

The Foundation's many-faceted program brings help and hope to millions of Americans who suffer from kidney disease, through research, patient services, the donor program, and professional and public information and education. Such activities are made possible by voluntary contributions from a concerned and generous public.

164. ***My brother finally went to see his doctor months after he began to see blood in his urine. He was diagnosed as having cancer, but claimed he never thought it was serious because the bleeding used to stop by itself. You would be doing your readers a real service to discuss this condition.***

Thank you for your concerned letter and your sound counsel. Cancer can be fought successfully only when we all realize that treatment is most effective when we can make an early diagnosis. Cancer of the bladder is a common disease of the urinary tract, second only to cancer of the prostate.

As many as 40,000 Americans this year alone will face the diagnosis that your brother now does. Most of them will be older, between the ages of 40 and 80, as the disease is seldom seen before the age of 40. Three out of every four patients will be men, possibly as the result of exposure to cancer-producing chemicals encountered in the workplace. Some of the tobacco tars that pass through the urine also may be a cause, for smoking has been shown to increase the possibility of developing this cancer. However, there is no evidence to show that the tendency to develop this disease is inherited.

The most common symptom is blood in the urine that stains the urine red. It may come and go as in the case of your brother, but usually there are other symptoms, such as frequent urination and pain and burning during urination. These symptoms serve as important signs to indicate the need for a medical examination.

The physician will check the urine for blood, pus and infection, as well as for cancer cells that may come from a bladder cancer. Kidney X-rays are indicated as well as a cystoscopy, which permits the physician to look directly into the bladder and search for tumors.

Bladder tumors tend to develop in groups and can recur after being removed, so this process may have to be repeated often. If the lesions are superficial, they may be removed quite easily. But cancers that have invaded the bladder wall will require a combination of surgery and radiotherapy. Bladder cancer also can spread to other parts of the body, which once again underlines the need for early diagnosis and treatment.

165. *I've been taking a medication for many years. It's called a diuretic. I know it is a water pill, but that's all. You've written in the past that people should ask questions about their medications. So I am asking you, what's a diuretic?*

I think I suggested that people ask their doctors about medications, but if you're asking me, I'm happy to be your doctor, at least for now. Simply put, a diuretic is a medication that increases the production of urine.

The kidneys are in charge of that function and manufacture urine in a two-step process. The first step is to "filter" the blood through the clump of capillaries and tubules that forms a structure called a glomerulus. This process produces a liquid that passes through the tubules of the kidney to reach the main tube (ureter) that goes to the bladder. As the liquid passes through the tubules, new chemicals are excreted into the liquid, while some precious chemicals and water itself are reabsorbed back into the body. The final fluid that passes down the collecting ducts is called urine.

The structure that includes a glomerulus, the tubules and the duct is termed a nephron, the basic anatomical and physiological structure that kidneys are made of. Now if you have all that clear, I can describe just how diuretics work.

Diuretics either increase the rate at which the glomerulus works, thus producing more of the basic fluid, or decrease the reabsorption that takes place in the tubules. Either action results in the production of more urine. Different chemicals that are used as diuretics act on different parts of the nephron system. So physicians choose carefully and prescribe the diuretic that is best for their patient's condition.

Diuretics may be used to prevent or eliminate swelling (edema), control hypertension and treat heart failure. The next question to ask your doctor is, "What am I taking this medicine for?" Sorry, I can't answer that one for you.

166. ***You wrote that you believe in one dose of medicine to cure a bladder infection. My doctor says you're wrong. Who should I believe?***

This is an area about which there is some obvious disagreement. In fact, a recent issue of a medical journal featured this question and had two doctors address it — one on the side of one-dose therapy for bladder infection, the other on the side of several days' therapy. Both sides presented valid arguments.

The one-dose method has the advantages of reducing the complications of longer-term therapy, such as stomach upset and yeast vaginitis. The cost is usually lower and taking one pill is more convenient than taking several a day for several days. Initial reports about this method of treatment indicated that cure rates were quite high. Now, with more experience with this method, we're seeing that only about 70 percent of patients are cured using the one-dose method. In young, healthy people, this is not a significant health risk: If the problem is not cured, it does not progress to a more serious one but instead creates uncomfortable symptoms.

Instead of the one-dose method, many doctors now favor a compromise between the one-dose and the longer, more conventional method. Three days of therapy are effective in most healthy patients, and the cost of this treatment is comparable to the one-dose cost.

Whether medication is given for one day or for several, it's important that the correct antibiotic be given. Sometimes the bacteria that cause the infection are not sensitive to that particular medication, and only a change in medicine will be effective in curing the infection. In people who have frequent bladder infections, this can be a common problem because the bacteria become resistant to certain antibiotics. The only way to know for sure whether bacteria are sensitive to a particular antibiotic is to run a culture and sensitivity test.

Any time an antibiotic is prescribed, whether for a bladder infection or any other problem, take all of it as prescribed. Don't stop taking it as soon as the symptoms disappear, because the bacteria are probably still present. Once the antibiotics are discontinued, the bacteria will flourish again and cause symptoms. Taking all the medications will help prevent this from happening.

If you have frequent bladder infections, you may want to evaluate several habits that may be a factor. Do you empty your bladder every time you urinate? Do you bear down after urinating, to ensure that all the urine is emptied from your bladder? Do you put off urinating? If it is difficult for you to get to a bathroom, whether because of your job circumstances, a physical limitation or maybe because you're traveling, you may be inviting a bladder infection. Find a way that you can empty your bladder more frequently. Do you drink at least eight glasses of water a day? Limit your intake of soft drinks and drink water instead. In females, after using the toilet, wipe from front to back. This keeps bacteria away from the urethra, which leads to the normally sterile bladder.

I still hold with the one-dose school of therapy, but am wise enough to know that no single treatment works for every patient. I'm also smart enough not to argue with a knowledgeable family physician who has examined the patient, knows the situation, and has the best interests of his patient at heart. In this case, your doctor is right.

167. *We're devastated. The daughter of a close friend has been diagnosed as having a Wilm's tumor. We think this is a fatal disease but do not wish to discuss it with the parents. Can you give us some information?*

Wilm's tumor is the single most common cancer of the kidney in children. There are no special symptoms to alert the parents or child, although a common sign is swelling of the abdomen or a lump that can be felt in this area. Blood appears in the urine in about 25 percent of children afflicted with this disease, but sometimes the quantity of blood is so little as to go unnoticed.

The disease can cause any one or all of the common symptoms of cancer: weight loss, anemia, fatigue and low-grade fever. It takes a good physical examination to put the doctor on the right track, but usually a battery of special X-ray tests will be necessary before the diagnosis is made.

There is some really good news for you. Treatment, which may combine radiation therapy with anti-cancer drugs, can achieve a long-term disease-free status (the equivalent of a cure) in more than eight out of 10 young patients. Newly developed surgical procedures now can be used in children and infants, adding to the chances of success. While side effects from these treatments can be expected, the successful outcome makes it all worthwhile.

You can obtain more information, and even a publication or two, by calling the Cancer Information Service at 1-800-4-CANCER. With all this knowledge, I'm sure you can offer important support to the parents of this child.

168. ***Please don't laugh at my question. I assure you it really happened and almost made me pass out. While passing my water, I noticed that my urine was definitely a green color. I have no other symptoms, and it happened only once more after that, but the color was less intense. Do I have anything to worry about? Will it happen again?***

If it has disappeared without any other symptoms or complaints, you most probably are out of danger. You probably never had anything to seriously worry about anyway.

The most common reason for green urine is the result of something you have eaten or ingested. Chlorophyll-containing breath mints when taken in large quantities are a frequent cause. There are a number of other substances in common medications that also may provoke a green color: guaiacol contained in many cough medicines, magnesium salicylate in Doan's Pills and thymol, which is an ingredient in Listerine mouthwash.

The most serious cause of green-tinted urine occurs from an infection caused by pseudomonas in the urine. The pus may contain a pigment (pyocyanic) that causes the green color. Methylene blue, which is used in some medical tests and treatments, when combined with the normal yellow color of urine produces a green color as well.

Now it's up to you to think back over the circumstances that preceded your colorful experience. Try to determine which of these possible causes might have been the reason in your case. If you don't repeat the experience, your green urine days are over.

169. *Is it possible for something to block the flow of urine and cause it to back up in the system? Could you explain these causes and if they are at all serious?*

The causes of urinary tract obstruction are many, and the resulting backup of urine is indeed serious and may cause permanent damage to the kidneys. Urine is produced by the kidney, and then flows down a tubelike structure called the ureter to the bladder. Here the urine is stored temporarily, until the bladder's capacity is reached and you feel the need to empty it through another tube (urethra) that leads to the outside.

Any stoppage in the urinary flow causes increased backup pressure to be exerted on the delicate kidney tissues and can impair their function. The solution is to discover the cause of the obstruction as rapidly as possible and relieve the blockage to once again allow the kidneys to perform their essential function.

170. *During a recent routine physical examination, my physician took a urine test as well as some blood for testing. As I understand it, the nurse did a "dipstick" test on my urine and found that it contained "protein." Now I am to start a whole new series of tests to see what is wrong. Can you tell me what this all means, and do you think it is serious?*

All normal urine contains some protein although the quantities are small, less than 150 milligrams during a 24-hour period. However, screening tests can detect higher levels and give some indication as to amounts.

The "dipstick" is a screening test, which uses a small strip coated with a chemical that changes its color in relation to the amount of protein present. A positive finding of the presence of higher than normal levels of protein in the urine (it's called proteinuria) is reported in as many as 10 percent of patients tested with this method.

In children, adolescents and physically active young adults, this may be a situation that is benign (not caused by a disease) and frequently disappears by itself. In some cases, it is the result of a false positive, which may occur when the urine is highly concentrated or when it is contaminated by certain antiseptics.

Protein found in the urine may be caused by some illness, such as infection and fever, and is not always the sign of kidney disease. However, while the presence of some protein in the urine on a screening test is not necessarily a cause for alarm, it most certainly demands an explanation, which may be afforded by additional testing and investigations.

In some cases the patient, under a physician's supervision, may be able to conduct a series of dipstick tests himself to see if the results continue to be positive or if there is some pattern to the findings. In other situations, more accurate methods of analysis are used to determine the amount of protein in the urine.

Along with a careful history and physical examination, further tests, which utilize X-rays and other procedures, may be used to determine the causes of the positive findings. You're well-advised to continue the testing to determine the exact diagnosis and complete any treatments that may be required.

171. ***My girlfriend is absolutely sure that bladder infections are a result of sex, and she almost has me convinced. I don't mean a sex infection, but the disease that causes painful urination and the feeling that you have to go constantly. Can you provide me with some answers?***

There are many causes for cystitis — and certainly not every case can be linked to a sexual act. But in women, the most frequent cause is when bacteria from the vagina find their way up through the urethra (the small tubelike passage between the bladder and the outside) into the bladder, where they rapidly reproduce and create an infection.

It can occur after sexual intercourse, though not necessarily so. When such an infection is seen after prolonged or repetitive sexual activity, it's called honeymoon cystitis. It's not included with the group of infections known as sexually transmitted diseases (STDs), and it can be treated successfully with antibiotics.

However, prevention is still the best medicine. Here are a few tips you can pass on to your girlfriend to help reduce the possibility of recurrence:

■ It's important to empty the bladder both before and after sexual relations.

■ Drinking a great deal of liquids produces more urine and washes out the bacteria more frequently.

■ Perfumed feminine hygiene products and douches may cause irritation that can lead to infection.

■ Birth control methods using diaphragms and foams may lead to more frequent cases of infection, and consideration should be given to changing these methods.

■ External sanitary napkins are preferable to vaginal tampons, particularly in patients with recurrent bladder infections.

If all these methods fail, a physician should be consulted to discuss the use of antibiotics prophylactically to prevent this condition from recurring. Trimethoprim sulfamethoxazole or nitrofurantoin in low doses have been used successfully in such cases.

172. ***I have a friend who has Reiter's disease. I'm considering a sexual relationship with this man, but I am concerned because I understand it is a sexually transmitted disease with no cure. Could you please provide information about the disease, including its symptoms and effects on both men and women?***

The symptoms that form Reiter's syndrome have four main elements: arthritis, urethritis (inflammation of the tube that carries urine from the bladder to outside the body) or cervicitis (inflammation of the cervix) in women, conjunctivitis (red eye) and small, painless, ulcerlike lesions usually found in the mouth or on the tongue or head of the penis.

Reiter's syndrome may result from bacterial infections to the digestive system, such as salmonella or shigella, but a sexually transmitted form occurs most frequently in men ages 20 to 40. This sexually transmitted form usually is associated with an infection by chlamydia trachomas and should be treated with antibiotics, tetracycline or erythromycin for at least 10 days. Both sexual partners should be treated at the same time to prevent the infection passing back and forth from one to the other. The arthritic symptoms receive the same care as any other form of arthritis, by using aspirin or other anti-inflammatory medications.

The other manner of transmission is called dysenteric. In this case, the syndrome develops after a bacterial infection of the intestines, which is usually caused by shigella or salmonella. Antibiotic treatment is effective in controlling the infection.

Few patients are disabled by chronic or recurrent outbreaks of this disease, which also may have an inherited element in its pattern, since it strikes more frequently at individuals who have a specific genetic marker (called HLA-B27).

173. *Can you tell me what makes urine smell really bad? I have had this for over a year and would like to be rid of it.*

In a healthy person who is properly hydrated, the odor of urine, while typical, is not considered offensive. However, there are many possible situations in which the odor of urine is changed, and the new odor may be displeasing to some noses.

Dehydration (lack of sufficient body fluid) can produce a concentrated urine with an intense odor that still is perceived as urinelike. Some diseases, such as diabetes (diabetic ketoacidosis), kidney and liver failure, also produce unpleasant odors. In some cases, the odor of urine is changed by medications that are taken on a regular basis. Certain foods also may provoke a change.

However, the most logical possibility in your case of prolonged bad odor is an infection in your bladder or urinary tract. The only sure path to an exact answer is a visit to your physician.

174. *I think I have discovered blood in my urine. At least it looks red sometimes. What could this be caused by? Is it possible that the color comes from foods I have eaten? I think I need help.*

You certainly do need some personal medical attention. There are about 100 causes for hematuria, which is the medical term for blood in the urine, most of which aren't serious. But any condition that makes you think you have blood in the urine requires some testing and evaluation.

Some medications and foods can cause darkened urine that doesn't contain blood. Foods such as beets, blackberries and rhubarb can redden the urine, as can certain antibiotics.

True hematuria can be caused by problems with the blood, the kidneys or the urinary system that collects the urine from the kidney and then excretes it (the ureters, bladder and urethra). People with blood coagulation disorders (hemophilia, sickle cell anemia) or who are taking anticoagulant drugs may have small amounts of blood in the urine.

Kidney stones, infections or tumors also can cause blood in the urine. A kidney stone can injure the ureters and urethra, which can cause bleeding. Kidney stones account for 20 percent of all cases of hematuria, while another 25 percent of cases are due to urinary tract infections. In some people, strenuous exercise causes minor trauma that creates hematuria.

175. ***A doctor visit following the sudden change in the appearance of my son's urine has given us another medical problem to deal with. The doctor called it something like "glomonephritis," but we were too frightened to understand all the rest. We don't know where it came from, nor do we seem to be doing too much about it. Can you please explain this disease for us?***

The correct spelling of this disease is glomerulonephritis, which is sometimes shortened to just nephritis, or it's called acute nephritic syndrome in some texts. It's an inflammation of the glomeruli, or filtering parts, of the kidney. Glomus means ball in Latin, which is a very descriptive name for these cells, since they form small balls or tufts when seen through a microscope. The condition is seen most frequently in children over the age of 3 years old — though it can occur at any age — and is more common in boys.

The first symptoms are a reduction in the amount of urine produced and a discoloration of the urine, sometimes described as coffee- or cola-colored, smoky or rusty. This occurs about seven to 10 days after a sore throat or skin infection (impetigo) caused by streptococci. In many cases, this infection may pass without serious symptoms and the nephritis appears without warning. Other frequently seen signs are fluid retention, with swelling of the face, eyelids and hands.

A urine test will show the presence of blood cells, white blood cells and protein, and special blood tests can prove a recent infection with streptococci. An elevated blood pressure also is commonly found and must be treated.

Usually by the time the nephritic syndrome develops, it is too late to treat the bacterial infection with antibiotics and there is no specific treatment for the glomerulonephritis. A low-salt diet is useful and protein in the diet also may be reduced.

When there is much edema, diuretics are used to reduce the volume of liquid in the body. The good news is that in the vast majority of cases the disease runs its course and healing is complete within three to 12 months after it all began.

176. ***Here is a question that has me very puzzled. After I had a few minor urinary problems, my doctor ordered some tests to help him figure out my problem. The results didn't reveal too much except the fact that I have a "horseshoe" kidney. My doctor's statement that it is nothing of consequence doesn't satisfy my curiosity. Can you offer me more information about this condition?***

As you know, most people have two kidneys. They're normally about the size of a child's fist, shaped like a bean and located against the back wall of the abdomen, one on each side of the spinal column. The lower end of the kidney is at the level of the lowest rib.

In some rare cases, however, because of a quirk of prenatal development, the lower ends of the two kidneys remain joined, which results in what appears to be a single kidney with the shape of a horseshoe. But in most cases there are still two ureters that lead from the kidney to the bladder, and each side of the horseshoe functions as if it were an individual kidney.

Most people with this congenital condition have no difficulties, but since the ureters must take a different route to the bladder than normal, they may be more prone to obstruction, which prevents urine from flowing to the bladder. And that can promote a situation that leads to frequent infections and kidney stones.

Frequently the condition goes undetected and unsuspected. However, when a special kidney X-ray test is performed, called an IVP (intravenous pyelogram), the pattern of the horseshoe kidney is seen on the X-ray. In this test, special liquid called contrast media is injected into a vein in the arm. This liquid is opaque to X-rays. As it collects in the kidney and then runs down the ureter to the bladder, it outlines the shape and structure of these organs.

The pattern produced by the horseshoe is unique, and the shape is quite like a horseshoe with the ends pointing upward. This alone is not a cause for alarm. Since your other tests must have been negative, your doctor's reassurance was in order.

177. ***My mother, who has been suffering with urinary difficulties, reports that her doctor told her that she has "female prostatic obstruction." Come on now, everyone knows that the prostate is found only in men! What is this, another medical put-on?***

No, it is not a put-on, and the doctor' explanation surely must have been accompanied by additional information. In certain cases of obstruction of the neck of the bladder, which can cause symptoms ranging from painful urination (dysuria) to complete bladder obstruction, the cause is thought to be the inflammation or growth of glandular tissue found in the area. It's known as Marion's disease or the bladder neck syndrome.

Because X-rays of the region show a pattern similar to that seen in men with prostatic enlargement, it also has been called female prostatic obstruction, although many authors dispute both the name and this explanation for the condition. However, surgical removal of the tissue yields good results.

178. ***My brother has been told he has a disease that causes cysts to form in the kidney. The doctor also told him it was inherited and therefore I might have it as well. Have you ever heard of this kind of illness, and would you share some of your knowledge with me? Thank you very much.***

I believe your brother has been diagnosed with a disease of the kidney known as Autosomal dominant polycystic kidney disease (ADPKD), which is also known as adult polycystic renal disease.

ADPKD is a relatively common familial disorder, which affects approximately one in 500 Americans. The possibility that you, too, may have the same condition without realizing it does exist, especially if you are younger than he is. Patients with the dominant gene have an almost 100 percent chance of developing the disease by age 80.

In individuals with ADPKD, the kidneys are abnormal from birth. Small cysts are present in the newborn and gradually grow larger with age. As the cysts enlarge, they press on the neighboring kidney tissues, which reduces the blood flow to these cells. The combination of increased pressure and diminished circulation causes these cells to atrophy and die. This reduces the kidneys' ability to function. But this is a slow process. It often can proceed without causing any obvious symptoms, and in some cases can go undiagnosed throughout the patient's entire life.

Most patients show no symptoms until their mid-20s or early middle adulthood. Because screening of asymptomatic individuals in families with known ADPKD is recommended, you might wish to consult with your own doctor. Ultrasound examinations, followed by additional studies in positive cases, frequently provide a diagnosis before the onset of symptoms.

Some of the symptoms that may be provoked by ADPKD are: blood in the urine, renal colic due to obstructing clots, pyelonephritis and hypertension. In advanced stages, there may be palpable abdominal masses, chronic renal failure, weight loss or brain hemorrhage from an aneurysm. Since chronic renal failure often occurs within 10 years of the onset of symptoms, you would be well-advised to start your own investigations now.

179. *As a physician, you must have heard about pyelonephritis, but it is a new and disturbing disease for us. I know it has to do with a kidney infection, but little else. What is it, and how do doctors diagnose and treat it?*

You are correct. It is an infection of the kidney, but the term pyelonephritis refers to the fact that the infecting bacteria strike both at the tissues of the kidney and the renal pelvis. The renal pelvis (from the Greek pyelos, which means pelvis) is a funnel-shaped structure that forms the upper end of the ureter, where it joins the kidney. The ureter, a tube-like organ, carries the urine from the kidney to the bladder.

The most common cause of pyelonephritis is a bacterial infection, and the most common type of bacteria is E. coli, which accounts for about 75 percent of these infections. The bacteria find their way to the kidney by ascending the ureter from the bladder, which they entered through the urethra (the tube that leads to the bladder from the outside of the body).

Certain conditions make it easier for the bacteria to reach the kidney, such as obstructions in the ureter, kidney stones, enlargement of the prostate gland, scars from previous infections of the urinary system and poor emptying of the bladder.

The infection is more common in women, especially during pregnancy, or in older women when they suffer from a "falling uterus." It also often occurs after catheterization of the bladder, as the tube inserted into the bladder provides a route for the bacteria to follow and enter the system. This is particularly true in patients who suffer from diabetes.

Usually the onset of the infection is swift, with chills, fever, pain in the flank, nausea and vomiting. In about one-third of the cases there is urination, frequently with pain. Often a tender and enlarged kidney can be felt by the doctor performing an examination. Testing the urine for blood and white cells, and culturing the specimen for the presence of bacteria can offer the final proof of the diagnosis.

Antibiotics provide effective treatment, which should be started as soon as the diagnosis is confirmed. While oral medications are usually adequate, they can be administered by intravenous drip if the infection is severe.

180. *Is it always necessary to be operated on for kidney stones? I mean a full blast procedure with all the risks of anesthesia and a big wound that takes time to heal. It scares me to death. I guess that's the wrong word to choose, but I'm sure you get the idea.*

Well, let me begin by telling you of the experience I shared with one of my patients. Ralph had become a statistic. He had become one out of every eight men in this country who, by the age of 70, will develop a kidney stone. He came to me in distress and pain. A while back, he would have had two choices: Either he would have waited and hoped that he would be able to pass the stone on his own (and that will happen in most cases) or invasive open surgery would have been performed.

Of course, surgery was and still is dictated by some hard and fast rules. The first is the size of the stone and its ability to be passed. Usually stones smaller than 4 millimeters (one-sixth of an inch) have a 75 percent chance of being passed. Other criteria are persistent pain or bleeding, partial obstruction, chronic infection and stones increasing in size. Well, Ralph had all these symptoms, but as a doctor practicing medicine today, I have some non-invasive techniques for the elimination of kidney stones that can be considered.

The first technique is called PNL (percutaneous nephrolithotomy). It involves the use of a needle to gain access to the kidney through the skin. A contrasting dye is instilled into the urinary tract through the needle to indicate the location of stones, which are removed with forceps. This procedure is not for patients with bleeding problems or those who have hypersensitivity to the contrast medium. A second procedure is called urethroscopy. It involves the use of a urethroscope and is for stones located in the ureter.

Answers from the Family Doctor (Questions 156-180)

The most recent procedure is ESWL (extracorporeal shock-wave lithotripsy, or just plain lithotripsy for short), which is a method first used in Germany in 1980 and approved by the Food and Drug Administration for use in this country in 1984. This method uses shock waves that pass through a large tub of water in which the patient is submerged. These shock waves break the stone into small sandlike particles. Once the stones have been reduced to this size, they can pass quite easily on their own during the next two to three weeks.

So, though Ralph was a candidate for removal of his kidney stones, he did not need open surgery. We discussed the best method for him and he was spared the lengthy hospitalization, the increased risk and the drain on his finances. What these three methods have in common are a good success rate and the ability to make a patient as good as new in a short period of time.

7.

The Digestive System, from Top to Bottom

Nothing is good for the body
but what we can digest.
What can procure digestion? – Exercise.
What will recruit strength? – Sleep.
What will alleviate incurable evils? – Patience.

FRANÇOIS-MARIE AROUET VOLTAIRE
French poet and dramatist (1694–1778)

We shall begin our journey through the ***digestive system***, which extends from the ***mouth*** to the ***anus***. Also known as the ***digestive tract*** or the ***alimentary canal***, this system has many parts, including the mouth, ***esophagus***, ***stomach***, both ***large*** and ***small intestines***, and two glands — the ***liver*** and the ***pancreas***. Its entire complicated structure is dedicated to ***digestion***, which is the process by which the nutrients in food are converted into the chemicals used in the body's metabolism. These basic substances then are absorbed into the bloodstream, while the unused or unusable materials are passed out of the body as waste.

Any trip down the alimentary canal, a voyage of nearly 11 meters (more than 35 feet), must begin with an exploration of the mouth, which is the entry portal for all food and drink. The mouth, its 32 adult teeth (eight incisors, four canines, eight premolars, eight molars and four wisdom teeth), the tongue, and three pairs of ***salivary glands*** (two submandibular, two sublingual and two parotid, which when swollen by a virus infection are known as the mumps) perform four functions that initiate the process of digestion:

1. The teeth, aided by the very strong, agile and flexible muscle called the tongue, chop the food into smaller particles by chewing, or *mastication*.
2. Then the particles are lubricated by the saliva, which is produced by the six salivary glands, to make swallowing easier. These six glands each day produce about 1,500 to 2,000 milliliters (about 1½ to 2 quarts) of saliva, which contains *ptylalin* (a digestive enzyme) that serves to change starch into sugar.
3. While the food is in the mouth, it is warmed or cooled to more closely approximate the body's temperature.
4. When the food is sufficiently prepared, the mouth initiates *deglutition* (swallowing) by squeezing and rolling the food mass (now known as a *bolus*) to the back of the mouth where we consciously swallow.

The bolus then passes down the *esophagus*, which is a muscular tube about 22 to 26 centimeters (9 to 10 inches) in length in the average adult and reaches from the back of the mouth to the stomach. The coordinated, rhythmic contraction of the muscles (known as *peristalsis*) moves the food down the length of the esophagus, through a circular muscle (sphincter) located at the entrance to the stomach. Sphincters act as valves, for when they contract they close a tube or opening in the body; when they relax, they permit the tube to open again. This muscle, the *cardiac sphincter* (so named because it is in close proximity to the heart), is responsible for letting the food into the stomach, then closing to keep it there. When it relaxes at the wrong time and allows the stomach contents to pass back up into the esophagus, *gastric reflux* occurs. This is the cause of the pains and other symptoms called *heartburn*.

The stomach is a bottle-shaped, thick-walled elastic sac made of smooth muscle. Though it can distend to accommodate a large meal, it does not shrink during a diet, as many people think. Under normal conditions, the stomach can hold about 1.5 liters (about 1½ quarts). The food stays in the stomach for about three hours, exposed to the secretions of the special cells contained in the tissues that line the stomach walls. This gastric juice includes *pepsinogen* (enzymes), *mucus* and *hydrochloric acid*. The mucus protects the walls of the stomach from physical damage as well as preventing the enzymes from digesting the stomach itself. The acid helps to activate the pepsinogen (changing it to *pepsin*), and together they act to digest meat and other proteins. The acid also kills any invading bacteria that enter the stomach along with the food.

The smell, sight and taste of food can help stimulate the stomach to produce more gastric juices. The nerve stimulation passes along the *vagus nerve* to the stomach and excites the cells that produce the secretions. The cells of the stomach also produce *gastrin* (a hormone) when stimulated by the presence of amino acids released by the digestion of proteins in the stomach. The hormone passes into the bloodstream and, in turn, stimulates the stomach to secrete more gastric juices. Since this process takes just a bit of time, your digestive juices can be flowing long after you have swallowed your last bite of food.

The blending process of food and digestive juices is brought about by the constant contraction of the stomach muscles, which produces a churning action that transforms the contents into a creamy soup called *chyme*. The chyme passes out of the stomach, a bit at a time, through the *pyloric sphincter*, which is located at the exit of the stomach. The chyme next enters into the first short, C-shaped part of the small intestine, called the *duodenum*. The name is derived from the Latin word *duodecim*, which means twelve, for the length of the duodenum is approximately 12 fingerbreadths or about 25 centimeters (10 inches). There the chyme is met by additional digestive enzymes that are coming from the walls of the liver, the pancreas and the intestines. Peristaltic waves push the chyme along at a rate of about 2 to 3 centimeters (about 1 inch) per minute as the digestive process continues. These waves of muscular contraction result from the contraction of the two types of muscle that form the walls of the intestine: an inner circular layer and an outer longitudinal coat. The peristaltic actions are controlled by the autonomic nervous system.

In the duodenum, the digestive juices from the liver are mixed with the chyme. The liver is the second-largest organ in the body (after the skin) and is located in the upper right corner of the abdominal cavity, neatly molded to fit into the space below the diaphragm and above the stomach. It weighs about 1.5 kilograms (3⅓ pounds). The liver is of spongy texture, filled with blood vessels and reddish-brown in color. It has two lobes: a large right lobe and a smaller left one. It has many diverse and important functions. Most of the food digested in the alimentary tract will pass through the liver before reaching other parts of the body.

The liver cells process the digested food, change it into substances the body will need, and then store the substances until they are required. The liver stores energy-rich *glucose* as *glycogen*, which can be rapidly converted back into its original form when needed by the body. The liver is responsible for turning *toxins* (poisons) into less harmful chemicals, a process known as *detoxication*. The liver processes amino acids and acts as the storage house for vitamins. It is engaged in so many chemical exchanges that form part of the metabolic process that a great deal of heat is produced, which is used to heat the blood as it passes through the liver at the rate of about 1 liter (about 1 quart) a minute. This is the heat that keeps the body warm and at the correct temperature for vital activities to proceed in a normal fashion.

The liver also produces *bile*, which is then stored in the *gallbladder*. Bile contains sodium bicarbonate, so it is alkaline, as is the pancreatic juice. This helps to neutralize the excess acid contained in the chyme. The bile also contains bile pigments (the result of the breakdown of the hemoglobin in old red cells), bile salts and cholesterol. Bile is important in the digestion of fat as an emulsifying agent, which means it breaks up the fat into tiny droplets that are processed more easily by fat-splitting enzymes. Bile flows from the liver to the gallbladder by way of the bile and cystic ducts, and it passes from the gallbladder to the duodenum by way of the cystic and common bile ducts. The arrival of stomach contents in the duodenum releases hormones produced in the duodenal wall. One hormone signals the gallbladder to contract and release its content of bile, while another hormone stimulates the production of digestive juices by the pancreas. This puts the digestive juices from both the liver and the pancreas in contact with the food at exactly the right time.

The pancreas spills its digestive juices into the duodenum as well. The pancreas is an endocrine gland as well as a digestive organ. It is a thin organ, about 12 to 15 centimeters (5 to 6 inches) long, snuggled within the curve of the duodenum. The pancreas produces three important digestive enzymes — ***trypsin***, ***amylase*** and ***lipase*** — that help to digest proteins, split fats and break down carbohydrates such as starch.

As the food leaves the duodenum, it enters the small intestine, which is the longest portion of the digestive system. It measures about 5 meters (16⅖ feet), arranged in tight coils in the middle of the abdomen. It is here that nutrient absorption essentially takes place. The walls of the intestines are lined with tiny fingerlike projections called *villi*, which in turn are covered with even smaller projections called *microvilli*. This increases the surface area of the intestines enormously, so that an area of almost 350 square meters (420 square yards) is available for absorption. This great area is necessary to cope with the 5 to 10 liters (1³⁄₁₀ to 2⅗ gallons) of food, water and secretions that pass through the intestines in a day's time. The dead cells shed by this surface each day weigh about 125 grams (4½ ounces), and this material passes out of the system as part of the stool. The walls of the small intestine secrete the enzymes *sucrase*, *maltase* and *lactase*, which break down the carbohydrates into simple sugars. The *erepsins* are intestinal enzymes that complete the digestion of proteins by converting them into the basic amino acids. Digestion continues all along the long path of the small intestines, including the next section known as the *jejunum* (from the Latin word for empty). During the passage, some of the nutrients enter the bloodstream by way of the villi, and this process (*adsorption*) is completed as the chyme enters the final portion of the small intestines, called the *ileum* (derived from the Greek word *eilos*, which means to roll up tight). The ileum continues for another 3.7 meters (12 feet) or so until it connects to the large intestine, or *colon*, by means of the *ileocecal valve*.

The ileum attaches to the large intestine at the bottom of the ascending colon, which is a pouchlike area known as the *cecum*. The dead-end *appendix*, which is useless in humans but important in the digestive system of animals that eat grass, also is attached here. The residues or wastes of the digestive process now travel slowly up the ascending colon on the right side of the abdomen, across the transverse colon to the left side and down the left side in the descending colon to the *sigmoid* and *rectum*, a journey of almost 1 meter (about 3 feet). The colon withdraws water and important salts from the wastes, leaving the semisolid waste (*feces*) to be excreted. A number of bacteria live in the colon and can produce vitamins and amino acids from the waste, as well as gas from the decomposition process, before it is eliminated. A large percentage of the feces is made up of dead bacteria.

As the feces passes through the sigmoid colon, which is an S-shaped section of colon, it enters the rectum, which is the final section that accounts for the last 40 centimeters (16 inches) of the digestive tract. The normal brown color of the waste comes from the pigments originally contained in the bile, which in turn were drawn from the hemoglobin contained in the red cells. The exit from the rectum to the outside is through another sphincter, which encircles the rectum at the anus. Normally the rectum remains empty, but as it fills with fecal material, the feeling of distention provides the desire to eliminate the waste (*defecate*). When too much water has been removed from the feces, it is hard and difficult to eliminate, causing *constipation*. Additional fiber in the diet plus additional liquids can soften the feces and make elimination easier to accomplish. Normal stool weighs about 250 grams (9 ounces) daily, of which 10 to 20 percent is bacteria.

We have come to the end of our voyage through the digestive tract. Hopefully your time has not been wasted, and you have absorbed some of the information presented during the trip.

Questions and Answers

181. *What is stomatitis? Where does it originate? Is there a cure for it?*

By definition, stomatitis is an inflammation of the mouth, and it often is a symptom of generalized disease. It has many causes and origins. Among the causes are infections, including streptococci, gonococci, yeasts and the viruses of herpes, measles and infectious mononucleosis. Trauma, dryness, irritants and toxic agents, hypersensitivity and autoimmune conditions also can provoke this unpleasant condition.

The lack of vitamins, particularly the B vitamins and vitamin C, can produce diseases such as pellagra, sprue, pernicious anemia and scurvy. When you realize that the excessive use of alcohol, tobacco, hot foods and spices, and sensitivity to toothpaste and mouthwashes also can produce the symptoms, it becomes apparent why diagnosis is difficult.

Of course, treatment depends upon accurate diagnosis. Antibiotics are quite effective against bacterial infections, and simply discontinuing the use of an irritant may bring lasting and welcome relief.

182. *I'm thoroughly confused. What I thought would be a simple yearly examination has now led to a diagnosis of a hiatus hernia. I had no symptoms and don't really understand about a hernia in my chest. Can you help me out?*

That is what annual examinations are for — to discover unsuspected conditions and deal with them before they advance too far. It isn't unusual for a hiatal (or hiatus; both terms are correct) hernia to be silent, which means without any symptoms or complaints from the patient.

Let's look at some definitions to help clear up your lack of understanding and to deal with your evident anxiety. Whenever an organ pushes through a wall of the body cavity that encloses it, that situation is called a hernia. In men, the common use of the term refers to the pushing of intestinal contents through the abdominal wall into the scrotal sac. In a hiatal hernia, the stomach is pushing through the diaphragm, which is a sheet of muscle that separates the abdominal cavity from the chest cavity.

In general use, a hiatus means a gap, cleft or opening. There is such an opening in the diaphragm that permits the esophagus to pass through from the chest cavity to attach to the stomach in the abdominal cavity. This opening has become enlarged, probably by an increased pressure within the abdominal cavity that may have been provoked by chronic coughing, straining, a sudden physical activity, pregnancy, obesity or as a result of some trauma.

Hiatal hernias occur in people of all ages and both sexes. Usually it's seen in middle age, and a small hernia can be discovered in most people over the age of 50.

In many cases, the cause is not clear, but that doesn't affect the type of therapy needed. For most asymptomatic cases like yours there is no treatment necessary as long as there are no complaints. It's unnecessary to change your diet, work or play habits or activity. You should be alert, however, to any changes that may occur. If new symptoms develop, consult your physician promptly.

183. ***I always preferred simple terms to explain medical conditions, but was surprised when I was told that I had dyspepsia. Although it's simple enough, I'm now afraid that my doctor is trying to conceal something from me. What does the word "dyspepsia" really mean? Is it a condition that can be helped? If so, what is the treatment?***

It may be confusing, but it's not meant to hide anything from you. The term dyspepsia means bad digestion. By definition, it relates to food or drink and their digestion. But digestion difficulties can be a symptom of more complex problems. Dyspepsia is a problem that plagues everybody from time to time. Some suffer it more often and more severely than the rest. If dyspepsia is a constant problem that causes you severe discomfort, it deserves attention.

But you and your physician are faced with a puzzling scenario when you have dyspepsia. The problem is so common, yet has so many variations, that it is hard to evaluate. Digestive discomfort can mean nothing more than overindulgence, or it can be the warning sign of ulcers, heart attack or gallbladder disease.

In light of the complex problems that can hide behind the upset stomach, your role as patient and chief observer of the problem becomes really important. Know as much about your complaint as you can, so that you can help your doctor decide which investigative avenue to take. Total evaluation of all the possible causes of dyspepsia is expensive and uncomfortable, and unnecessary if the two of you work together to investigate the most likely causes first.

Despite the best efforts of you and your physician, the cause of your dyspepsia may never be found. In this case, he probably will recommend that you avoid the foods that cause your problems and treat the symptoms with an antacid or acid antagonist like cimetidine or ranitidine.

To help your doctor evaluate your problem, ask yourself the following questions. Keep a simple diary for a while, so you can identify patterns of symptoms:

- Are your symptoms related to eating?
- Do the symptoms occur before, during or after eating?
- Do certain foods trigger different symptoms?
- Exactly what are your symptoms?
- Are you nauseated, and does the nausea progress to vomiting?
- Is there vomiting without nausea?
- Do you have pain, and where is it exactly?
- Are there tender spots, or is the pain vague and diffuse?
- Do you notice other symptoms that seem unrelated to your digestion?
- Have you had any weight gain or loss?
- Have you noticed any change in your bowel habits?
- Have your eating patterns changed?
- What emotions are you experiencing when you have digestive problems?
- Is there a family history of ulcers, gallbladder disease or other problems?
- What medicines are you taking?
- Do you drink alcohol or smoke?

Dyspepsia has been blamed for everything from bad marriages to the decline of entire empires. Its sufferers support a large industry of antacid manufacturers. The only problem that keeps people away from work more often is the common cold. Those individuals who haven't suffered a bout of dyspepsia yet probably will someday. And though it may be unpleasant, it most likely will not be dangerous.

However, the important thing to remember is that you should keep track of your symptoms and see your doctor if the problem is severe enough to interfere with your normal activities and good health.

184. *A problem with my eating has been diagnosed as being caused by something called "Zenker." I'm very concerned. Could you shed a little light on this situation for me?*

Zenker's diverticulum or pocket (or in medical terminology, a pharyngeal diverticulum) is a pouch in the esophagus that can trap food and mucus. It can cause difficulty with swallowing, problems with breathing, vomiting, hoarseness, lung abscess, inflammation, neck pain, coughing and, in rare cases, cancer.

Zenker's pocket is most prevalent in people over the age of 70. It occurs in men about three times as often as women. Although there is no known definitive cause, the most widely accepted hypothesis is that the pocket is the result of incoordination of the swallowing mechanism. This can produce abnormal pressure on an area of the esophagus, which can lead to herniation that forms a sac. Once that begins, the sac elongates as a result of gravity.

Surgery to remove the diverticulum is recommended for almost all patients with this condition. If the problem is left untreated, the complications can be extremely weakening. In rare cases, Zenker's pocket can recur after surgical removal, but this is the exception rather than the rule.

The only right way to deal with your concern, in this case, is to follow your doctor's counsel.

185. *I frequently develop the most awful sores in my mouth, which can make eating a painful and almost impossible task. After a time they go away, but I want to know what they are and what to do about them.*

You most probably suffer from canker sores (or fathoms stomatitis), ulcerlike sores that occur within the mouth. They are common and not fatal, but are nevertheless extremely painful.

Canker sores are present at some time in almost 20 to 50 percent of the adult population. Slightly more common in women, this problem seems to run in the family. We used to think they were caused by mouth viruses, but that no longer seems to be the case.

These sores start by causing a burning sensation from one to 48 hours before they appear. Then they form tiny blisters that break open, which leaves painful sores in your mouth. These will heal completely on their own without scarring in seven to 10 days.

I suggest applying Orabase (a type of ointment that is useful for conditions in the mouth) to the sore and avoiding foods with high amounts of salt or acid. Sometimes drinking with a straw may be helpful. Tetracycline mouth rinses, cortisone creams and numbing ointments also are acceptable means of caring for canker sores.

While most painful mouth sores are canker sores, sometimes they are not. So it's important for you to be checked by your doctor or dentist. This is especially true if you have many of these sores in your mouth, or if they're not painful but hang on for long periods of time.

186. ***It's a terribly embarrassing situation to ask a question about, and I wonder how you might answer it, but I bet a lot of people would be glad to have your advice. I suffer from gas and break wind at the most awkward times. Is this normal? What can I do about it?***

There's always an appropriate way to respond to a serious question, even when the subject is not one frequently discussed. I know you're right in thinking that many people will be interested in the answer. My mail proves that.

The medical word for the problem is flatulence, which simply means the passage of gas through the rectum. No one is exempt from this occurrence as the body produces from 400 to 2,400 cubic centimeters (24 to 146 cubic inches) of flatus (gas) each day, and the body must get rid of it one way or another. Most of the gas in our intestinal system comes from swallowed air, which frequently leaves the way it comes in when it's belched out. Air swallowing occurs when we eat rapidly, chew gum or have dentures that fit poorly. Additional gas comes from drinking soda, beer or any carbonated drink.

Any gas remaining after belching travels into the intestinal system to be joined by the gas produced during the digestion of food. The choice of foods may be part of the cause, since beans, cabbage, cauliflower, brussels sprouts and the now-famous bran are digested only partially in the small intestine. When the undigested particles reach the colon, a process called fermentation results in the production of still more gas. All of these are normal processes that produce enough gas to explain the problem. However, some medical conditions that involve digestive enzymes may be the cause, and your physician can help you sort that out.

If you have read all of this carefully, you will see that there are several things you can do. Have your dentist check your dentures for proper fit, stay away from gas-producing foods and stay away from carbonated beverages. Eat your food slowly, chew it well, swallow it carefully and take chewing gum out of your daily routine. Following these suggestions can do much to help. As for medications, simethicone may help, but the usual antacids offer little relief for your problem.

187. ***I thought it was only heartburn at first, but now after all the tests, I'm more confused than ever. My doctor has been trying to explain it to me, but I get lost in the big words. Can you explain "achalasia" to me, and what does "dysphagia" mean? He also mentioned something about "cardiospasm." Does this mean I have a heart condition, too? I had the nice nurse write down all these words for me, so I hope they're spelled right and that you can help me.***

You and the nurse did just fine, and I'll have no trouble explaining these words to you. All these terms have to do with a condition of the esophagus, which is the muscular tube that carries food between your mouth and your stomach. It's not clear to me just what your specific problem is, but perhaps understanding these words and just how your esophagus works will help clear up some confusion.

When you eat or drink and then swallow, the food is moved along through the esophagus by a special wavelike contraction, called peristalsis, of the muscles. The rounded mass of food (or bolus) is carried to the lower end of the esophagus, where it passes through a ringlike muscle called a sphincter into the cardiac portion of the stomach. So the word "cardio" here (as in cardiospasm) does not refer to the heart, and "spasm" refers to one of the special esophageal sphincter muscles, not the arteries of the heart.

Achalasia is another word that deals with the same problem. Literally it means a failure to relax, and it implies that the esophageal sphincter does not open sufficiently to allow the food bolus to pass through. When this happens, a pain occurs that mimics the pain of heart pain. It even can radiate into the neck and left arm, just as pains that result from certain heart problems do. Dysphagia is the term applied to pain or difficulty in swallowing.

The diagnosis of the condition often can be made when an X-ray called a barium esophagography (barium swallow) is performed. After you swallow a mouthful or two of barium liquid, the esophagus is seen to be widely dilated, as the sphincter muscle fails to open and all the barium is held back in the esophagus. In most cases, the causes of achalasia remain unknown.

188. ***Please explain what goes on during an operation to remove the appendix. My daughter recently was operated on. Now that all is well, we're curious to learn what happened.***

The appendix is a small, useless, dead-end tube near the start of the large intestine. It has no function and plays no role in the process of digestion. An inflamed appendix must be removed or it will rupture and infect the abdominal cavity, which can lead to peritonitis and possibly death.

The surgeon makes an incision on the right side of the abdomen through the skin, and then proceeds through the three layers of muscle that form the wall of the abdomen in this area, to enter the abdominal cavity. There the surgeon searches for the inflamed appendix and ties it off (closing it), if it hasn't ruptured, before cutting it off. Tying it keeps the infected contents from spilling into the abdominal cavity and spreading the infection.

After the appendix is removed, the abdomen is closed with sutures. If everything goes well, the patient stays in the hospital for a few days to a week and can resume normal activities in three to six weeks. If the appendix ruptures, strong antibiotics are used, and the patient may need a drain inserted at the incision. Hospitalization and convalescence will be longer in such a case.

Because a ruptured appendix is so serious, an appendectomy is performed in almost all patients with symptoms of appendicitis. About 10 percent of these people will have a perfectly normal appendix, but it's better to remove a healthy appendix than risk leaving a bad one in.

189. ***My sister says her husband is being treated with antibiotics to cure his stomach ulcer. It is certainly a new one on me, and we're wondering if she has it a bit mixed up. Or if possibly the doctor isn't telling her the whole truth. Do you have any way of finding out about this treatment and telling us about it? We would be most grateful.***

I think she has it right, and I doubt that the doctor is holding back any bad news. Peptic ulcers (or stomach ulcers, if you will) are the result of one of three main factors: the use of medications that irritate the stomach lining — most noted with nonsteroidal anti-inflammatory agents

(NSAIDs); cigarette smoking; or an infection caused by Helicobacter pylori (formerly known as Campylobacter pylori).

Some medical writers insist that inheritance plays a role or that life's stresses also may be a cause, but there's some controversy about this. The treatment of any illness depends upon its cause, so when the suspicion that H. pylori is present is proven to be true, antibiotics make an effective treatment.

It's probable that the ulcer is an indirect result of the infection and that the bacteria first interfere with some of the protective mechanisms of the stomach lining or actually damage the tissue before the ulcer develops. Some studies show that healing follows the use of antibiotics in such cases, while still other research papers fail to demonstrate the same effect. There are no such doubts about the relationship between cigarettes — which damage the gastric lining, increase acid secretion and change the blood flow — and the development of a stomach ulcer.

In addition, smoking slows the healing process. So patients who suffer an ulcer are helped by treatment, but if they continue smoking they will find that the ulcer develops again and again. An ulcer may be treated with several medications now available, and a cure may be obtained in 90 to 95 percent of patients who are adequately treated for a 12-week period. When ulcers do recur, an evaluation using an endoscope permits the physician to look into the stomach to determine the actual state of the disease.

190. *It took emergency surgery to save my closest friend, who suffered from "volvulus" — a condition I never heard of. Could you please explain what happened?*

Volvulus refers to a blockage in the stomach or intestine, which occurs when part of the organ wraps around itself. This can happen when stomach ligaments are weak or missing, or where fibrous bands and adhesions are present as a result of past surgery or inflammatory disease.

Acute gastric volvulus causes severe pain from trapped gas and fluid, and if left untreated it can prove fatal. The condition must be corrected as soon as possible, either through surgery or by passing a tube through the patient's nose and into the intestines to relieve the pressure.

Although the condition can be diagnosed by observing a patient, X-rays that use a contrast material, such as barium, to highlight the blockage on the X-ray image can reveal the site of the blockage.

191. ***I would like some information on esophageal reflux. I've been diagnosed as having this and have had the problem for two years. I do not eat any acidic or spicy food and do not drink coffee. I have a burning sensation in the chest and on the mouth and lips. I wonder if this is due to the disease. I would appreciate any information about treatment that you may be able to give me.***

Gastroesophageal reflux disease (GERD) refers to an entire group of digestive disorders with the symptoms you describe. This acid backflow (reflux) creates a burning sensation or heartburn behind the breastbone that occurs after eating or while lying down. This burning is caused by the acid contents of the stomach flowing backward into the lower end of the esophagus (the tube leading from the mouth to the stomach), where it irritates the tissues and creates the pain. It is difficult to state with certainty that your lip and mouth pain are from the same cause, but it is possible.

Initial treatment of GERD is conservative. Since the condition involves gastric backflow, lifestyle changes may be the cornerstone of good therapy. Modifying the diet, as you are doing, to exclude foods — such as tomato juice or orange juice — that irritate the mucosal tissue may help. Coffee frequently is named as a culprit, as are alcohol and chocolate. Decreasing or stopping smoking altogether is also helpful. Eating meals well before bedtime and elevating the head of the bed to prevent backflow are additional good tips.

Drugs called H2 antagonists — such as cimetidine and ranitidine, and more recently a new drug called omeprazole (which works in a different fashion from the others) — reduce gastric acidity and frequently are used to treat these disorders.

If these measures do not provide lasting relief, and when there is serious inflammation of the esophagus leading to hemorrhage and strictures from scarring, surgery to tighten the sphincter muscles of the esophagus may be indicated.

192. ***While we were sitting with a group of friends, my husband's stomach started to growl, which made enough noise to wake the dead. Talk about being embarrassed! I can't let this happen again, but I don't know what to do for my man. How can I make my husband's stomach shut up?***

The simplest answer I can provide is: Feed the poor man! The stomach muscles are always in action by contracting to push the stomach's contents through to the intestines and additional digestion.

But the sounds are magnified when the stomach is half-empty (only partially filled with fluids and gas). This is the condition the stomach is in after several hours without food. Drinking a carbonated beverage or swallowing air during an animated discussion also may increase the force of the contractions and the sounds they make. If meal time is close, with the wonderful smell of food in the air, the digestive juices flow more abundantly, and the muscle activity increases.

You might have your husband try some vigorous exercise to stop the contractions or provide him with a glass or two of water to drink, but the best bet is to put dinner on the table and start eating.

193. *I have been on medication to treat a stomach ulcer for some weeks now, and am feeling much better. However, my brother keeps telling me that the only sure cure is an operation, which is something my own doctor has never mentioned. Should I be following my brother's caution and seek the advice of another physician?*

Second opinions from another physician are a valuable resource when considering an operation recommended by your own doctor, but they're rarely necessary in a case such as yours. By your own admission, you're doing well on the medications your doctor has prescribed and are feeling better.

To be sure, follow-up examinations should be undertaken to determine the present state of your stomach ulcer. Gradually the ulcer should disappear completely under the effects of the medication. There are now quite a few very effective medications available. These medications lower the amount of acid produced by cells in the lining of the stomach and allow the ulcer to heal.

The ulcer is a sore in the lining of the stomach that results from an injury to the tissues, which may be caused by bacteria, some medications and alcohol, among other things. With successful treatment, this sore heals, and the symptoms that may be present disappear. An operation is not required under these circumstances.

However, ulcers frequently do recur. When they return often and then fail to respond to medications or if complications do occur, surgery will have to be considered as a method of treatment. The failure of an ulcer to heal is the most frequent indication for surgery, for such cases may turn out to be an ulcerating cancer. This requires careful evaluation using gastroscopy, which is a direct viewing of the inside of the stomach with a telescopelike instrument. During the procedure a biopsy, or tissue sample, may be taken and then examined under a microscope to determine its nature. Surgery is undertaken only when the indications are there, for it is not the most pleasant experience and has its own set of complications.

194. ***It seems as if you only answer questions that deal with exotic diseases no one ever has nor cares much about anyway. Why not use your knowledge to help us common people and talk about real subjects like constipation? I know I could use some assistance.***

Commoner or king, constipation can be a problem for anyone. You are right, it's a subject that should be discussed. However, for an understanding of the causes of this annoying condition, you must first understand how the large intestine, or colon, works.

After foods have been digested and the nutrients absorbed by the small intestine, the remaining waste reaches the colon, which is the last section of the intestinal system before the rectum. The colon moves the waste along with rhythmic contractions, called peristalsis, which drive the fecal material toward the rectum. At the same time, the colon reabsorbs the excess fluids, which makes the stool firmer and firmer as it reaches the last sections of the bowel. If the muscle contractions are slow or irregular, the stool spends too much time in the colon and too much water is removed, which forms a hard or dry stool. If peristaltic rhythm is too swift, the stool will be loose and watery, and leave as diarrhea.

Constipation is therefore best prevented by assuring that these contractions (called involuntary as we have no control over them) remain normal. They can be affected by illness, stress, poor bowel habits, lack of exercise and, above all, improper diet and eating habits. The object is to have the stool arrive at the rectum in a form that makes your voluntary efforts to pass your stool easy and normal.

Here are some tips for you:

- Eat at regular times, take pleasure in your meals and chew your food thoroughly.

- Make sure your diet contains sufficient bulk. Fiber is present in fruits, cereals, raw vegetables, and in cooked high-residue vegetables, such as corn, potatoes, spinach, string beans and turnips, to name a few.
- Be sure to include plenty of fluids in your daily diet.
- When the urge to move your bowels arrives, pay attention and try to move your bowels without straining; let nature proceed normally.
- Adding a brisk walk and sufficient exercise to daily activity might just make the difference that changes your problem of constipation into an unpleasant memory.

195. *At first it was thought my husband was suffering from a stomach ulcer. Now the doctor informs us that my husband has a disease with the strange name of Zollinger-Ellison, but that the treatment is the same. What does this all mean?*

The strange name comes from the discoverers of this syndrome, which indeed, closely resembles a stomach ulcer. It develops rapidly with pain that is difficult to control, ulcer formation and diarrhea as its principal symptoms, but the ulcers are found to be in different locations in the stomach than usually are found with simple peptic ulcers. Even with tests performed correctly, including X-rays and endoscopy (looking at the stomach through a special telescopelike tube), this syndrome cannot be distinguished from ordinary ulcer in more than 50 percent of the patients.

A tumor, called a gastrinoma, of the pancreas or wall of the duodenum causes Z-E syndrome. These tumors result in the increased secretion of gastrin into the blood, which stimulates the cells of the stomach to produce massive amounts of gastric acid. If a sensitive blood test for gastrin shows there are increased amounts, Z-E syndrome can be diagnosed.

The tumor, however, is hard to find. Arteriography, which may show circulation to the tumor, is the best test, but it discovers it in fewer than one case in two. Sometimes ultrasound can be used, but it, too, detects tumors in only 20 to 30 percent of the patients. The good news is that the same medications (called H2 blockers) that block acid formation in peptic ulcers work very well for Z-E. However, since a surgical cure is possible, an exploratory operation should be considered to locate and remove the tumor.

196. ***I know that a person with severe diarrhea loses lots of water from the body, and that liquids should be given. However, I'm not sure just what fluids are considered correct, or if the drinks that athletes use to combat dehydration by excessive perspiration are useful. Will you please provide this information?***

Not only is the water loss in acute diarrhea critical, but important elements, such as sodium and potassium, that function as electrolytes in the body also are lost. When the fluids and electrolytes are not replaced, dehydration may occur, which is even more dangerous than the diarrhea itself.

The goal is to replace all that is being lost, as well as to provide some basic nutrients. Old-fashioned tea and honey, and chicken broth (without fat) can work wonders. Gatorade or nondiet, noncaffeinated soft drinks are useful to assure sufficient fluid volume. Fruit drinks help provide additional carbohydrates, but avoid fruit juices that have a laxative effect, such as prune or apple juice.

You can prepare your own solution by following this recipe:

1 quart of water
¾ teaspoon salt substitute (potassium chloride)
½ teaspoon baking soda
3 tablespoons white corn syrup (Karo syrup)
1 packet of unsweetened powdered drink mix, or
concentrated fruit juice to taste

This will provide the exact electrolyte requirements in the right concentration. The recommended intake is about two quarts of liquid a day or up to three quarts if a fever and sweating are also present.

197. ***I'm writing to ask about crone or crone disease. What is it, and what is the cause of it? A few months ago, my brother was sick and he just told me that the doctor said that he had that disease, but he does not remember any explanations. He is 71 years old.***

Your letter caught my eye, because it expresses a concern that occurs in so many families who are interested in the welfare of each member. When the sick individual does not understand the nature of the disease, it's the right and obligation of any family member to seek the necessary explanations and gain the knowledge that can help provide the care needed to alleviate suffering and discomfort.

Your brother has Crohn's disease, also known as regional enteritis, which is one of a group of intestinal diseases classified as inflammatory bowel diseases. It usually starts with chronic diarrhea, along with abdominal pain, fever, loss of appetite and loss of weight.

In many cases, the first episode may mimic appendicitis and care must be used in making the diagnosis. However, a barium enema (X-ray) can clearly show the ulcerations in the walls of segments of the intestine. These diseased areas are limited and occur next to parts of the intestines that show no disease at all, which gives rise to the term "regional" used in describing the disease. A biopsy, in which a small piece of tissue is obtained for a microscopic examination, often is used to help make the diagnosis.

The disease occurs with equal frequency in both sexes, usually begins before age 40, and is more common among Jews with a tendency to be seen in members of the same family. The exact causes for any of the inflammatory bowel diseases remain unclear, although immunologic factors, infections and fiber-poor diet in developed countries all have been considered to play a role.

Without the knowledge of a specific cause, there can be no one therapy, so many are used, depending upon the severity and extent of the disease. These include steroid therapy (prednisone), antibiotics when infections do occur, anti-diarrhea medications and special diet. When all else fails, surgery may be considered to remove the portion of bowel that is affected.

You may obtain additional information by contacting the Crohn's and Colitis Foundation of America (CCFA) at 444 Park Avenue South, New York, New York 10016-7374, or call 1-800-343-3637. The CCFA is a source of a great deal of up-to-date and valuable advice.

198. *Is there any difference between "diverticulitis" and "diverticulosis"? It seems as if the doctor uses both of the words like they mean the same thing. It's very confusing. Please help.*

The two terms can be confusing. Diverticulosis is a fairly minor problem, and a great number of people have it without knowing it. In about 15 percent of cases, it progresses to a more serious problem called diverticulitis. Because of this, it's important to control the milder diverticulosis, so that it doesn't progress to the more serious situation.

Diverticulosis is a condition of the colon. The healthy colon has rings of muscle that push waste along and eventually out of the body. In the person with diverticulosis, the walls of the colon develop tiny pouches that stick out of the outside wall of the colon. The pouches are called diverticula and usually form near the end of the colon in the sigmoid region. Some experts say that a low-fiber diet leads to this problem, because the muscles of the colon must be stronger to push less bulky wastes along the colon. The pouches form as a result of the increased pressure.

One out of 10 Americans over the age of 40 has diverticulosis. Most of these people have no symptoms. However, if the colon wall becomes thick enough to slow or block passage of stool, tenderness in the lower left side of the abdomen, cramping and bloating may occur.

If the little pouches become inflamed, diverticulitis results. The inflammation may result from stool becoming trapped in a diverticula, or the weakened colon wall may tear and become infected. The infection requires medical care, because it will create fever, pain and abdominal swelling. Sometimes the colon is obstructed by the infection and swelling; then a real emergency results.

Treatment of diverticulitis depends on how severe it is. Antibiotics, rest and medicines to calm the colon often are prescribed. Although your doctor normally might recommend a high-fiber diet, he may ask you to avoid fiber until the colon is healed.

To prevent diverticulosis from turning into diverticulitis, eat a diet high in fiber, which includes fruits, vegetables and plenty of water. Regular exercise also helps keep the colon healthy.

199. ***I'm having trouble finding material to read about a surgical condition called "peritonitis." I know it is a serious situation, and I wish to know what causes it and how it should be treated.***

First, a definition or two: Peritonitis is an inflammation of the tissues that line the abdominal cavity and cover most of the organs, such as the intestines, that are located there. Although the inflammation can be caused by chemical irritation or by traumatic irritation, the most common cause is an infection, caused by either E. coli or streptococcus fecalis, although other infections can and do occur.

Peritonitis may develop in a number of ways. It can result as a complication of an operation. For example, bacteria can escape from inside the intestine when two ends of the intestine have been sewn back together after the removal of a section containing cancer. Or if any organ of the abdomen or pelvic cavity becomes infected and forms an abscess, the rupture of the abscess may spread the infecting bacteria over the peritoneal tissue, which causes an acute peritonitis. This occurs frequently in pelvic inflammatory disease (PID). Another more obvious cause may be that of a penetrating wound of the abdomen, such as in a stabbing or automobile accident.

The treatment requires the elimination of all infecting organisms, which may sometimes necessitate surgery to remove the source of the infection. Removing a ruptured appendix is a good example.

The mainstay of all treatment, however, is the effective use of antibiotics, which are usually given intravenously in high dosages to assure the complete eradication of the bacteria. The treatment may require more than one type of antibiotic, and the choice will depend upon the type of bacteria that is the culprit, for peritonitis is a serious condition that requires intensive treatment. Fortunately many potent antibiotics are available, meaning that the chances for the patient are excellent.

200. *I've had flare-ups of severe abdominal cramps. After a series of tests and X-rays, my gastroenterologist told me I have something that he called a "successful women's ulcer." He put me on a high-fiber diet but would prescribe no medication. Have you ever heard of such a thing?*

Yes. The so-called successful women's ulcer (SWU) is actually very common, but it's really a misnomer, because it's not actually an ulcer. The condition could be called more correctly irritable bowel disease.

SWU may occur in up to 25 percent of working women at some time, especially in women who are meticulous and overachievers. The symptoms of SWU are a burning or stabbing pain in the abdomen, nausea, diarrhea, constipation and indigestion. The symptoms are the result of intestinal spasm caused by stress.

Irritable bowel disease is best treated with a high-fiber diet and stress management programs. High-fiber foods, such as unprocessed cereals, breads and beans, create more bulk in the digestive tract. The added bulk prevents the painful intestinal spasm, because it keeps the muscles from fully contracting. In addition to the high-fiber diet, your doctor might have suggested some stress management techniques, such as meditation, biofeedback and reading. Learning to relax fully is really the key to ridding yourself of this problem.

201. ***Except for the fact that it is something like an appendix, we know nothing about a condition called "Meckels." Can you explain what a Meckels is, what the symptoms of the condition are, and what treatment is advised? Does the fact that one child may have this mean that his brothers and sisters are also likely to have Meckels? Neither my husband nor I has ever been suspected of this, and we're all quite confused.***

Properly identified as a Meckel's diverticulum, this condition results when a tube called the vitelline duct fails to disappear during the growth of a fetus. In the early stages of fetal development, this tube connects the primitive intestines to the embryonic yolk sac.

As other means are established to provide nutrition to the fetus, this duct normally closes and then disappears. When this process stops before the duct is absorbed fully, a small portion of the tube may remain, forming a sac or diverticulum. This occurs in about 2 percent of the population, is twice as common in males as in females, and leaves a diverticulum that is about 5 centimeters (2 inches) long.

Two types of tissue most commonly are found lining the sac: gastric tissue (like the lining of the stomach) and pancreatic tissue (similar to that found in the pancreas gland). The gastric tissue is by far the most common and is the most important type of tissue from a practical point of view, since it can ulcerate just as the stomach lining can, causing pain, hemorrhage and perforation. The presence of the diverticulum also may create a situation that leads to intestinal obstruction, which is seen in about 25 percent of adult patients and is also most common in children.

The diagnosis is difficult, since symptoms can mimic many more common ailments. But a technetium radionuclide scan can detect the presence of the gastric cells in an abnormal position and is successful in making the diagnosis in about 80 percent of the cases.

Once the diverticulum is found, the treatment is surgical, which means removal of the unnecessary structure. The presence of Meckel's diverticulum in one child has no relation to the possibility of its presence in your other children, as this is not considered to be an inherited condition.

202. ***Am I correct in assuming that fissures and fistulas are the same thing? When discussing my problem, the physician didn't seem to describe a fissure differently than he discussed a fistula.***

Both anal fissures and anal fistulas cause pain to the rectum and anus, but that is where their similarity ends.

An anal fissure is an open vertical tear or wound that usually is located in a straight line along the back wall of the anus. In most cases, it is caused by passing a large, hard stool, but fissures also can be caused by severe diarrhea. Fissures are painful, especially during and immediately after a bowel movement. This pain causes sufferers to try to avoid bowel movements, which in turn aggravates constipation. There may be some bleeding during the bowel movement, but it is not profuse.

The way to treat an anal fissure is to lubricate the anal canal and avoid constipation. The best lubricant is a nonmedicated emollient suppository. A good way to soften stools is to eat a high-fiber diet and perhaps take a fiber supplement. Chronic fissures may need to be surgically corrected.

Anal fistulas are abnormal passages that connect the inner surface of the rectum (anus) to the skin's surface. They are the result of an abscess, or acute infection, in one of the anorectal glands that surround and open into the anus.

An unopened, swollen abscess is one cause of anal pain. The anal fistula is usually painless except before the abscess opens, and it may heal by itself after the abscess drains. An unopened abscess should be drained completely by a physician. In most cases, antibiotics are not needed. Once the abscess is drained, the fistula may disappear, but chronic fistulas can develop and should be removed surgically, even when they cause no pain or symptoms.

As you can see, chronic anal pain should not be left undiagnosed and untreated. This condition warrants a physician's attention.

203. ***I know we're getting only half the information we need from our daughter-in-law, but we fear that her description of my son's condition is wrong. She keeps telling us about cirrhosis, but we fear that she means it is cancer. Are they the same thing?***

I'm sure many individuals have thought of the same question, and the answer is no. Cirrhosis is a condition of the liver that follows a wide variety of chronic and progressive liver diseases. The result of these diseases is to scar the liver so that the normal architecture — the pattern of cells within the liver — is disrupted. Although the liver tries to heal itself by growing new tissue, this tissue, too, is of an abnormal pattern.

In the United States, alcohol is the most common cause of cirrhosis, while chronic hepatitis is the most important cause of cirrhosis in other countries. In cirrhosis, the liver is large, but as the disease progresses, the liver may shrink and become smaller than usual. A cirrhotic liver does not function well. Patients experience the symptoms of fatigue, malaise and loss of vigor, although these findings sometimes can be associated with other diseases. As for cancer of the liver, here the pattern and form of the cells themselves change and take on specific appearances that can be diagnosed by using microscopic techniques.

Primary liver cell cancer develops in 5 to 20 percent of patients with cirrhosis, although it also can occur in people who have never had an underlying liver problem. To look at it another way, cirrhosis is present in 40 to 80 percent of all patients who have primary liver cell cancer, but the two diseases, although occurring in the same individual, are different. I'm sure your daughter-in-law is telling the truth, but in a manner she hopes will not cause you any extra worry.

204. *My physician has discovered that I have gallstones, even though they're causing me no pain. What are gallstones made of, and how did I get them?*

You're not alone with your stones, for an estimated 25 million Americans have them, and that's about 10 percent of the population. In addition, you're one of the lucky ones who have "silent" stones, not one of the 500,000 patients who will have their gallbladders removed to treat their painful condition and to prevent serious or even life-threatening complications of this disease.

Gallstones form when chemicals that usually are dissolved in the bile precipitate out, forming crystals that cling together to make stones. There are two main types: stones formed from cholesterol (in about 80 percent of the cases) and pigment gallstones formed from bilirubin and other compounds.

The typical sufferer is a woman who has been pregnant, is overweight, consumes a lot of dairy products and animal fats, and is past the age of 50. However, 20 percent of Americans of both sexes over age 65 have gallstones. Heredity plays a part as well, since there is frequently a family history of the disease. If this description comes close to fitting you, you now have an indication of where your collection of unwanted stones came from.

205. ***What is the name of the disease that is like ulcerative colitis but happens in the rectum? Where does it come from, and how can it be treated?***

Ulcerative colitis is an inflammatory disease of the inner lining of the large intestine, or colon. Ulcerative proctitis and proctosigmoiditis, on the other hand, are similar inflammations of the rectum and of the final curve of the colon that leads to the rectum.

The symptoms of these two diseases include rectal bleeding and mucus in the stool. Ulcerative colitis is not to be confused with proctitis caused by infection, which is frequently transmitted through sexual contact.

Medical experts disagree on the nature of ulcerative proctitis and proctosigmoiditis. Some clinicians say the two are a mild, limited form of colitis. Others argue that they're completely separate diseases. However, it has been shown that if the disease hasn't spread to the rest of the colon after six months, then it probably never will. Furthermore, the prognosis for proctitis and proctosigmoiditis is better than the outlook for colitis. Patients with the more limited disease rarely need to be hospitalized or treated with system-wide corticosteroids. Therefore, it can be important to distinguish between the diseases.

In any case, ulcerative proctitis is generally fairly mild. Since most of the colon is not affected, normal stools usually are formed. In fact, a patient with the disease may even be constipated. Treatment involves medication for the inflammation and hydrocortisone or corticosteroid foam enemas.

206. ***I've been having abdominal pain for months now. My gynecologist has run dozens of tests and has found nothing wrong. He sent me to a gastroenterologist who tells me that he suspects "irritable bowel syndrome." Please tell me about this. Is it life-threatening?***

Irritable bowel syndrome (IBS) is uncomfortable, painful and can produce stress and depression, but it's not related to cancer and is not a fatal condition. The classic symptom of IBS is a change in bowel habits. At least half of all IBS patients complain of constipation. Others suffer from constipation alternating with diarrhea.

In most cases, some of the pain eases up after a bowel movement. The discomfort might be noticeable again 30 minutes to an hour after eating.

As many as 60 percent of IBS patients suffer from frequent headaches, and some may have urinary problems.

Management of IBS includes adopting a high-fiber diet. Your doctor will have to look into what medications you might be taking that could exacerbate your pain. Cutting down or cutting out your intake of coffee, tea and sodas may help lessen the frequency of the diarrhea. Also, it's very important for those afflicted with IBS to learn how to relax and to lessen stress factors in their lives.

207. ***Does the color of your stool reveal anything about the state of your health? I have a friend who gives me a daily report on this aspect of her life, and she has almost got me believing it is something everyone should do. Is this true, or is her behavior just bizarre?***

I've never seen a study about such habits, but I would suspect that most people take a passing notice of the state of their bowel movements, without paying it a great deal of focused attention. Although the color may vary normally from light to dark brown, which results from the bile content of the stool, there are other factors that can influence this color, and some do have a medical significance.

Food may play a large role. Beets and carrots, especially, when eaten in large quantities, impart their own hue to the stool. But a colorless, pale gray to white stool signifies a blockage in the flow of bile, and a very dark brown to black color indicates an excess flow of bile — both of which require medical attention. A black tarry stool is sometimes the result of bleeding in the intestinal system and denotes digested blood. However, iron pills and stomach preparations that contain bismuth also produce a black color.

It is therefore not the color alone that may be important, but the history of food or medicines taken in the past 24 hours, as well as the general state of the individual, that may give meaning to the stool color. Frankly speaking, I doubt that it deserves a daily report or excessive attention.

208. ***I have an ongoing problem with my bowels, and have been most diligent in following instructions from my physicians (I now have more than one). I've been through a barium enema and a sigmoidoscopy, and now a colonoscopy is being suggested. My problems are real ones, and I will go forward, but can you tell me the reasons this test may be necessary?***

You sound like a reasonable patient, and your physicians appear to be doing a step-by-step evaluation of your problem. That's fine. It's the best way to get to the answers you need for a diagnosis and proper treatment. I can't second-guess your doctors, nor would I want to, so my answer will be straight from the textbook. Please don't interpret any of these indications as a diagnosis; that you must obtain directly from your personal counselors.

Colonoscopy is an excellent procedure for diagnosing difficult cases of bowel trouble, since it enables the physician to view directly almost the entire length of the colon. It's particularly valuable to clarify findings of a barium enema that may have been too indistinct to interpret with any degree of certainty.

It's possible to obtain tissue samples during the colonoscopy (a biopsy) that may be analyzed under a microscope. When chronic, slight bleeding is the worrisome sign, the exact site may be located through the scope. Should the source of the bleeding be from a small polyp, it can be removed easily during the examination. Some individuals with chronic situations, such as ulcerative colitis and inflammatory bowel disease, may require colonoscopy to discover the extent of their disease, or whether changes that could lead to malignancy are occurring.

Many physicians develop methods of evaluation and diagnosis that use their personal skills most effectively, and they will recommend procedures that are of the greatest benefit to their patients. You apparently have come a long way, and hopefully the answers you seek are just around the corner.

209. ***My brother was diagnosed recently as having a condition called "hepatitis C." I had never heard of this disease and found little in my reading to increase my knowledge. Can you tell me where this disease comes from, and what it might mean to the future well-being of my brother?***

It's not surprising that you have not heard much about this type of hepatitis, since it's the least well-known type of hepatitis. Hepatitis C is caused by a virus and affects about 170,000 Americans each year. Formerly, it was known as "hepatitis non-A, non-B," until testing techniques were developed that could distinguish this particular disease form.

Hepatitis C can strike as an acute hepatitis or develop into a long-lasting, serious, chronic form. Symptoms are variable, from no symptoms whatsoever, to sufferers who experience vomiting, fever and abdominal pain. Many patients experience varying amounts of fatigue, weakness and headache. Although hepatitis C is seen in people who are considered high risk — intravenous drug abusers, sexual partners of infected individuals, and those who have received transfusions of whole blood or blood products — many cases occur in people with no clear risk factor.

Hepatitis C is never a disease to be dealt with lightly. Close medical supervision and treatment are required, but in many cases it disappears by itself after about six months.

210. ***I am writing on behalf of my boyfriend. He says he has a hernia, but he refuses to have it checked. Over the years it has gotten bigger and is now the size of a softball. He believes as long as he can push it back he'll be all right. Please give me any information you have, because I don't know anything about the subject at all.***

It's obvious from your letter that your boyfriend doesn't have a clear understanding of his condition either. And he may not be the only one, since hernias are quite common in the general population, with about 15 people out of 1,000 bothered by the problem.

A hernia occurs when a loop of bowel or intestines pushes through an abnormal opening. The most common is the indirect hernia, which accounts for 50 to 75 percent of all hernias. This type of hernia usually develops in men under the age of 30. In this case, the gut pushes through a weak point in the sheet of tissue that lines the inner abdominal wall (the abdominal fascia) and passes through a canal into the scrotum. Although there may be few symptoms, the swelling is noticed easily. As the opening becomes larger, the hernia may seem to grow.

When the intestines push through the muscle wall of the abdomen as a result of a weakness and produce a bulge in the groin area, it's termed a direct hernia, which is seen most frequently in men over 40. Although this bulge may be pushed back easily or held in place with belts, the danger lies in a hernia complication known as incarceration, in which the gut becomes stuck in the position. Emergency surgery may be required to correct the situation. Incarceration also may cause the circulation to the trapped intestines to become blocked, in which case the bowel becomes strangulated and can die easily, becoming a life-threatening situation.

Repair of the hernia is the answer, and it's one of the most common surgical procedures performed. The patient will need time for recuperation, from two to three months, while the surgery heals, during which activities will be increased gradually from walking to full exercise.

211. *Is it possible for a person to develop cirrhosis though he is not a big drinker? Please explain a bit about cirrhosis, for we have been given little information by the doctor.*

Cirrhosis is actually a group of diseases that cause serious damage to the body's largest internal organ — the liver. As cirrhosis progresses, normal liver cells are replaced by scar tissue. The disease is often fatal, because the liver provides the body with very important functions. The liver is involved in producing blood-clotting factors, blood proteins, bile and more than 1,000 different enzymes, as well as performing many other crucial roles.

Alcohol abuse is by far the leading cause of this disease, which kills more than 30,000 Americans a year. However, there are several other conditions that lead to cirrhosis.

A small percentage of people who suffer from chronic hepatitis develop cirrhosis. Diseases such as hemochromatosis, in which the body does not handle iron properly, and Wilson's disease, in which the body handles copper abnormally, can cause cirrhosis. Congenital and inherited conditions also cause this liver disease.

Cirrhosis also can be caused by conditions in which the body is not able to use sugar properly, or by deficiencies of specific enzymes in the liver. In rare cases, a severe reaction to drugs or environmental toxins, some forms of heart disease, parasitic infestations or obstruction of the bile ducts can cause scar tissue to form on the liver.

When cirrhosis of the liver begins, it's often silent, showing no signs or symptoms. But eventually the sufferer may experience a loss of appetite, nausea, vomiting, weight loss, itching, an enlarged liver, increased sensitivity to drugs, vomiting of blood, abdominal swelling and jaundice. Many patients never develop any symptoms, but lab tests may discover the disease when the tests are performed for other ailments.

Further deterioration of the liver often can be stopped if proper treatment is started immediately after cirrhosis is diagnosed. In the large majority of cases of cirrhosis due to alcoholism, the easiest way to stop the disease is total abstinence from alcohol and a wholesome diet complete with needed nutrients and vitamins.

212. ***Recently a friend told me of a new procedure for removing gallstones that doesn't involve major surgery. She didn't have the details down too well, but mentioned something about a 1-inch incision near the belly-button and a tube inserted to suck out the gallbladder or stones, and that the patient only had to stay overnight at the hospital. Can you give me some real information about this?***

Here's the real inside story, but hold onto your hat, because the name of this new surgical procedure is a doozy. It's called laser-assisted laparoscopic cholecystectomy and, as you indicated, it removes the diseased gallbladder through a small incision made in the patient's navel (or belly-button) instead of the large incision in the abdomen used for standard gallbladder surgery.

Laser-assisted laparoscopic cholecystectomy must be performed under general anesthesia and takes about one hour. Actually, four small incisions of 2½ centimeters (1 inch) are needed for the procedure. Besides the one at the navel, another is made beneath the breastbone and two more below the ribs. Through these incisions the surgeon will place the laser, used to cut the gallbladder away from the liver, and the laparoscope, an instrument that permits the physician to see what is going on. The other incisions are needed for inserting instruments that can grab the gallbladder and move it about.

Although standard gallbladder surgery is safe and effective, the larger incision of about 10 to 15 centimeters (about 4 to 6 inches) causes greater pain and requires both a longer hospital stay and a longer time to heal after surgery. With this procedure, the patient is out of the hospital and back to work in about a week's time.

However, there are still situations in which the standard operation is preferable: when previous operations may have left adhesions and scars that make additional surgery more difficult to perform, or when a gallstone is blocking the tubes leading from the gallbladder to the small intestine. You may want to check with your local hospital to see if it's equipped to perform this latest innovation in gallbladder surgery.

213. ***I have an itch in my bottom (anus) that I can only describe as "ferocious." I thought it was piles, but my physician assured me this is not the case and that I have nothing to worry about. What can it be, and what can I do?***

Questions about this distressing condition, called anal pruritus, are frequent. Your physician is correct, too. Hemorrhoids, or piles, alone are not one of the causes of this itch. Actually, in 40 to 70 percent of cases, no cause can be found. In such cases, the condition is labeled idiopathic or primary. This diagnosis is made when a careful history and physical examination fail to turn up any skin disease or findings in the anorectal area.

When a cause is found (secondary pruritus ani), 25 percent of these patients have conditions such as fissures, ulcers and skin tags, while 65 percent suffer from skin disorders such as dermatitis, psoriasis and bacterial or fungal infections. The remaining 10 percent have other disorders, such as diabetes, or have developed the condition as a result of diet.

When a local condition provokes an itch, patients scratch as a response, exchanging the "weak" pain we call itch for a more endurable "strong" pain. However, this scratching can break the skin, which leads to more irritation and, of course, more itch-scratch reactions.

More than any other factor, moisture in this area can lead to the development of a skin irritation, which leads to a chronic situation. Though opinions vary, here are a number of good tips for ending the cycle of itch-scratch-itch:

- The use of icy cold compresses can provide cooling and immediate relief. If itching is more severe at night, a pitcher of ice water can be kept by the bedside.
- Proper cleansing after a bowel movement can be accomplished by patting (not wiping) with a moistened tissue, followed by careful blotting and drying.
- Avoid any foods that seem to bring on attacks.
- Since stress seems to worsen the condition, a good plan for stress management should be a part of the treatment program.

214. *I recently had a bowel examination during which polyps were discovered in my colon. My doctor promptly removed them. Does this mean they were cancerous?*

You and many others share this condition, since polyps of the colon are the most common type of polyp found in the digestive tract. There are two types of polyps: pedunculated, which are attached to the wall of the intestine by a thin stem or stalk, and sessile, which are attached by a broad base.

Although polyps occur as a single lesion in most patients, some individuals with an inherited syndrome may have literally hundreds of polyps growing. The most common type of colon polyps are classified as hyperplastic (excessive growth of normal tissue) or as adenomas (benign growths of glandular tissue).

While hyperplastic polyps probably remain benign, adenomas are considered to be precancerous. These classifications are the result of a microscopic study of the tissue. To take no chances of leaving any possible cancerous growths behind, all polyps are removed and then classified.

Ask your doctor for the tissue report of your polyps to find out just what they were. The probability is that they were benign, and your operation prevented a dangerous cancer from occurring. As I so frequently stress, prevention — in this case, removing all polyps — is just about the best kind of medicine there can be.

215. ***I used to think the subject of hemorrhoids was mildly humorous — until I developed them. Now I dread the possibility that I may need surgery to rid myself of the problem. Do you think this may be needed?***

Hemorrhoids are really just dilated veins. They can be internal, external or both. If you have small external skin tags that are painless, ignore them. If they're swollen, bed rest and sitz baths may help. Ice packs at the onset of swelling may provide relief, but heat is better when swelling is severe. If external hemorrhoids are recurrent and interfere with daily life, then surgical excision may be your only hope.

Internal hemorrhoids occur in four degrees, which range from painless, unobtrusive ones to those that protrude from the anus. No treatment is necessary for mild cases unless there is pain or swelling, in which case the hot baths and bed rest may be all that is required to remedy the situation. Occasionally, injection therapy, which uses liquids that cause the veins to close by scarring, may be prescribed.

For the more severe types, excision of the hemorrhoid or tying it off with an elastic band (elastic band ligation) can provide the solution. A combination of internal and external hemorrhoids may require removal, depending upon the symptoms. For all kinds of hemorrhoids, a diet that contains more bulk plus the addition of stool softeners will reduce straining and make the condition a bit easier to bear.

8.
The Special Concerns of Women

There is a woman at the beginning of all great things.

ALPHONSE DE LAMARTIN
French poet (1790–1869)

The design and structure of the special female organs provide the exact accommodations for three most essential functions: conception, pregnancy and childbirth. These are extremely complex functions that far exceed the responsibilities of the male reproductive system, which focuses all its actions on the simple production of a single type of cell — the sperm cell. However, the female reproductive system must not only produce the primary cell contributed by the female to reproduction, called the egg (or *ovum*), but also provide for the protection and nurturing of the fertilized ovum over a nine-month period as it develops into a new life. Even then the duties are not finished, as the milk secreted by the breasts (*mammary glands*) is required for the continued nutrition of the newborn. Yet the marvelous adaptations seen in the anatomy and physiology of these organs are equal to the task.

The female reproductive system includes the *ovaries*, *Fallopian tubes*, *uterus*, *cervix* and *vagina*. These can be divided into internal organs and external organs. The internal organs are involved more closely with the reproductive functions, while the external organs relate more closely to the sexual role. In addition, the breasts, which are actually a modification of the sweat glands, play a substantial role in supporting the new life by providing the nutrition needed by the baby but, in the woman, may be the site of certain problems unique to the female sex.

The ovaries are a pair of small, egg-shaped glands located in the lower abdomen, one on each side of the body. Though the actual position of the ovaries is quite variable, they usually are found about 10 to 13 centimeters (4 to 5 inches) below the waist, putting them about midway down (or up) within the pelvic cavity. The ovaries are about the size of a shelled almond, grayish-pink in color, and measure about 3.75 centimeters (1½ inches) in length and 1.9 centimeters (¾ inch) wide in the adult woman.

In addition to producing eggs on a more or less regular schedule from puberty to menopause (when a woman is about 11 years old until she's 45 to 55), the ovaries also produce two female hormones: *estrogen* and *progesterone*. The estrogen is responsible for controlling the secondary sexual traits, such as the growth of body hair and breast development, as well as ovulation and menstruation. Progesterone acts on the endometrium to prepare the uterus for pregnancy, and contributes to breast enlargement during pregnancy and to the production of milk after the birth of the child. Together these two hormones control the menstrual cycle.

Unlike the testicles in the male, which produce the male hormone at constant levels, the ovaries' production of estrogen and progesterone fluctuates through the monthly cycle. It is their interaction, with differing levels of each, that affects the production of eggs and the growth and shedding of the lining of the uterus (*endometrium*), which results in the monthly flow (*menses* or *menstruation*) or the *period*. The hormone production of the ovaries is, in turn, regulated by hormone secretions from the *pituitary gland*, which is located at the base of the brain. Both physical and emotional stress can affect the amounts and kinds of hormones produced by this "master gland." These hormones then affect the regularity and length of the menstrual cycle.

At birth, the ovary contains all the primary eggs (*oogonia*) it will ever have — from 250,000 to as many as 1 million — but only about 500 ever will develop into mature ova during a woman's lifetime. There are a number of compartments within the ovary called *Graafian follicles*, which contain egg cells in various stages of development. These follicular cells secrete the estrogen that influences the buildup of the endometrium, which is the tissue that lines the uterus. When an egg is released and fertilized, the follicle is transformed into a *corpus luteum* (white body), which continues to secrete the hormone progesterone for about six months.

After the mature egg is released from the ovary in a process called *ovulation*, it must travel a short distance to the entrance of one of the Fallopian tubes (*uterine tubes* or *oviducts*), which serve as a transport system to move eggs from the ovary to the uterus. These tubes are about 10 centimeters (4 inches) long and about as thick as a pencil, but the central passageway is as thin as a needle. The Fallopian tube is not connected directly to the ovary, but has, instead, a wide, trumpetlike opening, which is equipped with fingerlike extensions (*fimbriae*) that help ensnare the egg and direct it into the opening of the tube. The ovum is swept along on its travels by the special cells that line the tube, which are equipped with *cilia* (hairlike projections) that push the ovum down the duct. The muscles of the Fallopian tube also aid by contracting, which creates peristaltic waves to propel the ovum. During this passage, the tube secretes various substances that provide nourishment for the egg. Fertilization takes place within the Fallopian tube when an ascending sperm meets a descending ovum. It takes about three days for the egg to travel from the ovary to the uterus, and fertilization may take place only within the first 24 hours of this journey.

The Fallopian tube connects to the uterus (womb), which is a single organ located in the middle of the body, between the bladder (which lies just in front of the uterus) and the rectum (located behind the uterus). The uterus is a pear-shaped organ about 6.25 centimeters (2½ inches) long in the nonpregnant female. It has a thick, muscular wall that is lined by a blood-rich tissue called the endometrium. These muscles provide the "push" needed to propel the baby from its prenatal home into the outside world. The muscles of the uterus are constantly contracting and relaxing slightly. This activity increases during a sexual orgasm and tends to suck the sperm into the uterus. This same muscular activity helps to expel the endometrium that is shed during menstruation.

The uterine wall has little endometrial tissue lining on Day 1 of the new menstrual cycle, following menstruation. By Day 5, the lining begins to build up in preparation for receiving a fertilized egg, should one exist. Between Day 14 and Day 20, the endometrium is at its thickest, as this is the time during which conception (fertilizing an egg) is most likely. If no fertilization occurs, the endometrium is shed during Days 24 through 28 (menstruation), and the cycle starts again.

The uterus is held in place by strong fibrous ligaments that form the floor of the pelvis and are aided, as well, by the muscles in the region. The uterus is attached to the sides, front and back of the pelvis by eight ligaments with names that describe their shape or function: the *round*, the *broad* and the *suspensory* ligaments, which are strong, cordlike structures of dense fibrous tissue.

At the bottom of the uterus is the cervix, which forms a passageway between the interior cavity of the uterus and the vagina. The cervix is normally very small and provides just enough space to permit the menstrual fluids to pass out, but far too small to permit a tampon to penetrate into the uterine cavity. Much of the time the cervix is blocked by a mucus plug secreted by glands that line the walls of the cervix. During birth, however, the cervix stretches wide and opens sufficiently to allow the baby to pass through into the birth canal, or vagina.

The vagina is normally a small organ, fashioned like an elongated S-shaped tube, and is about 10 centimeters (4 inches) long in the adult woman. In the resting state, there is little internal space, since the vagina's walls actually touch each other. However, the muscles of the vagina are able to stretch during intercourse or childbirth and then return to their previous size. In addition to muscles, the vagina contains a rich network of *capillaries* (blood vessels) that fill with blood when a woman is sexually stirred, much as a man's penis fills with blood and becomes erect during an aroused state. The additional blood in the vagina's blood vessels results in a higher blood pressure, which causes the mucous lining of the vagina to secrete a fluid that provides the lubrication for the sexual act.

The external sexual anatomy includes the *mons pubis*, *labia majora*, *labia minora*, *clitoris* and the *vestibule*, or opening to the vagina. The mons pubis is composed of a pad of fatty tissue, which lies just below the skin at the base of the abdomen. During the process of puberty, the mons pubis becomes covered by curly hair. The labia majora, or outer lips, are two folds of skin that enclose the other external structures of the genitals. The labia minora, or inner lips, are two smaller skin folds that also contain a rich network of blood vessels. Normally a pink color, they turn darker, displaying a variety of deeper colors during sexual stimulation. The clitoris, often compared to the penis in the man, is made of spongy erectile tissue that becomes firm when the woman is sexually stimulated. Normally it is covered by a fold of skin called the clitoral hood. According to sex researchers Dr. William Masters and Dr. Virginia Johnson, the clitoris is a unique organ in the human anatomy, for its major function is to provide a pleasurable sensation during sexual activity.

Just below the clitoris and above the opening to the vagina, there is another opening, or orifice. It is the entrance to the urethra, which is the small tube that connects the bladder with the outside. The urethra's location here, plus its tiny dimensions, allow bacteria to enter easily from the outside and travel through the urethra, making the bladder — and indeed the whole urinary system — vulnerable to infections.

The vestibule contains the thin, sheetlike membrane called the *hymen*, which partially blocks the entrance of the vagina and is seen in women who have not engaged in sexual activity. However, active participation in sports also can stretch or break the membrane and cause it to disappear. Special glands called *Bartholin's glands*, which contribute secretions that help to lubricate the vagina, also are located here. These secretions, along with those produced by cells within the vagina, also assist in cleaning the vagina naturally.

These external structures often are referred to collectively as the *vulva* (from the Latin word for a "wrapper" or "covering"), since they cover or shield the entrance to the internal organs.

While not a part of the reproductive system, the breasts are considered to be a secondary sexual characteristic for women. The breast consists mainly of a round mass of glandular tissue, which is actually a modified form of sweat gland separated into lobes. Each breast has 15 to 20 lobes, which end in a small duct that leads to an opening in the nipple. Around the glandular tissue is a covering of fat tissue, and it is the amount of this tissue that determines the size of the breast. The full development of the glandular system is seen only during pregnancy, at which time the glands become congested in preparation for secreting the milk that will nourish the newborn. The breast is formed around a framework of dense connective tissue. This framework runs from a layer of ligaments that lies beneath the breast into the breast itself, and provides the breast's firm consistency.

There is great variation in the size and the form of the breast. But using a well-nourished woman who has not given birth as an example, the location of the breasts on the chest can be placed between the second or third rib, down to the sixth or seventh rib, and extends from the outer edge of the *sternum* (breastbone) to the skin fold under the *axilla* (armpit).

The nipple is surrounded by a pigmented area called the *areola*, about 3.75 centimeters (1½ inches) in diameter. The areola is lubricated by sebaceous glands, which are located within the dermal layer of the skin. During pregnancy, the pigmentation increases and the areola becomes larger and darker in color. This pigmentation usually fades after the pregnancy is over.

No chapter on the special problems of women would be complete without considering the period of *menopause*. Also known as the *climacteric*, it arrives some time between the ages of 40 to 60, usually around age 50 for most women. It marks the time when the reproductive years come to an end as the ovaries stop producing the female hormone estrogen. The menstrual periods become increasingly irregular, flow is reduced, and finally all menses cease. For many women this would be more than acceptable if it weren't for all the other symptoms associated with this time of life.

Both physical and mental symptoms complicate the life of the menopausal woman. Most common are the *hot flashes*, a feeling of flushing that covers the face, neck and chest, accompanied by intense sweating. They last for a few minutes, but they can recur several times a day. Other physical symptoms include headaches, joint pains, pounding heartbeats and the drying of vaginal secretions. The mental symptoms of depression, irritability and anxiety can coincide with a decreased ability to concentrate and insomnia.

The menopausal experience is variable from one woman to the next, with some 25 percent experiencing no symptoms and another 25 percent finding the symptoms extremely difficult to bear, while about 50 percent experience some problems that are, for the most part, bearable. The condition can last from but a few months to more than five years. The good news is that treatment with estrogen (ERT for estrogen replacement therapy) offers relief for many women.

The complexities of the female reproductive system and the difference in female physiology from that of the male has been known by scientists for hundreds of years, and by just ordinary folks for tens of thousands of years before that. But it is only during the past decade that these distinctions have received attention in the research area. While formerly all new medications were tested uniquely on males, the latest studies include considerations for their use in the special needs of women. And that bodes well for the medical and health care of women in a new, enlightened era.

Questions and Answers

216. ***I've finally made the important decision to start taking birth control pills. But I'm still full of anxiety. What should I worry about as I start to take this medication?***

I'm not sure you should worry about anything, but you should know all the facts. Make an intelligent decision based on those facts, then stay in touch with your body to be sure your choice is a good one for you.

You've probably heard a lot about the dangers of birth control pills, but birth control pills are safe for most women. In fact, for some women, they're safer than a pregnancy. If you're younger than 35 years of age, don't smoke and are in generally good health, you probably can take birth control pills without problems. It's always smart, though, to see your doctor regularly and immediately report any changes you notice in your body.

If you smoke, you need to find another method of birth control, because the chances of complications (mainly blood clots) with the pill dramatically increase for women who smoke.

Generally, birth control pills are safest for young women. Women over 40, particularly those who have other risk factors, should use birth control pills with caution.

In selecting a birth control pill, your doctor will choose the one that offers the lowest possible dose of estrogen combined with the least potent dose of progestin that will be effective for you. This offers the benefits of fertility control with the fewest side effects. Recent improvements in birth control pills have lowered the effective doses of hormones that they contain. Women vary widely in what combination of hormones they can comfortably and effectively take in a pill. Breakthrough bleeding, or vaginal spotting between periods, is a sign that the dosage may not be high enough.

When you take birth control pills, it's especially important that you see your doctor regularly. Report any headaches, blurred vision or other symptoms you may have. Common side effects that are also important and should be reported are breast tenderness, weight gain, and nausea and vomiting, but those side effects usually require only a small adjustment in dosage.

Birth control pills offer you no protection against venereal disease or AIDS, so do not rely on them for this important part of your sexual health.

In years past, it often was thought that women should take breaks from the pill about once a year for a couple of months, to allow themselves to cycle naturally without interference. This is no longer thought to be important. Most physicians do not advise their patients to stop the pills, unless a problem is noticed.

Birth control pills are a most effective way to control your fertility, and they're safe if used carefully. This is no different for any other drug — an informed patient is a healthier patient. Intelligent use of birth control pills will protect you from both pregnancy and the pill's side effects.

217. ***I examine my breasts regularly and have never found anything abnormal until yesterday, when I noticed a slightly bloody discharge coming from my right breast. Is this something to worry about? I'm 34 years old.***

It's always a good idea to report changes in your breast condition, such as lumps or discharges, to your doctor. Though most changes are benign, bloody nipple discharge warrants extra-careful attention. It can be a warning sign of a breast tumor.

Among the many benign causes of a reddish nipple discharge are pregnancy, certain drugs, or benign fibrous tissues or cysts within your breast tissue that can produce bloody fluid. The most common cause is a benign breast tumor, but the chance that the tumor could be malignant ranges from 7 to 10 percent. However, this chance of malignancy increases for a woman found to have a breast lump or abnormal breast X-ray findings, for a woman over 50, or for a male with this symptom.

To help your physician diagnose the cause correctly, take careful note of your symptoms. Was the discharge grayish-green or red? Did it come from one breast or two? Has this ever happened before? What kinds of drugs or medications are you taking?

Your physician will examine you for lumps, skin dimpling or other nipple abnormalities, and may require mammography, or breast X-ray. If the cause of the problem is not discovered by these means, exploratory surgery must be considered as the next step in treatment. If a tumor is found, whether benign or malignant, then it can be removed.

Remember, most often the original source of the problem is a benign tumor, but don't take any risks — see your doctor immediately. The principle of early treatment for the best results definitely applies in this situation.

218. ***It seems that every day there is another story in the newspaper that tells of a woman being beaten by her husband or boyfriend. I am deeply touched by the misery that results from such situations, but can't help wonder why these poor women stay with these beasts. Surely, all they have to do is to get out to protect themselves. Why do they stay?***

These are complex situations dealing with human feelings and emotions, which are different in each case. I'm sure many people feel as you do, but unfortunately wife beating usually does not start at the beginning of the relationship, but rather after strong ties have developed and children have come along.

This tragedy can occur in families from all walks of life, the rich as well as the poor. And it is pure fiction that some women "ask for it," as there is nothing specific in the actions of these women that seems to provoke the violence, and nothing they can do to prevent it.

In many cases, the attacks begin during a first pregnancy, when the man feels threatened by the new life that now occupies the feelings and attention of the woman, attention that up until then was his exclusively. Although his remorse may be acute after the battering, with promises and actions of love and consideration, the beatings occur again, with a cycle of increasing tension, a beating, and a period of remorse and repentance by the abuser. The woman is trapped in this pattern, as she hopes that the situation will change for the better and remain that way.

Once the protective environment of the home is broken, battered women doubt that anyplace is safe. In many cases, the woman has no financial resources necessary to make that break, particularly when there is no supportive family to turn to, and when there are children who must be clothed and fed. With the man's threats still ringing in her ears, she fears retaliation if she shows any signs of leaving.

Education can be an effective source of help. Once these victims learn that domestic violence is against the law, and are helped to identify the resources available in society to help them, they can escape from their living hell.

219. *I have been required to return to my physician on several occasions, because my Pap smear is a "two." He keeps treating me and then takes another smear. I'm afraid I have cancer, because I don't understand what's going on. Can you help?*

You most probably do not have cancer. Since 1941, when Dr. George Papanicolaou published his paper describing the value of cervical smears to detect cancer of the uterus, the technique has been used routinely to discover early abnormal changes of the cells of the cervix (the entrance to the uterus).

The cells are scraped from the cervix by the physician, placed on a glass slide and then stained. When these cells are examined under a microscope, the subtle changes from normal can be detected and graded against a classification of results that allows an interpretation to be made.

There are five such classifications, from I to V (we use Roman numerals, as Dr. Papanicolaou did):

- Class I means there are no suspicious cells that reveal any changes. This is interpreted as negative for cancer.
- Class II (as in your case) means there are some changes in the cells

that could be caused by an inflammation, but are not considered to be changes that are due to or lead to cancer. When the inflammation is treated and has cleared up, usually the cells return to normal.

- Class III is made up of cells that show mild or moderate changes that are suspicious of cancer, but for which a diagnosis cannot be made with certainty.
- Class IV is used to indicate that a cancer has started in the cervix.
- Class V tells of malignancy and invasive carcinoma, which has attacked the uterus.

There are varying recommendations as to the frequency that the test should be taken. It is a test that must be performed correctly to obtain results that are accurate. The best time to obtain cells for examination is at Day 14 of the menstrual cycle, when the hormone effect of estrogen is at its maximum.

Any patient with a classification of Class III or higher should have a biopsy of the cervix performed, since this is a more reliable test and affords a more dependable diagnostic interpretation. When inflammatory changes are noted, the Pap report may signal the presence of an infecting bacteria, which can help the physician determine the treatment.

Most physicians agree that a Class II smear should be repeated three months after treatment. It looks like your doctor is following this appropriate course.

220. *Although my menstrual period comes regularly enough, I think it's much heavier than what many of my friends experience. Does this indicate anything is wrong? What should I do about it?*

If you're concerned about bleeding too heavily, discuss it with your physician. The only way to know whether there is something wrong is to evaluate the situation thoroughly. You will need to keep a careful record of the pattern and amount of bleeding. Take special note of the times you bleed and any activity that seems to have triggered it. This information will help your physician determine the cause of the bleeding, as well as whether it is excessive.

Many different conditions can cause excess bleeding, and each one has a different treatment. Your physician will want to be sure you don't have a platelet (small cells found in the blood) disorder. Platelets are important to the body's clotting mechanism, so anything that interferes with their action will cause increased bleeding. Do you take aspirin for menstrual cramps? Some people are particularly susceptible to aspirin's anti-platelet action.

In evaluating your heavy bleeding, your doctor will examine your uterus to be sure it is free of tumors, both malignant and benign. If all other problems are ruled out and you simply have heavy bleeding during your menstrual period, your doctor may treat you with a medication that works as a prostaglandin antagonist. This medication will work against the prostaglandins your own body produces, and thus help to slow blood flow.

A D & C (dilatation and curettage) provides no decrease of blood flow except in the cycle directly following the procedure, so it offers no long-term benefit. Methylergonovine, which is effective in slowing blood flow in women who have just had babies, has no effect on the amount of blood lost during the menstrual period.

Any occasion when there is an exceptionally heavy flow and a possibility that you might be pregnant is another time when a trip to your physician is truly in order.

221. *I know there are many good commercial douche preparations on the market, but my mother insists that her home remedy for the situation is still better than the rest. She also insists that it is a must for every woman. Is douching twice a week with a vinegar and water solution bad for you?*

There really is no need to douche that regularly, but at the same time, there is no evidence that it is bad. A mild vinegar douche using white vinegar and lukewarm water will make the vagina more acidic, which can affect the microbial and pH balance (amount of acidity or alkalinity).

Douching will not prevent vaginal infections, and it could increase your risk for them by washing out good microorganisms that normally are found in the vagina and throwing off your normal vaginal pH. The pH of the vagina varies with the menstrual cycle and age, but it's usually neutral to moderately acidic.

A healthy vagina is a self-cleaning organ. If you're douching because you think it is necessary for hygiene, you're wrong. Normal discharges from the vagina do not have an odor until they come into contact with bacteria on the skin. Normal washing of the perineum should prevent odors. A vaginal discharge with an odor is a symptom of an infection and should be checked out by a physician.

222. ***My grandmother died of breast cancer, my mother has had it, and I'm afraid I'll get it, too. I have a condition called fibrocystic breast disease, which I'm told is very common. It scares the living daylights out of me to have this lumpiness in my breasts. What can I do to prevent this from happening?***

Besides cutting down on the amount of fat in your diet, there is little that can be done to prevent breast cancer from developing. With careful monitoring of the breasts, however, you can avoid tragic consequences of breast cancer by catching it in its earliest stages.

The presence of fibrocystic breast disease does not mean you will definitely get cancer. In fact, the majority of women with this condition are not at a significantly increased risk for cancer. About half of all women have some signs of fibrocystic breast disease, which is characterized by breast pain, lumps or cysts. These lumps and cysts are generally benign.

However, you should take more caution than most because of the history of the disease in your family. Major risk factors of breast cancer include being over the age of 50, never having children, early age at start of menstruation, late menopause, atypical cells in a breast biopsy, previous history of breast cancer, or having a mother, sister or daughter with the disease.

Your best weapon in fighting breast cancer is early detection. This means you should find a good doctor you can feel comfortable with over the years. By seeing the same doctor, you enable him or her to note changes that might be suspicious over a period of time.

The initial examination for a breast complaint should begin with a careful history. This includes giving the physician information about the presence of any mass, pain or nipple discharge, and any changes associated with menstruation, pregnancy, local injuries or medication that could have hormonal effects.

If you've had previous mammograms with another doctor, you should see to it that the new doctor receives copies of the reports. A base-line mammogram should be given to every woman between ages 35 and 40. It should be repeated every two years until age 50, and yearly after that.

Your doctor must do an extensive physical examination. In many cases, the benign breast lumps need no treatment. In some cases, aspiration of the lump is necessary. This involves the doctor inserting a needle while applying suction. Any bloody fluid that is removed should be examined. Anything suspicious requires biopsy. Some researchers have found that you can lessen the symptoms of fibrocystic breast disease by eliminating caffeine from your diet (although there is some controversy about this). Nowadays, however, this isn't very difficult because there are many decaffeinated products on the market, including decaf coffees, teas and cola beverages.

As I have insisted so many times, the answer to questions on breast diseases, particularly breast cancer, lies in the philosophy of early detection and rapid treatment as the best defense.

223. *Is it possible to treat vaginal and urinary tract infections with just one dose of medicine?*

Many vaginal and urinary tract infections can be treated with one dose of medication, but not all. This is an important development, because these infections are among the most common conditions seen by physicians. And one-dose treatments greatly reduce medical costs and the risk of side effects.

Single-dose treatments can be used in four types of genitourinary infections: candidal vulvovaginitis (yeast vaginitis), trichomonal vaginitis, bacterial vaginosis and cystitis. In candidal vulvovaginitis, 89 percent of women who were treated with one vaginally administered dose of clotrimazole were cured. Similar cure rates were found with other medications for bacterial vaginosis, trichomonal vaginitis and the bladder infection cystitis.

The drawback to a single-dose treatment is that it may not clear up every case. Still, for uncomplicated cases of genitourinary infections, single-dose treatments should be considered, particularly when the infecting organism has been identified and the selected medication has a record of being effective against the diagnosed infection.

224. *Can you please provide some easy-to-understand explanations about the causes of endometriosis? I would like to learn more about this very strange disease.*

Although several controversial theories exist, it would appear that endometriosis is the result of occasional "retrograde," or reverse, menstrual flow, combined with an immune system problem.

This reverse flow occurs in many women occasionally. When it does, the menstrual fluid escapes upward through the Fallopian tubes into the abdominal cavity. From the abdominal cavity, the fluid can travel to other parts of the body. The endometrial tissue, which normally lines the uterus, has now located in an abnormal place within the body and follows the same pattern of monthly growth that it would in the uterus. But because this tissue has no escape as does the tissue in the uterus, it can cause problems by accumulating. An immune system defect, which would prevent the body from correcting the problem, can make the situation even more severe.

Endometriosis is more common in higher socioeconomic groups. An estimated four per 1,000 women ages 15 to 64 are hospitalized with the problem each year in the United States. Women with first-degree relatives who have had endometriosis have a seven-times greater chance of having the problem themselves. Patients who start menstruating at an early age are at higher risk as well.

Infertility, pelvic pain, low back pain, or menstrual irregularity or discomfort may be signs of endometriosis. The only way to make a positive diagnosis is to examine the abdominal cavity and obtain small samples of the suspicious tissue (biopsy). This is accomplished through a laparoscope, which is a thin telescopelike instrument that is inserted through a tiny incision around the navel.

Once diagnosed, endometriosis may be difficult to treat, but there are effective medical and surgical methods that can be used help correct the problem.

225. *I've noticed a peculiar and persistent itch in my right nipple. I don't recall when it started, but it hasn't just gone away with time. What could cause an itchy nipple? I'm beginning to become concerned.*

When a woman has a persistently itchy nipple, it could be nothing serious, but it also might be a symptom of the breast cancer called Paget's disease. This type of cancer shows itself as a skin rash on the breast, but the rash really represents a cancer in the tissue that lies beneath.

Even if there is no visible change, if you have this problem, you should have your doctor check it. A physical examination and mammography (breast X-ray) can reveal any lumps or other causes for concern. If you're pregnant, your doctor may choose to perform an ultrasound examination instead of mammography. In addition, a small biopsy that is performed under local anesthesia can be done safely, even if you're pregnant.

These tests will determine whether the cause of your itchy nipple is benign, or provide the early detection that is so important for effective treatment of a more serious condition.

226. ***Though I had my uterus removed many years ago, my doctor still insists that I have a Pap test from time to time. I ask him why I need this test now, but he just smiles and tells me to take his advice. Do you think there is any need for this in a woman in my present condition?***

I wish you had provided me with more information about your "present condition" and had told me the reason for your hysterectomy (removal of the uterus). This information is essential in judging the value of a Pap test for women who have had this operation.

It may well be that though your uterus was removed, the tip of this organ, called the cervix, was left in place. This is called a subtotal hysterectomy and was practiced widely in the United States before 1960. There are still many women alive who had this surgery. In such situations, continuing the practice of regular Pap screening tests is considered essential, as cancer may develop in the tissues of the remaining cervix.

While there are no absolute rules concerning the continuing of Pap tests after hysterectomy, some useful guidelines do exist. Continued Pap smears are not considered essential 1) if the hysterectomy was performed for a benign condition (non-cancerous), 2) if all of the cervical tissue was removed, and 3) if there is documentation that the Pap smears of the cervix taken prior to surgery were all normal.

Obviously your doctor must have all that information available to him or her, if such a decision is to be made. Without all that documentation, most physicians would feel that prudence demanded that the Pap test be continued. It certainly is the best way to be sure. Anything doctors can do to diagnose cancer in the earliest stages, when treatment is most effective, is to be recommended.

227. ***My girlfriend is a real fanatic about bathrooms. I have known her to hold herself in for hours to avoid using a public restroom, even in the finest restaurants. She claims that they are a breeding ground for all sorts of sexual infections and refuses to use them. Now she has***

me wondering. Is this true, and what precautions can be taken to prevent such infections?

I remember the first time a patient told me that his sexual infection was acquired from a toilet seat, and that he was just an innocent victim. It wasn't true then, and it isn't true today.

The bacteria and viruses that are responsible for sexually transmitted diseases (STD) need hospitable environments in which to grow. That includes moisture, warmth and a good supply of nutrients, among other ingredients — certainly not the surroundings to be found on a toilet seat. Most toilet seats today are made of plastic and do not provide an arena in which bacteria can grow. In fact, the bacteria soon die on the dry plastic surface.

In addition, most bacteria or viruses that are strong and virulent enough to provoke an infection in the body require large numbers of organisms to establish a foothold. The body's own defenses are usually enough to control just the few cells that might survive a period of time on a toilet seat.

Using paper seat covers, which sometimes are provided, or scrubbing down the seat with hot soapy water may help. It certainly would give the user more peace of mind, but the truth is that the STDs — syphilis, gonorrhea and others — require direct sexual contact for transmission. That old "toilet seat story" is but a feeble alibi for other actions. Personal cleanliness is a fine attribute, but neither you nor your girlfriend (nor anyone else) has much to fear from a toilet seat.

228. ***Are vaginitis and yeast infection the same condition? How is it treated? I'm puzzled and am sure that many of your readers may have the same questions.***

Many women are confused about this situation, so the answer to your questions can help a lot of women. Actually, yeast infection is only one type of vaginitis, which is defined as any inflammation of the mucosal tissue that lines the vagina.

The causes of the problem are many and can include infections, changes in hormone balance, mechanical irritation and even allergic reactions. There are three major types of infection: bacterial, yeast (it goes by the name of candidiasis in medical circles), and trichomoniasis.

About 20 to 40 percent of all vaginal infections can be attributed to a yeast infection. The most common complaint is one of itching in the vaginal area. Other problems may include redness and tenderness of external tissue, and pain during urination and intercourse. The discharge is usually thick, white and cheesy in nature. Symptoms like these usually demand attention from a physician, who can determine the cause.

Once the cause is clear, a choice of medication can be made. When a fungus is the cause, for example, the prescription of an anti-fungal agent, such as terconazole, in either cream or suppository form, can cure the infection rapidly and alleviate the symptoms. Then it will be up to you and your physician to try to determine the source of your infection, so that you can take all the steps necessary not to repeat past mistakes and avoid the reccurrence of this most uncomfortable situation.

229. *My gynecologist says she feels a biopsy of my cervix is necessary, but has told me that she can perform this in her office. Do you agree that this is OK? Doesn't this need to be done at a hospital?*

A cervical biopsy, which is done to check the opening of the uterus for cancer and other conditions, can be done easily in your doctor's office. In some cases, treatment also can be done in the office, and you can go home immediately afterward.

If your situation is proceeding as most do, your doctor already has done a Pap test, which is a quick screening for abnormal cells in the cervical tissue, and the results came back positive for abnormal cells. She now wants to take a biopsy of your cervix, in order to get a better idea of what is going on. The tissue sample, which is smaller than a nail clipping, will be evaluated by your doctor and a pathologist.

For the biopsy, you'll be in the usual exam position, with your feet in the stirrups. Your doctor will wipe away the cervical mucus, and she may use a special viewing device, called a colposcope, to take a close look at the vagina and cervix. The biopsy will be taken from any spots on the cervix that look abnormal. If you notice any bleeding after you go home, call your doctor.

If the biopsy shows there is no cancer and the area of abnormal cells is small, your doctor may use cryotherapy (or freezing technique) to treat you in the office. You're in the same position as for the biopsy. Your doctor uses a device to freeze and kill the abnormal spots. Two days later, on a return visit, the site will be cleaned. A thin watery discharge may last for about two weeks after the procedure, but then it usually disappears by itself.

230. ***I know it's not normal, and I don't know where to turn for help. I experience a great deal of discomfort and pain during sexual relations. I'm a young woman and realize that this shouldn't be happening. Why is it? Help!***

You may be embarrassed to talk to your doctor about this condition, but keeping quiet about it and hoping it will go away is not going to work. Pain during intercourse, or dyspareunia, is uncomfortable to talk about, but worse to suffer through in silence.

There are several possible physical and psychological causes, and both types may have a hand in causing the pain. Describe the pain or discomfort to your physician. Tell him or her how long you've had the pain, what it feels like, and when and where it occurs. Also note whether the discomfort is only at the opening of the vagina or deeper within.

In older women, pain during intercourse may be due to the drying of the vagina that occurs after menopause. However, some younger women have a chronic lack of lubrication even when they're sexually aroused. This can be treated easily by using a lubricant. Vaginitis also can cause pain during intercourse, since the walls of the vagina may be inflamed and irritated. Pelvic inflammatory disease, endometriosis and tipped uterus all can cause discomfort during deep penetration.

Pain during intercourse also may be caused by a severe involuntary muscle spasm known as vaginismus. This spasm may be caused by a psychological fear of sex, perhaps due to sexual trauma or because a physical problem has made sex painful. Behavioral and psychological therapy can help with this problem.

Without doubt, pain during sexual relations is not something that a young woman must or should try to live with. Please don't take this brief information as the last word, but gather up your resolve and courage, make a few notes on paper to help, and see your gynecologist now.

231. ***My girlfriend swears it's true and that she uses it, but before trying it myself, I want to check with you. Is it true that Coca-Cola can be used as a contraceptive? Are there any dangers to using it?***

The only time Coca-Cola is effective as a contraceptive is when you drink it instead of having sex. All kidding aside, this is an old story that refuses to die. Some women have used Coca-Cola as a douche after intercourse in hopes that it will kill sperm.

In a laboratory (not a woman's body), some formulations of Coca-Cola do kill sperm. But in a woman's body, sperm make their way to the oviducts, where they can fertilize an egg, almost immediately after intercourse. Many physicians feel that any douche used after intercourse only pushes sperm farther through the reproductive tract, thus enhancing their chances of fertilizing an egg and causing pregnancy.

The side effects of the Coca-Cola douche are unknown, but there are some reports of increased infections in women who use it. If the Coca-Cola is shaken and allowed to spew forcefully into the vagina and possibly the uterus, additional, potentially serious, side effects can result.

If you're in need of an inexpensive, safe and effective contraceptive, talk with your physician or your pharmacist. There is a wide variety of products on the market, any of which is a wiser choice than the Coca-Cola douche. Show this answer to your friend. You will be doing her a favor.

232. ***I would be very grateful if you could address the problem of endometrial cancer. Could you please explain the causes of this disease? How is it diagnosed? Any other additional information would be most appreciated.***

Cancer of the endometrium (which translates from Greek as "inner mucous membranes of the uterus") is the most common cancer occurring in the female reproductive tract. It ranks third in cancers that affect women, after breast and colorectal cancers.

Women most likely to develop endometrial cancer are those who have not had children, are obese, have diabetes and/or high blood pressure, and reach menopause past the age of 52 (delayed menopause). A family history of breast or ovarian cancers may be another risk factor. Women with all of the above have very high risks of such cancers.

About 28,000 new cases are diagnosed each year. Endometrial cancer usually is seen in postmenopausal women, and the peak incidence of this disease is between the ages of 50 and 60. It is possible that as many as one-third of all cases of postmenopausal bleeding may be due to endometrial carcinoma.

Women who have taken progesterone therapy (including oral contraceptives) for long periods and those who menstruate somewhat infrequently seem to have fewer endometrial cancers than others in their age group.

Because endometrial (as well as cervical) cancers are the most common cancers associated with abnormal bleeding, endometrial biopsies and Pap tests are extremely important in establishing the correct diagnosis.

A large number of postmenopausal women who bleed abnormally develop malignancies of the reproductive tract (which involves Fallopian tubes, uterus, cervix, vagina and/or vulva). Therefore, physicians are alert to these possibilities and will use both Pap smears and biopsies of all suspected areas (as well as other diagnostic tools) to seek out these cancers.

Women who suffer endometrial cancer often develop breast and colon cancers. That provides us with another important reason to recommend regular checkups: to detect these conditions early when treatment may be most effective.

233. ***Though most of my girlfriends confide that their monthly periods are like clockwork, mine are never on time, never seem the same, and seem all wrong. I'm becoming very anxious and wonder if there is anything you can tell me about my condition. What can be done to help me?***

It's hard to tell from your question exactly what the problem is. It sounds as if you're complaining of irregularly spaced menstrual periods. If that's the case, you and your doctor probably will want to evaluate whether you're ovulating properly, since normal menstrual bleeding follows ovulation by two weeks if fertilization does not occur.

There are a variety of ways to determine whether you're ovulating. Many women identify a change in the cervical mucus when ovulation occurs. Some women spot slightly and feel a pain in the lower abdomen when the ovary releases its monthly egg. This has been given the descriptive name of *mittleschmertz*, which is German for "middle pain."

Basal body temperature rises by about a half-degree Fahrenheit at ovulation. It remains elevated until menstrual bleeding begins. Taking your temperature each morning with a basal body temperature thermometer (carefully following the directions) will help to tell you whether you're ovulating.

There are also several self-test kits on the market that can tell you whether you're ovulating. Be sure to use the tests properly for the best results. If your doctor feels your problem warrants more investigation, he may perform blood tests to check your hormone levels. Hormonal therapy can be ordered to solve the problem, but hormones should be prescribed carefully.

If you're not ovulating, what could the problem be? Stress, which is the culprit for so many other ills, can shut down ovulation. Emotional stress and physical stress, such as that induced by extreme exercise or illness, can change your hormonal levels enough so that ovulation is stopped until the problem is resolved. Women with anorexia nervosa often stop ovulating.

Obese women often stop ovulating until they lose weight. Body fat can produce estrogen, and the excess upsets the body's hormonal balance. The result is no ovulation, irregular periods and an increased risk for cancer of the lining of the uterus.

Women with abnormal thyroid function, especially those with a low thyroid production, often do not ovulate. Treatment with thyroid medication usually solves this problem.

Some women who do not ovulate have polycystic ovaries. Polycystic ovaries are enlarged and contain many partially mature but unreleased eggs. Drug therapy usually can correct this problem.

Tumors of the ovary or adrenal glands may cause ovulation problems, but they're rare. If no other problems are found, this possibility should be checked.

Not ovulating or irregular ovulation obviously causes fertility problems. Ovulation problems that are causing infertility sometimes can be treated successfully with hormonal therapy.

As you can see from my answer, irregular periods can be more than just a nuisance. If you're experiencing irregular menstruation, you should be evaluated thoroughly and completely, because menstrual problems may be a signal that something else is wrong.

234. ***I'm a 26-year-old, shy, married woman. I think I have a minor female problem for which my doctor has advised a complete pelvic exam. I'm too embarrassed to ask anyone else, so could you please tell what the doctor will be doing during the exam? What instruments will he use, if any, and will it be painful?***

I'm happy to outline the procedure for you. To start with, you most certainly will have the comfort and reassuring presence of a female nurse during the examination, for few physicians conduct this examination without such assistance. While your position on the examining table may not be the most comfortable, it's certainly not painful. It allows the examination to be conducted rapidly and yet to provide the information about your condition that your doctor is seeking.

First there is an external examination, which is mostly visual. The physician performs the internal examination using a lubricant on the gloved examining hand. With one hand on your abdomen and the fingers of the other in the vagina, the physician can determine the status of your uterus and the presence of abnormal masses. Then the doctor inserts a speculum, which holds the walls of the vagina open, permitting the physician to examine the cervix and obtain cells for the all-important Pap test.

While at times the procedure may be uncomfortable, it's never painful. With a little distracting conversation, the exam is over in no time. This is truly an important examination, and you're well-advised to proceed with it.

235. *As compared to some of the women who work with me, it seems that I get sexually aroused more easily than they do. Does this mean that there is something wrong with me?*

Not necessarily. First, it's really up to you to decide whether you have a problem. You say you're easily aroused. If you have a cooperative partner (that is, someone to have sex with), then it is not a problem. If your arousal interferes with daily life, distresses you or if you have no outlet, you have a problem.

Bear in mind that sexual appetites differ from person to person. Also remember that "nice" women do get sexually aroused. A fallacy held over from the Victorians said that "ladies" don't enjoy sex. That has changed as society has changed and new ideas about life become the order of the day.

If your easy arousal (or hyperlibido) is causing a problem, there may be a physical (as opposed to psychological) reason. A genitourinary infection can cause irritation that may be mistaken for arousal. In men, priapism (a persistent erection that has no sexual cause) often is mistaken for arousal. Neurologic problems, such as encephalitis or a head injury, also can cause hyperlibido. Curiously, a side effect of untreated syphilis can be nerve damage in the brain leading to hyperlibido.

Certain endocrine diseases, such as hyperthyroidism, can cause hyperlibido by elevating blood levels of the thyroid hormones and testosterone. Treatment for hyperlibido depends on the cause.

If there are no physical causes and you're worried about your own sexuality, a concerned and skilled counselor or physician may provide the answers you seek.

236. *What is a "hysteroscopy"? I have heard of this in reference to the examination of the female organs and would like to have more information upon which to base a decision.*

A hysteroscopy is a relatively new and successful method of examining the uterine cavity. The procedure involves the use of fiber optics for a reliable, strong light source, carbon dioxide gas to distend the uterine cavity for complete internal visibility, and an endoscope (a telescopelike instrument) with a 5-millimeter (less than ⅕-inch) diameter that allows the physician a wide-angle view of the entire cavity.

Hysteroscopy is valuable for both the diagnosis and management of many gynecologic disorders. It's commonly used to search for causes of abnormal uterine bleeding, but it also can confirm conditions such as polyps, myomas and endometrial cancer. Because of its diverse application, the hysteroscopy also can be used to obtain a biopsy of a suspicious lesion or to remove intrauterine tumors.

As a diagnostic tool, the hysteroscope is useful for many reasons. It can be used in the physician's office with minimal inconvenience and discomfort for the patient. The procedure, which frequently takes less than five minutes, has few risks and a low complication rate. In addition, no special preparations or medications are required for the examination. However, when the hysteroscope is used for an operation, it's usually performed in an ambulatory surgical center, and some anesthesia is required.

Despite its high success rate and low risk factor, hysteroscopy is not easy. It utilizes techniques that require training and experience. The endometrium is injured easily, and there's always the possibility of introducing infection into the uterine cavity, especially when using a gaseous medium such as carbon dioxide.

It's therefore necessary for a physician to master the techniques of hysteroscopy before attempting it. However, with today's knowledge, training can be acquired readily and accurately. Learning how to regulate the gas pressure properly and to manipulate the instrument carefully can be accomplished easily with practice. With these problems solved, hysteroscopy promises to be a major means for gynecological diagnosis and therapy.

237. *I need to know the difference between a "myomectomy" and a "hysterectomy." It's probably only a difference in terminology and they're really the same thing, but my medical dictionary didn't make it clear enough. Please help.*

No, they're not the same thing at all, even though both are surgical operations, both deal with the same organ (the uterus), and both terms frequently occur in the same discussion. A hysterectomy refers to the surgical removal of the uterus (*hystera* in Greek means uterus).

Frequently, the uterus forms benign tumors of muscle and fibrous tissue. This is a condition commonly referred to as fibroids or a fibroid uterus. These tumors are called myomas, since *mys* in Greek means muscle. A myomectomy refers to the surgical removal of these tumors.

When a patient suffers from this condition, the surgeon has two choices. If the tumors are small but create problems such as cramps and bleeding, only the tumors need be removed — hence myomectomy. But when the tumors are large, continue to grow and cause suffering and pain, particularly when the patient no longer wishes to bear children, a hysterectomy may be performed to solve the problem. A well-informed patient will have a choice in the decision, provided these terms are not "Greek" to her.

238. *My problem has been irregular menstrual bleeding. Now it seems I'm to have a D & C. I suppose I should know what this means, but I don't. Would you please tell me what I should know?*

A D & C (dilatation and curettage) is a relatively simple diagnostic and therapeutic procedure. The neck (cervix) of the womb (uterus) is expanded with a tool called a dilator, and the lining of the womb is scraped off with a spoon-shaped instrument called a curette. The lining then is studied in the lab to rule out any abnormal pathology, such as a benign or cancerous tumor.

Although a D & C is used less frequently than it once was (to spare the patient the risks and costs of surgery), a physician still will recommend it for a few specific clinical situations. For instance, a D & C is used to clean out the uterus and/or reduce the amount of bleeding after a miscarriage. A D & C is also the best way to obtain an accurate diagnosis if a potential problem is detected by biopsy in the office, if the patient is experiencing abnormal uterine bleeding, or if the office work-up does not yield enough tissue for evaluation.

239. ***I encounter a burning pain, which is severe at times, in the right lower abdomen for one to three days. It occurs halfway between my menstrual periods each and every month. Three different doctors have found nothing wrong, and all said the pain is from monthly ovulation and is normal. I find this hard to believe. I certainly would appreciate any comment you can offer on this condition. I'm 40 years old.***

With very few exceptions, you offer a classic history of a patient who suffers with a condition known as *mittelschmerz*. This German word describes a "middle pain," or pain that arrives each month at the time of ovulation.

In almost all women, ovulation occurs 14 days before the onset of the next period, and for women with a 28-day cycle, ovulation occurs at exactly the midpoint of their menstrual month. During ovulation, when the mature egg separates from the ovary to begin its journey through the Fallopian tube to the uterus, the ovary may bleed at the point of egg separation.

Though an insignificant amount of blood escapes, it can fall on sensitive tissues nearby, where an inflammatory reaction produces the pain. It is normal, in your case, and may be controlled by using an anti-inflammatory analgesic, such as ibuprofen.

240. ***I'm disturbed by the information that I've read about chlamydia. Because of its sensitive nature, I'm unable to get the information I need about the symptoms of this infection and its treatment. You could be doing a lot of people a real favor if you would please discuss this.***

Chlamydia is a sexually transmitted disease (STD) that affects men and women. It's the leading cause of pelvic inflammatory disease in women, and the major cause of non-gonococcal urethritis in men. This infection can lead to ectopic pregnancies and sterility. Three million to 4 million Americans have chlamydia.

Part of the problem with chlamydia is that, unlike with most STDs, a sufferer usually doesn't show any symptoms. Eighty percent of women with chlamydia are asymptomatic, while up to 20 percent of men have no symptoms. When a symptom does appear, it's usually a discharge from the penis or pain during urination in men. In women, the only clue may be a vaginal discharge. The only sure way for a physician to diagnose chlamydia is to test for it.

A complicating factor with chlamydia is that it is often not alone. Many cases of chlamydia are accompanied by other STDs, notably gonorrhea, genital warts or other types of vaginitis. An important factor in diagnosing chlamydia is sexual history. A new sexual partner within the past two months increases the risk of chlamydial infection being present.

Barrier contraceptives, such as a condom or diaphragm, give some protection against chlamydial infection, but this protection depends on consistent use. The usual treatment for chlamydia is the antibiotics tetracycline or doxycycline. Women who are pregnant may be given erythromycin as the medication of choice. The sexual partner also should be treated at the same time, otherwise reinfection will occur.

241. ***It's not something I feel I can discuss with my doctor, but a recent hysterectomy has brought about some unwanted and unexpected changes in my sexual desire. All my previous feelings have changed, and I'm afraid I have become a wife with a perpetual "headache." Is this a normal result of my surgery, or can I be helped?***

It is neither a "normal result," nor one you have to accept. Help is only a conversation away, if you just consult with your physician. It's not that this situation is unusual, for surgery of this type has both a physical as well as an emotional impact upon your life, but there are no lasting effects that must discourage you from your normal fulfillment.

To be sure, intercourse may be painful if the wound has not healed completely, and it should await your follow-up visit with your surgeon. Even if you had your ovaries removed, hormone replacement can restore normal vaginal secretions.

You need reassurance and knowledge that this operation is not the end of your sexual life. Many deeply entrenched myths surround this surgery, including the one that normal relations are no longer possible. Even husbands may feel strange if not afforded the opportunity to express fears and doubts. You both need an opportunity to open up and discuss your feelings. You and your husband are entitled to request a counseling session with your doctor, who can provide you with answers to relieve your anxiety and to end your "headaches."

242. ***I've kept away from coffee and tea for years, as well as other caffeine-containing beverages, because I was told that it could make the lumps in my breast more tender. During a recent checkup with my family doctor, he told me not to worry about this, as the story isn't true. Is this something new, or have I been laboring under a misconception for all these many years?***

I would consider this information to be under the category "relatively new." The story about caffeine and tender breast lumps (fibrocystic breasts) has been around for quite some time. It was considered good advice until recently.

The basis for this "no caffeine" counsel was a research paper published more than 15 years ago. It reported that a small group of women did indeed experience increased breast pain that was associated with caffeine. However, when other researchers tried to reproduce these results in other investigations over the years, they were unable to arrive at the same conclusion.

With little evidence to support the theory, your doctor is on the right track. However, it's easy enough to find out if the theory is true in your case. Drink a few cups of coffee as an experiment. If your breasts become tender, don't drink any more coffee.

243. ***After I gave my boyfriend all there was of my love, he left without an explanation or even a good-bye. I'm left feeling empty and worthless. I know I can get lots of advice, but they're just words. Surely a doctor must have some medicine, some pill to help me through this terrible time? Won't you please help me?***

If I tell you that you're not alone, it's to make you realize that everyone reading your letter can remember a similar experience in their lives. We all have suffered the almost unbearable pain of losing the affections of a loved one in the manner you describe. Yet, look around — we are all still here.

The wounds have healed and become less painful, more bearable. You seek medication from me as if it could be a magic cure, and that is just not possible. I dread when my patients become dependent upon chemicals to blunt the normal emotions and feelings that are a part of daily living. It seems so easy to "pop a pill" and feel better, but the trap is there. Soon we use the same way out when an expected job promotion does not materialize, or when the term paper we labored on so long comes back with a "C" instead of the "A" we felt we deserved.

Living these days takes a bit of courage and the firm belief that things do change and we can make them better if we work at it. I don't know how Ann Landers might handle your question, but I suspect she might share my feelings. You're far from worthless. If you were here, I'd give you a big hug and hope that it might rekindle your own self-esteem. But the only medication I have to prescribe in your case is "time." It has cured more cases like yours than all the pills on the pharmacy shelf.

244. ***I have trouble with menses. I finally found a physician with an answer, but it made no sense to me. The physician labeled my problem as "DUB." What does this mean, and where does it come from?***

DUB stands for dysfunctional uterine bleeding, which means bleeding from the vagina that is excessive or that is unrelated to your normal menstrual cycle. Most women with DUB are either teenagers who have just started to menstruate or older women who are undergoing menopause.

Normal menstruation takes place every 21 to 35 days. Most women lose 20 to 60 milliliters ($\frac{3}{5}$ to $1\frac{4}{5}$ ounces) of blood over the entire period. Anything more than an 80-milliliter ($2\frac{2}{5}$ ounces) loss during a period is considered excessive. But estimating your own flow is not easy. If you're suddenly soaking through pads or tampons at a faster rate (six pads a day when you usually use three, for example), you should suspect excessive bleeding.

The bleeding you experience is not related to menstruation, but at the same time, there is no other diagnosable problem. So, in a way, DUB is a diagnosis left after all the others have been eliminated. Other causes of abnormal vaginal bleeding include pregnancy, pelvic diseases, blood coagulation problems, thyroid problems, uterine cancer and benign uterine tumors.

To diagnose DUB, your physician will need a history of your menstrual cycle: at what age you started having periods; what your normal cycle length is; whether you've ever been pregnant; and what other signs of a menstrual cycle (such as breast swelling or premenstrual tension) you feel. He or she will give you a pelvic examination, a pregnancy test and a Papanicolaou test (Pap smear) to check for certain types of cancer. You may be asked to take your basal body temperature every morning for a month to see whether you're ovulating.

In about 25 percent of teenagers with excessive bleeding, blood coagulation problems are present. Other symptoms are easy bruising or bleeding from the gums while brushing teeth. If coagulation is normal, lack of ovulation may be the problem, and a physician will prescribe oral birth control or progestin pills to regulate the menstrual cycle.

In an older woman, especially if profuse bleeding occurs, a physician may choose to perform a dilatation and curettage, which is a minor surgical procedure in which the uterus is dilated and its interior is scraped and examined for signs of endometriosis. Endometriosis can be photocoagulated with a laser, but older women who have had as many children as they wish may consider a hysterectomy. DUB not related to endometriosis also may be controlled by taking various types of hormones.

245. *I have just gone through a long and painful divorce, and am now trying to get my life back in gear. I am still young and a talented businesswoman, but now find that I have become a "pushover" for sex with my dates. Is it possible that this is due to my recent divorce, or do I need professional help?*

A divorce is never pleasant, even when both parties agree to the separation. In cases where a person feels rejected or displaced, the need to restore self-esteem and repair damaged pride may take the form of excessive sexual activity. The brief but sometimes intense relationship serves to make you feel wanted, attractive and to release some of the sexual tension that has built up. It also serves to combat the depression that follows any change in lifestyle.

Surely counseling can help, before this becomes a habit that can permanently damage your already disrupted life. And please, during this time, remember the rules of safe sex in order to reduce some of the other risks, such as infection.

9. The Special Concerns of Men

Whoever considers the study of anatomy,
I believe, will never be an atheist.
The frame of man's body, and coherence
of his parts, being so strange
and paradoxical, that I hold it be
the greatest miracle of nature.

LORD EDWARD HERBERT
English philosopher (1583–1648)

Almost all the systems in the body play multiple roles in carrying out the life processes. Though there may be a primary function, the secondary and associated tasks are also well-defined. The male reproductive system, however, is designed with but a single purpose: to produce sperm cells and transport them to the female. At the same time, the external male genitals play an evident and distinct role in sexual activity and behavior, because reproduction cannot take place unless sperm cells are delivered to the female reproductive tract in a healthy condition that permits them to make the journey required to reach the ovum.

The male reproductive system consists of just a few major organs. They are the ***testes*** (testicles), the ***prostate***, the ***seminal vesicles***, the ***vas deferens***, the ***epididymis*** and the ***penis***. Although the bladder empties through a duct that runs through the length of the penis and so is connected to the reproductive system, the bladder is considered part of the urinary or excretory system, which is described in Chapter Six.

The two testes, which are housed in a pouch of skin called the *scrotum*, are located outside the body. This is necessary because, in order for the testes to function properly, they require a lower surrounding temperature than that of the body. Only when the ambient temperature is several degrees below the normal body temperature of about 98.6 degrees Fahrenheit can the testes perform their most important function, which is the production of sperm cells in a process known as *spermatogenesis*. If the temperature within the scrotum increases by only a couple of degrees or so above normal, the process of sperm production may be seriously impaired, which reduces the number of sperm produced or increases the number of abnormal forms. This can result when the scrotal temperature is increased by heat coming from outside the body itself, such as occurs when bathing in very hot water, or from elevated temperatures produced within the body, such as a fever associated with an acute infectious illness, for example. To help keep the temperature down, the skin of the scrotum contains numerous sweat glands that assist in the cooling process.

Each testicle measures about 5 centimeters (2 inches) long and 2.5 centimeters (1 inch) wide, and is suspended from the body and held in place by a *spermatic cord*. Attached to this cord is a muscle (the *cremaster*) that can pull the testes closer to the body, nestling them in a more protected area. The reflex that produces this action (*cremasterian reflex*) can be elicited when the inner surface of the thigh is scratched or scraped. Thus, during running or fleeing from danger in an anthropological sense, the testes are pulled back from exposure and potential injury. Muscles within the scrotum (*dartos muscles*) also help this action when they contract.

This contracting mechanism also is brought into play when the temperature in the scrotum becomes too cold, thus drawing the testes closer to the higher-degree warmth of the body.

Within the scrotum, each testis is enclosed in a thick, protective capsule called the *tunica albuginea*. Within each of the testes is a network of tightly coiled tubes called the *seminiferous tubules*. There are 400 to 600 tubules in each of the testes, and each tubule is about 75 centimeters (nearly 30 inches) long. If all these tubules were uncoiled, they would stretch to almost 1.6 kilometers (one mile) in length.

Spermatogenesis takes place within the seminiferous tubules. The primary cell, called the *spermatogonia*, divides (*mitosis*) into two primary *spermatocytes*. Each contains the full complement of 46 chromosomes. When these divide (*meiosis*), the number of chromosomes is halved, and each new cell, called a *spermatid*, contains only 23 chromosomes. This cell then produces a *sperm cell* or *spermatozoon*.

Each sperm cell is made up of two parts: the *head* (which includes the *nucleus*) and the *tail*. The nucleus contains all the genetic information included in the 23 chromosomes that the sperm contributes to the 46 chromosomes contained in a fertilized ovum, or egg, which leads to another life. The other 23 chromosomes come from the egg itself. The tail is composed of protein fibers that can contract in an alternating rhythm, which causes the tail to move from side to side, just as a fish's tail does, to propel the sperm forward. From head to tail, the sperm cell measures only about 0.05 millimeter (two-thousandths of an inch).

Sperm production occurs fully by age 16, even though it can begin before a boy reaches puberty. The male is able to continue the production of sperm throughout his entire adult life. Men can produce about 200 million sperm each day, of which about 20 percent are either dead or abnormal. These abnormal forms are incapable of fertilizing an egg. Sperm production slows with advancing age, with fewer sperm produced and higher percentages of abnormalities noted. Despite this, men in their 70s or 80s often are able to father children, though fertility usually has peaked much earlier in the life cycle.

In addition to sperm, the testes also produce the male hormones, or androgens, in the large cells called the interstitial *cells of Leydig*. These cells are located between the seminiferous tubules. These hormones are carried by the bloodstream and circulate throughout the body, affecting various organs. The principal male hormone is *testosterone*. As it becomes active at the beginning of puberty in the adolescent male, it promotes body growth, particularly muscle mass, changes the vocal cords, which deepens the male voice, and promotes the growth of body hair: facial, axillary (armpit) and pubic. When testosterone causes excessive secretion from the skin's sebaceous glands, acne may result. Just as with the production of sperm, the manufacture and secretion of the male hormones begin about the time of puberty and continue throughout life.

Since the production of male hormones decreases slowly over a long period of time, men do not experience the same intense symptoms that menopause causes in women. However, there is a male "change of life" similar to menopause. Since the term *menopause* relates to the end of the menses, or monthly cycle, it is not applicable to male physiology. In the male change of life (*climacteric*) the symptoms are milder, but can include the same hot flashes and heart palpitations women experience. These symptoms can be mistaken for signs of a heart attack.

Answers from the Family Doctor (Questions 246-275)

Let's now continue detailing the sperm's journey through the male reproductive system. Before the sperm cells reach the penis, they pass out of the testes into another system of ducts called the epididymis. Although the epididymis itself is only about 3.8 centimeters (1½ inches) in length, it's so tightly coiled that it would measure about 6 meters (20 feet) if drawn out as a single strand. The sperm cells remain in this duct system for about two weeks, where they mature. They then pass into a longer transportation duct called the vas deferens, where they can survive for another month to six weeks before they begin to degenerate and die, and are reabsorbed. The operation performed to render a man sterile, called a *vasectomy*, is named for this duct, because the procedure consists of severing the vas deferens and tying off the ends so that the sperm cells cannot complete the journey from the testes to the penis.

After leaving the vas deferens, the sperm cells continue their journey to the penis, traveling through or past a number of internal organs: the seminal vesicles, the prostate and *Cowper's glands*.

The seminal vesicles are two membranous pouches thought to act as storage organs for the sperm. Much as the gallbladder does for the secretions of the liver, the seminal vesicles serve as reservoirs for the mature sperm until the time arrives for them to make their way through the urethra and out of the penis. Another essential function of the seminal vesicles is to produce a thick, sticky, protective secretion that forms part of the semen. This liquid also includes the nutrient *fructose* (a type of sugar), which is vital to activate the sperm.

The prostate gland, a small doughnut-shaped organ, is located at the base of the bladder and encircles the first part of the urethra (also known as the ejaculatory duct). It measures about 3.8 centimeters (1½ inches) across and 3.2 centimeters (1¼ inches) vertically. It's enclosed in a firm, fibrous capsule. The prostate secretes an alkaline fluid to combat the acidity of the secretions in the vagina. As a man ages, the prostate may become larger, which is a condition known as benign prostatic hypertrophy. When this occurs, the new tissue mass presses down upon the urethra and may block the passage of urine from the bladder out of the penis. This causes a condition known as urinary obstruction, which may be treated with a variety of surgical procedures or recently developed medication.

Close to the prostate are the two Cowper's glands, each about the size of a pea, one on each side of the urethra. Their size diminishes as age advances.

The major function of these three internal organs together is to produce fluids that will provide the sperm cells with a nourishing and balanced environment when they leave the man's body and enter into the woman's body. Only a very small proportion of the male ejaculate (also called semen) actually is made up of sperm cells. Although a single ejaculation contains from 3 to 5 milliliters (.09 ounce to .15 ounce) of semen, the greater part is composed of the seminal fluids secreted by the internal organs. The seminal fluid contains various proteins, fructose and other chemicals important for the sustenance of the sperm cells. Because these three internal organs continue to function in a male who has had a vasectomy, he will produce about the same quantity of seminal fluid — even though no sperm are present — as a fertile male. Although seminal fluids are not absolutely necessary for a man to be fertile, these fluids permit the sperm cells to survive for a longer period of time within the acidic environment of the vagina.

In the final phase of the journey that will take them out of the body, the sperm cells pass through the urethral duct, a fibroelastic tube that runs from the bottom of the bladder through the center of the penis to its tip. The penis contains a large number of arteries, veins and small blood vessels that form a specialized tissue, known as erectile tissue, that is fashioned into three hollow, spongelike cylinders. The urethra runs through one of these cylinders called the *corpus spongiosum*, and ends in the *glans* (the tip of the penis). The other two spongelike tubes are called the *corpora cavernosa*. A central artery passes inside the center of these two tubes and brings blood to the erectile tissue. When a male has an erection, these spongy tissues fill with blood and become firm. Unlike the penises of a number of other mammals (whales, for example), the human penis has no bones.

Erection is produced solely by the relaxation of the blood vessels within the penis. For this to occur, specialized muscles contract around the veins in the corpora cavernosa and corpus spongiosum and hold back the flow of blood, causing the spaces within the three spongelike cylinders to become engorged with blood. At the same time, the blood vessels all relax to contain this added volume of blood. Thus when a man is under emotional or physical stress, he may experience some difficulty achieving a firm erection, because the blood vessels may not relax enough, preventing the corpora from filling sufficiently.

Ejaculation occurs during sexual excitement, when all the fluids that form the semen and contain the sperm cells are propelled down the urethra and discharged suddenly out of the tip of the penis. Although as many as 300 million sperm may enter the vagina, only a few hundred will make it through the uterus to the Fallopian tubes, and only one sperm cell will fertilize the egg. It takes about two hours for the sperm cells to travel from the vagina to the Fallopian tubes. The sperm are propelled by the swimming motion of their long tails and are aided by contractions of the muscles forming the walls of the uterus and vagina.

When the final, single sperm cell penetrates the wall of the ovum, conception takes place. And that is a story for another chapter.

Questions and Answers

246. ***My husband has a terrible job, but at least he's working. Every day the stress seems to get worse. There's more pressure to get things done and less help to share the load. And doom to the man who tries to suggest changing things. So my husband keeps his mouth shut and comes home every night ready to explode. Sometimes he does. I just tell myself it may be doing him some good. Can holding in the anger harm his health?***

The suspicion that anger held in against one's nature could cause physical harm has been the subject of a great deal of research over the years. There's been much work, yet few answers and little agreement among scientists.

At one time, the idea that a Type A personality — aggressive, compulsive, hard-driving, tense — had a greater risk of heart attacks was accepted commonly. But gradually research that isolated each of these Type A characteristics reduced the conviction that these factors were linked to heart disease. Even hostility, which remained the last emotion still considered a risk factor, cannot be tied conclusively to heart attacks.

However, recent studies on anger, particularly suppressed anger, seem to indicate that it may be a valid emotional risk factor as a cause of heart disease. A bit surprisingly, it may be more of a danger for women than men. And it still isn't clear whether venting anger, or "blowing up" as some would have it, really does any good.

Unleashing anger does make some people feel better, but the energy used in venting anger does little to help solve the problem. Recognizing anger, and trying to control it by keeping cool, calm and clear about the issues, may be helpful to some. Yet men who experience daily anger as part of the job — bus drivers, for example — do have increased medical problems, increased death rates from heart disease, and are more susceptible to diseases of the gastrointestinal tract.

I know jobs are hard to come by, but continuing the search for another position may offer some mental relief for your husband. Just the idea of landing a new job may provide the hope that change eventually may come, and this may rid your husband of the stress he now must endure.

247. ***I'm a young man — too young to start balding. But the hair loss is now pretty visible, and I'm confused by all the advertising for hair products that I see on television. Are any of them proven really to help hair grow? I don't want to spend my hard-earned bucks for nothing.***

You pose an excellent question, one that applies as well to many types of advertising for health products on television. The secret is in the listening.

The ads I've seen do not claim to promote new growth in so many words, but tell of "stopping the loss" of hair through "natural means." By this they mean that their product is not a medication in the sense that it acts on a disease process through chemical means, and therefore it is not approved by the Food and Drug Administration. "Natural means" could refer to a cleansing process that might help the general scalp condition, but these claims are never quite clear.

The one product that does have scientific evidence to back its claims, and FDA approval, is Rogaine (minoxidil is the generic name), which is produced by the Upjohn Company. Minoxidil has been used in the control of high blood pressure. It also was found to promote hair growth in balding men. Rogaine is indicated for male pattern baldness of the top of the head (vertex).

The medication, obtained with a doctor's prescription, will cost you about $2 a day, must be used continuously for life and is most effective in younger men, men with balding of less than 10 years' duration, and men whose bald spot covers less than four inches.

And it doesn't work on everyone. About one-quarter of men using the medication over a period of one year displayed no growth, or growth of only very fine hair (vellus).

You can obtain more information from the manufacturer by calling the Rogaine Hot Line, 1-800-635-0655, from 9 a.m. to 8 p.m. Eastern time Monday through Friday. An attentive and polite representative will answer all your questions.

248. *All this talk about condoms has me baffled. How do you use them?*

This question, in one form or another, is a most frequent one in my mail. Despite the enormous importance of preventive measures to control the spread of sexually transmitted diseases, particularly AIDS, information of the type sought here seems difficult to obtain. In the interest of the health of those who need this information, and trusting that it is understood that the information I'm providing is medical in nature and implies no moral judgments, I shall answer this question as precisely as possible.

Condoms are sheaths of very thin rubber (latex) that fit closely onto the penis and prevent the escape of semen. They are an old and reasonably effective form of birth control. More importantly, in these days, latex condoms are effective in reducing the spread of sexually transmitted diseases, including AIDS.

There are two types of condoms: latex or rubber condoms, and natural condoms made of sheep gut. Only the latex type has been shown to stop the transmission of the AIDS virus. In order to be effective as either birth control or disease protection, a new condom must be used each and every time you have sex — no ifs, ands or buts.

A condom comes rolled up. It's placed on the head of the erect penis, leaving a bit of space at the tip to catch the semen. Then the condom is unrolled down the shaft all the way to the base. A condom must be in place before intercourse. After intercourse, the male partner must withdraw carefully to avoid dislodging the condom, after which it may be removed and disposed of.

The American College of Obstetricians and Gynecologists estimates that condoms cost about $30 a year and are 90 percent effective at preventing pregnancy. Most failures are due to forgetting to use a condom or tearing it while putting it on. Additionally, they are almost universally recommended as a means of promoting "safe sex" and preventing the spread of sexually transmitted diseases.

249. *I suffer from an inability to complete the sex act because I cannot ejaculate. I overheard a conversation about a new procedure that uses an electric shock that helps, but didn't want to come forward and ask about it. Do you know anything about this?*

It is difficult to interpret the conversation you overheard from your letter, but it's possible that they might have been talking about a process called electro-ejaculation. This method is used to obtain sperm from men who are unable to ejaculate, and can be used in artificial insemination procedures for their wives. It's a method long used in veterinary medicine.

An electrical probe is inserted into the rectum, and an electrical impulse is used to produce the contractions necessary to expel the semen. This semen then is preserved, concentrated and used for insemination. It's not a procedure that can aid in intercourse. It's useful for those individuals whose inability to complete the sex act is due to neurological problems caused by spinal cord injury, multiple sclerosis or advanced diabetes mellitus, as well as other conditions.

250. ***I'm having a terrible problem with a condition that makes small, pus-filled bumps crop out all over my face. I try to be careful when I shave, but this only makes it worse. I wash carefully and only use my own electric razor, but nothing seems to work. I notice this condition more among men of my race than in whites, and would like to know if this is the cause. What can be done to treat the problem?***

The name of the condition is pseudofolliculitis barbae, if I don't miss my guess, and it's the most common skin problem seen in black men aside from pigmentation disorders. The description of its appearance and its relationship to shaving are the clues.

The condition occurs when the cut hairs curve back on themselves and become embedded in the skin. It's these ingrown hairs that provoke the reaction that creates the pustules you noted.

The first action is to stop shaving, and you may have to quit for four to five weeks. This will provide enough time for these hairs to grow out. At first it may look worse, but it's the best way to rid yourself of the problem. Then throw away that razor, for cutting hairs below the skin surface may be the problem. Use a safety razor for better results.

You also might do well to check with your own physician. In some cases, acne can be the correct diagnosis, for which medical treatment is available.

251. ***At a recent business convention, a colleague I've run into over the years confessed to me that a recent hospitalization was for a fracture of his sexual member. I know that there's no bone there to break, so I find his story difficult to believe. What do you think really happened to him?***

The penis contains three spongelike tubes — one corpus spongiosum and two corpora cavernosa, which are surrounded by a very strong fibrous tissue sheath called the tunica albuginea. When blood fills and expands these tubes during sexual arousal, this sheath becomes thinner and more prone to injury.

If some type of forceful trauma occurs during an erection (an accidental fall or unexpected blow directly to the erect penis), the tissues of the tunica, corpus spongiosum and corpora cavernosa can be torn. This condition is known as a fractured penis, and there are many articles in medical literature describing it.

This condition is considered a medical emergency, and it's extremely painful, as you might well imagine. The treatment of choice is surgery, which is necessary to find the area of the tear, remove the accumulated clotted blood and repair the tear. When these tasks are accomplished in a timely fashion, the function of the organ is preserved. Hospitalization of two weeks is average, and good results are achieved in about 75 percent of cases treated this way.

252. ***Perhaps this question is too difficult to answer, for I have never seen anything about it, but I certainly could use some information about losing my sexual abilities. It's not something you can just go out and talk about, but I'm sure there are many men who have similar questions. What causes this, and is there anything that can be done to help?***

Yes, this is a difficult question to respond to. Not only because it has a complicated answer, but because problems of a sexual nature always should be treated on a very personal, one-to-one basis. Each of us is very special and unique, and there is no place in medical care where that is more evident than in this area.

However, in the hope that I can be of some help, here are some important general considerations. The causes of the inability to perform a sexual act, or impotence, fall into two main categories: psychogenic and organic. Stated more simply, it means that the problem can stem from the mind and how we think about things, or it can be the result of physical changes in the body. More often than not, there is a bit of both involved.

The physical mechanism that allows a man to achieve an erection followed by ejaculation involves both the central nervous system (the brain) and the peripheral nervous system (the nerves that run throughout the body; in this case, particularly those that lead to the penis). The vascular system is involved, both arterial and venous. The endocrine system, which produces the hormones in the body, must function properly, and the penis must be anatomically intact. All of these systems can be tested in various ways to assure their ability to function and to contribute to the desired action.

To detect the state of the patient's mind requires a careful history, with many questions about attitudes and feelings. More often than not, the man's sexual partner should be consulted, for she too has important insights and information to offer. Most importantly, the man should realize that with today's technologies, virtually every man with this problem can be helped in a way that returns a satisfying intimacy to his life and his relationships.

When the diagnostic work-up leads to the conclusion that there is something organically wrong, the solution will depend upon the problem. Medications may be appropriate to restore hormone levels to normal in individuals whose problem results from levels that are too low. External vacuum devices are useful in many cases. They create a negative pressure around the penis, thus drawing blood into the spongelike erectile tissues in the penis. Once the penis has become erect, a constricting band around the base of the penis helps to maintain rigidity. In some cases, the patient can be taught to self-inject certain medications into the sex organ to initiate an erection. In other cases, a penile prosthesis is the answer, either semirigid rods or inflatable devices that can produce the desired rigidity and allow a normal relationship.

In each case, the needs, personal lifestyle and specific diagnoses will be the factors that are considered in the choice of treatment. But all of this requires you to take the first step and consult your own physician.

253. ***Maybe this question is not suited to dinner table conversation, but I hope you'll be able to provide an answer. It's certainly a misery for those of us who suffer with jock itch. What is it, where does it***

come from, and most important of all, what can I do about it? Hurry, please, for it always gets worse during hot weather. I hope you can find the right words to reply to this question.

I certainly will find the right words and choose them most carefully, as well. The medical name for this "misery" is tinea cruris. This annoying problem can be caused by a number of fungi and yeasts. Typically this skin condition affects the folds in the groin and the inner thigh, and sometimes this scaly, itchy rash may extend to the buttocks. The rash forms ringlike shapes on the skin, and it's often crossed with scratch marks.

Hot weather can make the condition worse, because body moisture and tight clothing favor the growth of the organisms. Keeping clean and dry can help prevent the development of jock itch. Use body powder or even a hair dryer (set on its lowest temperature) to keep the region dry. Once the organism is identified, there are a number of medications that can help you fight this infection. Check with your physician or pharmacist.

254. ***Several years ago I read that a birth control pill for men would be available in the near future. Well, the near future is here, but where's the pill? I think it's time for men to be as responsible for birth control as women are. Can you tell me what has happened in this field of research, and when we can expect to see the new product? Thank you.***

While there still may be a birth control pill for men available in the future, it may be further down the line than you were led to believe, maybe as long as 10 to 20 years. Don't blame the scientists. The male biology is quite different from that of women, and it's this distinction that is the basis of the difficulty.

All that's necessary in a woman's biology to prevent a pregnancy is to prevent the release of one egg per month. In a man, it requires interfering with the production of sperm, which is something that occurs on a continuous basis in men from puberty until death.

At present, research is centered on the male hormone testosterone. This male hormone must be present in order for the production of sperm to take place. However, scientists can inject a synthetic testosterone that the body interprets as real, shutting down the production of the real hormone and effectively stopping the man's sperm production. But this takes an injection each week.

Another mechanism also is being explored. For testosterone to be produced, the brain secretes a stimulating hormone called gonadotropin releasing hormone (or GNRH, for short). That in turn sets off the production of the male hormones required for sperm production. Using a chemical with a similar formula (called an analogue), the secretion of testosterone can be stopped. With the end of sperm production goes male fertility and, unfortunately, his sexual desires as well. This process requires a daily injection to be effective.

The long-range effects of both these methods have yet to be fully determined, although fertility returns once the regular injections are discontinued.

These injections have not been approved for general use and are still merely experimental. It seems that for the foreseeable future, responsible men will have to rely on condoms or surgery (vasectomy) if they want to undertake the responsibility for controlling the onset of pregnancy.

255. ***In talking with several women recently, I gather that their husbands have lost interest in, and ability to perform, sex after being diagnosed with hypertension. The common denominator seems to be their medicine. The men apparently are reluctant to pursue the problem. As a doctor, what route would you take to correct this problem? These men are not too old!***

Nowhere have I seen the power of communication more dramatically demonstrated than in your question, with all its implications. Sharing information makes us all wiser and sometimes leads to the discovery of problems that are frequently not discussed, and from there to solutions.

Male impotence may stem from many causes, both physical and psychological, but there's no question that medications are frequently the culprits. While the prescribing information may fail to take note of this unwanted side effect, there isn't a textbook worth its cost that doesn't include an impressive list of medications that reduce sexual ability.

The largest number is found under the heading of antihypertensives, with psychotropic medication (both anti-depressives and anti-anxiety agents) next in line. Central nervous system depressants, including alcohol, sedatives and narcotics, all are there as well.

Now for the right route to take. Let's use the same technique to solve the problem that led to its discovery: communication. If your husband suddenly has found himself deprived of powers he had possessed formerly and is unaware that his medications may be doing him in, he must be suffering emotionally from this unexpected loss of his manliness. This is kept locked up inside, frequently denied, but usually not addressed openly.

By sharing your knowledge (and this answer) with him, you can take the first step on the path that can lead to the solution you seek. The next step involves the physician, who has heard all this before. But since not all men have the same side effects from a medication, the physician is unaware that this problem now exists and must be informed. The last step is a change in medication to one that still will control the hypertension but will not generate this problem. There are several medications to choose from.

I hope this answer will cause many readers to stop and think whether they may be unknowing passengers in the same boat.

256. ***I recently heard a story about a man who developed rather large breasts. The word to describe it sounded like "gymnast," but I know that can't be correct. Could you please discuss this condition and give me the right name?***

You're pretty close. The correct medical term is gynecomastia, and it comes from two Greek words meaning "woman" and "breast" — thus, breasts like a woman. Gynecomastia means any benign glandular enlargement in the breasts of males.

It's a relatively common disorder, with several causes, such as obesity, aging and a reaction to certain drugs. Only rarely is gynecomastia caused by a serious medical problem. In adolescent males, it can be a very difficult emotional and psychological problem to deal with.

All normal adult male breasts contain most of the major elements found in female breasts. Everyone's breasts are sensitive to hormones, so male breast enlargement may be associated with an overabundance or lack of certain hormones.

In many adolescent males (one study suggests about 20 percent of men in this age group develop gynecomastia), breast enlargements develop and after a while disappear. Yet, sometimes the enlargements do not go away. When that occurs, medical decisions need to be made rapidly before psychological damage is done to these young men.

Approximately 60 percent of all men from 45 to 60 years old will develop some breast enlargement. Incidences of gynecomastia in adult men appear to increase with age. It's most often observed between the ages of 50 and 60. As many as 30 percent of all adult males will have some evidence of gynecomastia at some point in their lives, and more than 90 percent of them experience enlargement of both breasts. Nevertheless, breast enlargement on only one side of a man's chest is seen.

There virtually is no evidence that directly links gynecomastia to breast cancer. Male breast cancer is rare, and it accounts for less than 1 percent of all cancers in men. However, any enlargement in men or women should be examined by a physician. Also, if there is bloody discharge from a nipple or a firm, nodular mass within the breast area, a medical examination should be made immediately.

Some things are known to cause gynecomastia. Among them are: overconsumption of alcohol, kidney diseases, diseases that cause a decrease in male hormone levels, severe changes in eating patterns, thyroid malfunctions, certain tumors, all forms of estrogen — including estrogen in hair preparations and vaginal creams — Tagamet, Aldactone, Nizoral, and the digitalis-cytotoxic drugs (a few are Crystodigin, Lanoxin and Velban).

When gynecomastia is caused by drugs, the condition often develops rapidly and usually will disappear shortly after the drug's use is stopped.

Other things that many scientists suspect cause gynecomastia include: lung diseases, chest injuries, psychological stress, marijuana, heroin and some anti-depressant drugs.

Treatment for gynecomastia includes discontinuing the use of drugs and other substances that might cause it, treating any physical condition that could have produced it, and possibly performing surgery to remove excess tissue.

257. ***My husband was the greatest of men when we met. Through 10 years of marriage, he has been struck by several disappointments. His only solution has been to drink, and I believe he now has liver trouble. We used to solve a lot of his problems together, as husband and wife, but he now fails at that as well. Would injections of male hormone help him regain his powers and self-respect?***

There are many aspects to your problem. I wish we could have a talk to explore the many reasons why it has become this serious, but that will have to remain in the hands of your own family doctor. However, I will give you information that answers your specific question.

In a recent research project conducted at the University of Copenhagen, 67 percent of the 221 men who suffered from alcohol-induced liver disease (cirrhosis) complained of sexual dysfunction. Attempts to treat their condition with male hormone (testosterone) failed to improve their sexual performance.

However, when the amount of alcohol consumed was reduced, the men reported significant improvement in their ability to function. They also reported continued improvement at six-month, 12-month and 24-month follow-ups.

Testosterone will not solve your husband's problem. The answer is to attack the causes of his drinking problem and to return him to sobriety, health and vigor.

258. *We have tried unsuccessfully to have a child for three years. I have gone through all the tests, and now my husband realizes that he, too, must be tested. What are the chances that the problem may be with him, and how will they discover it?*

Infertility affects 15 percent of marriages, and studies estimate that a male factor is responsible in one-third of these cases. Through careful, sympathetic evaluation, the underlying causes often can be pinpointed and corrected, which leads to successful pregnancy for many couples.

First, the doctor must gather a complete sexual history of the couple. He or she will note any factors that may affect or inhibit pregnancy, such as the frequency of sex and its timing in relation to the woman's menstrual cycle. Lubricants, douches or other substances used in conjunction with sex may have a spermicidal effect and may be preventing the sperm from reaching the uterus.

One factor that reduces fertility in the male is cryptorchidism, which is the failure of one or both of the testes to descend into the scrotum during childhood. If this condition remains uncorrected past the age of 5, irreversible changes take place in the testes that reduce their fertility. Mumps orchitis, which is an inflammation of the testes, also negatively affects their reproductive ability; if both are infected, sterility may result.

Miscellaneous infections, emotional or physical stress, certain medications and even the treatment of hernias can impair fertility. To get the complete picture, it's necessary for the doctor to examine the genitals, with an eye toward any physical abnormalities in the structure of the penis or the scrotum.

An analysis of the semen yields the most important data regarding fertility. Since semen takes 75 days to develop, at least two samples should be taken, at two- to three-week intervals. The various characteristics of semen (the sperm's volume, shape and degree of movement) can vary tremendously between samples. Semen volume in an ejaculation is usually between 1.5 and 5 milliliters (45-thousandths and 15-hundredths of an ounce). The density of spermatozoa present should be above 20 million per milliliter (.03 ounce). Their degree of movement, or motility, should be active in at least 60 percent of the sperm observed under a microscope within two to three hours after the sample is taken.

Oval sperm heads are considered normal in such an evaluation; large, small, tapering, duplicated and amorphous heads also may be present. Fertile semen contains 10 percent abnormal forms and between 60 and 70 percent normal forms.

These tests may reveal the presence of azoospermia, a deformation in the testes that prevents the creation of healthy sperm. Patients who test abnormal in all these characteristics are likely to have varicocele (a collection of dilated veins in the spermatic cord), which is most responsive to surgery.

Hormones are less likely to play a role in infertility, but they can be tested if semen analysis fails to yield answers. A biopsy of testicular tissue is reserved for isolated cases.

In unraveling these questions, emotional support from the spouse and physician is critical in resolving the psychological and physical stress that results from infertility.

259. *There are times when I know that I'm going through a change of life similar to the one my wife experienced. She just laughs and says that men can't get hot flashes any more than they can have babies. I maintain that men can get hot flashes, too. What do you say?*

Men most certainly can. In both men and women, hot flashes are caused by the decreased production of sex hormones. In women, hot flashes are controlled most often by the biological clock and begin when menopause sets in. In men, however, the biological clock does not play as big a role. Hot flashes usually occur in men who have had a testicle removed, usually because of cancer.

A report published in the *Western Journal of Medicine* said many men mistake the symptoms of hot flashes for those of heart attacks. The symptoms of hot flashes are intense sweating, heart palpitations, fainting spells and a flushed color in the face, neck and chest. These are the same symptoms that women get, only women experience them more frequently and with greater intensity than men.

Typically, men who experience hot flashes are middle-aged or older. Since this same group of men is at highest risk of heart attack, doctors should ask possible heart attack victims if they've ever had a testicle removed or had many hernia operations, which also can lead to hot flashes. Such an inquiry at the initial stages of treatment could help prevent a possible misdiagnosis.

This may not be the cause of your particular episodes, but it seems reasonable to believe that your experiences, while not as common as in women, may be experienced by many men, in modified forms.

260. ***Could you please be so kind as to explain male sterility due to mumps contracted during puberty? I have been married to my husband for six years, and I haven't been able to get pregnant. How does this illness affect the male's reproductive system, and is there any cure for it?***

Mumps is a disease that is found worldwide. By 15 years of age, more than 90 percent of people who live in urban areas have blood tests that reveal they have been exposed to the disease. Mumps most often occurs in children between the ages of 5 and 9, but those statistics are changing due to the use of a mumps vaccine that was first available for use in 1967.

The cause of the infection is a virus that is passed through contact with secretions from an infected individual's nose, mouth or throat. About one-third of the time, the disease proceeds with no symptoms at all, except for a slight fever and malaise. However, the most noticeable feature of the full-blown attack is the swelling of the parotid gland located in the cheek, as well as other salivary glands.

Mumps also may affect the testicles of men past puberty in 10 to 20 percent of the cases. Then it's called orchitis, or inflammation of the testicles. It may affect one or both sides. According to some articles in the medical literature, it rarely causes sterility, and according to other experts, it may produce sterility in as many as half the cases.

The viral infection attacks the sperm-producing cells and destroys them, leaving the testicle atrophied or shrunken. Fortunately, the cells that produce the masculine hormone testosterone are not affected, so levels of male hormone remain normal throughout life. Once the damage has been done, there is no treatment available to regenerate the sperm-producing cells.

When the problem is sterility, a complete work-up must be performed to determine the number of sperm present and their activity, and to evaluate the potential for fertilization. If the findings indicate that sperm vitality is not the problem, you, too, must be examined for possible problems that stand in the way of pregnancy, which should then be treated and corrected as well.

Although a history of mumps is important in fertility problems, it must not be considered the culprit until all the possibilities have been examined.

261. *Would you please answer a question that I can never bring myself to discuss with my own physician? I experience a sharp pain at my climax during sex. What should I do? I'm a 28-year-old male.*

You can start by finding a doctor you can confide in, for only his evaluation is going to provide you with the personal answers you seek. There are many reasons for painful ejaculation. You'll be comforted to know you're not alone; this is not an uncommon problem.

Though it's difficult to guess at the cause in your case, here are a few possibilities. Sometimes the pain is caused by an obstruction, bacteria or inflammation. Other times, it's simply caused by certain medications that have been found to cause painful ejaculation. Accurate diagnosis and treatment depend upon a thorough history, examination and lab evaluation. Your doctor will need to know at what point the pain actually occurs — before, during or after intercourse.

It's also crucial to be able to tell the physician exactly where the pain occurs — the glans, penile shaft, scrotum or perineum. Once your doctor determines the cause of your problem, effective treatment can begin and will rid you of both the physical and emotional pain that are bothering you.

262. ***I've been to several doctors, received some treatment and explanations, but still find it difficult to understand what is happening to my sexual organ. The condition is called "Peyronie's Disease," and I would be most grateful for any help or explanation. I can't be the only one suffering from this, and perhaps you can help lots of men who suffer from this condition.***

You're not alone. It's rare that a week goes by without some letter requesting information on this most distressful disease of adult men. Peyronie's disease is an affliction of the male organ that causes the erect penis to curve, which occasionally causes painful erections and prevents normal function during intercourse.

Anatomically, the penis is composed of three long, spongy tubes (a corpus spongiosum and a pair of corpora cavernosa), each enclosed in an elastic sheath or covering. For reasons still unknown, these sheaths may thicken as the tissue becomes fibrotic (scarlike), and then shorten. The affected section of the sheath loses its elasticity and can't stretch properly during erection, so the penis bends in the direction of the scarred area.

Treatment is difficult and not always successful. Local injection of corticosteroids (cortisonelike medication) may help, but doesn't work when the medication is taken orally. The scarred area can be removed surgically and replaced by a graft, but that may result in even more scarring during the healing process. Some symptomatic relief can be obtained through the use of local ultrasound treatments. There are cases when, after many months, the disease just goes away by itself. I truly hope you fall into this last classification.

263. ***I'm too discomfited to ask this question of my own doctor. Unfortunately, it has happened to me more than once, and I know others have had the same painful experience. Can you tell me what to do when my penis gets caught in the zipper?***

Here is a case when prevention is truly the best medicine. However, it does happen, and I do believe the answer may be of interest to many. The first bit of advice is to consider this an emergency. While not fatal, it's probably best attended to by someone who can take all the precautions necessary.

It likely won't require any major surgery, but a bit of anesthetic cream and perhaps a sedative can make the rest of the procedure easier to endure. Once your member is numb, the zipper is eased down, a fraction at a time, until all the sensitive skin is free. The wound may require dressing or another application of anesthetic ointment. Cold applications to the area for the first 12 hours following the accident will prevent swelling and help relieve the discomfort.

264. ***During a recent office visit, my doctor took a number of blood tests, though I had no complaints other than a bad cold. I now must visit again, for one of the tests, a prostate test, has been found to be abnormal. Still, his nurse assured me that it may not be anything to worry about. Would you please tell me what is going on? I'm losing sleep just worrying about what might be in store for me.***

It's most probable that the test in question is a new screening tool called the prostate-specific antigen (PSA), which is recommended as part of a general prostate evaluation for men over the age of 50. It tests for a specific chemical (antigen) that is produced by the cells of the prostate.

When the results show elevated amounts of this antigen, it may indicate the presence of cancer cells, which produce large quantities of the substance. However, since the same antigen is produced by normal cells, a man with an enlarged prostate due to benign enlargement (hypertrophy) also may be found to have an elevated test finding. That is why the nurse said you may not have anything to worry about.

When this test is used appropriately as a screening tool, an elevated finding requires additional testing to determine whether a cancer is really present. In addition to a digital rectal examination, an ultrasound test or a biopsy can be used to fully evaluate the situation and make a correct diagnosis. So a return visit to the doctor's office is in order, as is additional investigation.

While the test is not as specific as we all would like, and a false negative can cause worry and loss of sleep, an early diagnosis is so important in fighting cancer of the prostate that we can rationalize the use of this test as a general screening procedure in middle-aged men. Only when prostate cancer is detected at its early stages (before it has had a chance to spread to other parts of the body) can the surgical removal of the diseased gland provide the desired cure. Take heart and follow through, for ultimately that is the best course to take to obtain the best results.

265. *What's an orchitis? I'm not sure the word is correct, but I have a personal interest in the condition.*

It's a relatively uncommon infection of one or both testes. Orchitis usually is seen in adults, and frequently it's one of the more painful aspects of a mumps infection. Twenty to 30 percent of mumps patients get orchitis of one testis about a week after they have contracted the mumps virus. However, syphilis and even tuberculosis can bring on this condition.

A person who suffers from orchitis initially has a sudden high fever, followed by extreme pain in the testicular area. Soon he is nauseated and vomiting. The scrotal area becomes bright red and filled with an abnormal amount of fluid. The infected testis is hard to the touch, swollen and terribly tender. (Patients with this condition are notoriously "testy." Do you think this is where the adjective comes from?)

Bed rest is recommended along with some cold packs and perhaps painkillers. It's best to support the scrotum by elevating it to relieve pressure upon the testicles. Antibiotics can be used if bacteria are identified as the cause of the infection. In severe cases, a cortisone drug is prescribed to relieve pain, or surgery is performed to reduce testicular pressure.

Half of all orchitis victims whose condition stems from mumps lose the function of the infected testicle. Sterility, however, is rare in spite of this loss. It's obvious that this is a serious condition, and a personal interest demands a personal consultation with your own family physician to determine the implications for you.

266. *We have been trying to have a baby for almost a year now with no results. We both have done a lot of reading, and the information has been encouraging. However, we still lack knowledge about possible problems with the sperm. What causes unhealthy sperm, and how can the situation be corrected?*

It's only in recent years that the biology of human sperm has gained the attention of researchers. As a result, there is little knowledge about sperm health. We do know that about 8 to 10 percent of apparently normal men, who have no history of any inherited disease, will show abnormal sperm. In some cases, the sperm do not have the normal number of chromosomes, while in others they seem to have some of the genetic information in the wrong places.

It's still not clear just how these changes would affect conception and pregnancy. The best information available seems to indicate that exposure to toxins in the workplace, alcohol abuse, smoking and exposure to radiation may play important roles in fertility problems. The results of these health hazards are seen in miscarriages, stillbirths, low birth weight, congenital defects and child developmental problems.

Until you have identified your fertility problem, if in fact any does exist, the rules for healthy living provide good guidelines for you. Smoking is not acceptable for many reasons, and this is yet another. Moderation in the use of alcohol, and abstinence from all drugs are recommended. If medications are required, discuss with your doctor their effects on reproduction. Proper nutrition, exercise and relaxation should form part of your life's schedule as well. Some recent studies have shown that sperm are harmed by the molecules called free radicals that circulate in the body, and a man can reduce this damage by including additional vitamin C in his diet.

Experience tells us that when you keep your levels of anxiety to a minimum, increase your patience and follow the rules of healthy living, problems like yours seem to resolve themselves.

267. *I'm worried about cancer of the prostate. Please explain its causes and treatments.*

Prostate cancer is the most common malignancy found in older men. Usually it's first discovered during a rectal examination as a symptomless lump or swelling in the prostate gland. The nodule is most often small (less than 2 centimeters or 4/5 inch in diameter), hard, irregular in shape and self-contained. Other indicators of prostate cancer are unexplained bone pain in the pelvis and lower spine, and bladder problems such as painful urination, dribbling and straining to void that might indicate an obstruction.

While the exact cause of this type of malignancy remains a mystery, the predictable way it progresses helps the physician make an accurate and quick diagnosis so that proper treatment can begin. Blood tests, a needle biopsy, X-rays of the kidneys and the urinary tract, and computerized tomography pictures (CT scans) of the lower abdomen to see if the lymph nodes are involved are useful components of a complete work-up that may be performed to define what stage the carcinoma is in. These stages range from (A) diseased tissue with no lumps, to (B) lesions confined to the prostate capsule, to (C) tumors that cover the outside of the capsule, and finally to (D) disease that spreads to other body parts.

Treatment varies according to the severity of the condition and other factors. These include the patient's age (young men tend to develop fast-growing cancers), his desire to remain sexually potent, and other medical problems he may have. For instance, early stage A cancers are without symptoms. They are discovered when tissue removed during operations for enlarged prostates considered benign are examined under a microscope. No further treatment may be necessary, unless the patient is under 55 and the cancer cells seem advanced, in which case radiation therapy is suggested. Stages B and C require either a complete surgical removal of the prostate gland or intensive radiation therapy, which reaps a similar result. The symptoms of stage D (advanced) disease can be lessened with hormone therapy as well as surgery. Though the manner and timing by which these therapies are implemented remain controversial, the goal is to reduce symptoms and make the patient more comfortable.

New advances in treatment are being developed every day. For example, a new surgical technique called a subcapsular prostatectomy (or partial removal of the prostate gland) seems to be successful in halting some cancers without causing the patient to become impotent. Unfortunately, long-term results are not yet known.

The Food and Drug Administration recently approved a new treatment called Zoladex, which is manufactured by ICI Pharma. It's an injectable hormone that acts on the pituitary/sex gland system and reduces the production of testosterone to levels that result in a medical castration. Zoladex is administered by your physician in a single injection each month. It can reduce tumor size and improve urological symptoms and bone pain.

The Prostate Cancer Education Council (PEC) and the National Institute of Cancer (NCI) have developed helpful brochures about prostate cancer that can be obtained by calling NCI's toll-free hot line, 1-800-4-CANCER, or by writing to Prostate Cancer Education Council, JAF Box 888, New York, NY 10116.

268. ***My husband had a lump in his testicle. After my prolonged nagging, he went to see the doctor. The doctor held a light behind the testicle and said he could see light through it, so it was only a cyst and nothing to worry about. A couple of years later, without any reason that we can figure, the testicle has swollen to three times its size and has remained swollen. The doctor has said by phone that if it doesn't hurt, don't worry about it. These diagnoses sound pretty cavalier to me. I would like my husband to go to a second doctor. What do you think?***

I suppose we're operating here on the principle, "If it isn't TOO broken, don't fix it," but your desire for a better explanation is certainly valid.

Let us first assume that the mass is in the scrotum or sac, rather than in a part of the testicle. Such cysts are common and are known as hydroceles. They are filled with a clear, sterile fluid, which results from overproduction or reduced absorption of the fluid produced by tissues within the scrotum. This fluid production may become increased when an inflammation exists, such as following an infection or trauma. Light can shine through these cysts, as the doctor demonstrated during your husband's examination.

Another type of cyst found close to the testes is a spermatic cyst, or spermatocele. It lies adjacent to the epididymis, the structure that stores sperm. The spermatocele contains sperm. It likewise allows light to pass through. Telling this cyst apart from a hydrocele is often quite difficult.

However, most doctors do agree that if these masses are not too big and do not cause pain and discomfort, they're best left alone. Needle aspiration, which draws off the fluid into a syringe, is at best temporary and may result in an infection. The only totally effective treatment for removing these liquid-filled cysts is surgical removal, and from the sound of it, old-fashioned nagging isn't going to convince your husband to undergo an operation he really doesn't need.

269. ***Why don't you ever respond to people who write to you with their sexual problems? You must get loads of letters like that, because most people like me are too ashamed to talk to their doctors. Or are***

you just like most other doctors who clam up when the subject comes up, because they're embarrassed and just don't want to talk about it?

I have no difficulty either talking to patients about their intimate problems or writing about sexual problems. Frankly, most of the letters I receive are either too individualized or too intimate to be published. When there are subjects of general interest, I do try to include them, for it is clear to me that there is a great deal of interest about the subject and not a great deal of clear thinking or easy-to-understand explanation.

Now in defense of my profession, I believe that most family physicians are skilled in discussing personal sexual matters, because they have had special training in their residency programs, or because their professional experience and study have provided a good deal of valuable insight. I realize that many patients have difficulty opening up to their doctor on this matter, but if only they would take the first step they would be well served.

If the physician has the skills necessary, the problem may be solved easily at this stage of medical care. If not, then opportunities for care can be obtained through referral to another doctor or to an agency that has the specialized knowledge needed to deal with the situation.

Sometimes patients have difficulty in finding the right words and think they need to explain their condition in highfalutin medical jargon. Nothing is further from the truth. A sincere story, honestly told, is all you need to convey the problem to your doctor. There can be no shame where there is no guilt, and judging guilt certainly is not within the scope of my profession.

270.

Please give me an update on Proscar, the new drug that is supposed to shrink the prostate. I want to use it, but my doctor says, "Let's wait; it's too early to see what side effects it will cause," etc. He also says the expense is pretty steep for a senior citizen. How expensive? I need to start on this pill as soon as possible.

The Food and Drug Administration approved this drug for the treatment of benign prostate hypertrophy (BPH) in 1992. Proscar (finasteride is the generic equivalent), manufactured and distributed by Merck, is the first of a new class of drugs known as 5-alpha reductase inhibitors.

Proscar is approved for use in cases of symptomatic BPH, and it's probably most effective in mild to moderate cases. BPH (or prostatism) can be seen in almost 100 percent of men over the age of 80, and prostate changes can be discovered in about 50 percent of men by the time they reach 60.

But the course of the condition is variable and unpredictable. Many men remain without symptoms, some show slow progression, and others remain stable. Some lucky ones even show a regression of the condition. However, about 400,000 men a year have symptoms severe enough to require surgery.

The prostate is a small gland located at the base of the bladder. It surrounds the tubelike urethra, which carries urine from the bladder out of the body. The prostate's function is to produce semen, which transports sperm during ejaculation.

The prostate reaches normal size during puberty. Then the prostate remains stable until after the age of 45, when the tissue begins to change and grow, causing the prostate to increase in size. The enlarging prostate squeezes the urethra, producing the symptoms that characterize BPH. These symptoms include difficulty in starting urination (hesitancy), a weak urinary stream, dribbling after urination, and frequency or urgency during the sleep period. Sometimes urination is painful. These symptoms of obstruction of the urethra often can become more severe if a urinary infection develops, which is one of the common complications of BPH.

Hypertrophy of the prostate tissue is related to the actions of the active form of testosterone called DHT (for 5a-dihydrotestosterone). The new drug interferes with the process that transforms testosterone into DHT. This leads to a reduction in the size of the prostate gland. The maximum effect of the medication occurs after three months of oral therapy. The daily recommended dose is 5 milligrams a day, which is a single tablet. A decrease in the prostate's size, averaging 12 percent, can be expected after four weeks of treatment, and the maximum decrease in size is about 28 percent. These amounts are usually enough to reduce symptoms, with up to 90 percent of patients showing significant improvement in their urinary flow after one year.

Side effects seem to be minimal, with most patients having no problems. When reactions such as headache do occur, they seem to be mild and transient. Data concerning long-term reactions to the medication is expected to be reported soon.

As to expense, the average cost of 30 5-milligram tablets (a one-month supply) at four pharmacies I called in my local area was $60. You would have to price them in your locality, where the price might differ considerably from mine.

271. ***Several years ago at the request of my first wife, I had a vasectomy. Times have changed, however, and now my second wife wants to be a mother. She's encouraging me to have an operation that will permit me to father a child. I was told originally that reversing the operation was impossible. Can you offer me any help or suggestions?***

Your first surgery must have taken place before the development of newer techniques. At that time, there was but a slim chance of reconnecting the cut portions of the vas deferens (the tube that normally carries the sperm). Attempts at that time resulted in poor pregnancy rates of 5 to 30 percent. This is easy to understand when you consider that the operation requires constructing a leakproof connection in a tube with an inner opening of only 0.3 millimeters (twelve-thousanths of an inch).

With the newer microsurgical techniques, the chances of a successful outcome are greatly improved. Now, the passage of sperm through the reconnected vas deferens is noted in more than 95 percent of the cases, and pregnancy rates are up to 63 percent. There are some factors, however, that can reduce these numbers somewhat.

The longer the time between the original operation and its reversal (repair), the greater the chance that some damage has occurred in the epididymis, which is an elongated, cordlike structure in which the sperm are stored and mature. If a secondary obstruction has developed there, the operation to correct it is even more difficult.

After a vasectomy, antibodies to sperm develop in the individual. These titers (levels) of antibodies may persist after the corrective operation (although the antibodies usually disappear after a time), which lowers the chances of pregnancy. Such a condition is often successfully treated with corticosteroids.

During the operation, the surgeon can take a sample of the sperm located in the testicular side of the vas (tube). If they are normal, healthy sperm with tails, there is a high probability that your operation will bring you and your wife the desired outcome.

272. ***When I married my gorgeous hunk of a man, I never suspected that some of his bulges were the unnatural result of steroids. I love the man, not the muscles, and want a baby to complete our family. However, we have been unsuccessful, and the doctor suspects it's the***

medications. Is it true that muscle-building hormones can destroy a man's ability to father a child?

I think the most powerful part of this response are the words in your question: "I love the man, not the muscles." Perhaps when your husband reads your sentiments, the muscles will be less important to him and he'll seek medical help. But the frightening facts are that among the many unwanted and dangerous side effects of anabolic steroids (the kind of hormones that build muscle) are several that have a direct bearing on a man's fertility.

The use of these steroids not only diminishes the number of sperm to the point of nonexistence, but it can provoke abnormal forms as well. The sperm that are produced are less active than normal, and the man's ability to father a child is severely affected.

In addition to reproductive difficulties, steroids can cause hair loss, baldness, acne and provoke severe alterations in mood and temperament. Athletes on steroids are aggressive and irritable, perhaps an advantage on the field of competition but definitely a handicap in marital situations. And many athletic associations have banned the use of steroids completely. Besides, cholesterol imbalance, liver tumors and hepatitis have been associated with the use of these chemicals.

Unless your husband's livelihood depends upon an overdeveloped body, it's hard to imagine a reason for the misuse of these steroids. The good news is that their effects on sperm production and sperm activity seem to be reversible, and a return to normal can be expected when the drug's use is discontinued.

It may be time for your husband to take a good look at his priorities and look to the future. A visit to his physician also might help, for I'm sure his doctor can provide him with more information dealing specifically with his problems.

273. ***A lump in my scrotal sac is bothering me. Is this a sign of cancer of the testicle? It isn't painful. Maybe it's my imagination, but I think it's growing. What does this mean?***

Although testicular cancer is relatively rare, it is a leading cause of cancer death in men between the ages of 15 and 34. It's more common in whites than in blacks or Hispanics, and extremely rare in men over 45.

The first symptom may be a painless lump that you discover while taking a shower or during sex. It can become painful or swell in the course of a few days or even hours. Sometimes the first symptom is back pain.

If your doctor finds a lump or irregularity on the surface of your testicle, he might first treat you with antibiotics, because the greatest probability is that an infection is causing the problem. But a follow-up visit is a must.

If the symptoms persist after antibiotic therapy, the next step is an ultrasound study of the testes to detect any lesions or tumors. Both testicles will be studied so they can be compared to see if there are any abnormalities. If a tumor is found, your doctor also will want to conduct a CT scan and chest X-rays to determine what stage of progress the disease is in. Staging (which evaluates how far the disease has progressed) is important to determine the precise treatment required.

Testicular cancer grows very rapidly, so it's important to detect and treat the problem as early as possible. When detected in the earliest stage, 95 percent of patients can be cured; in the second stage, more than 90 percent, and in the third stage, 75 to 80 percent. Once you have been cured, you will have to watch the other testicle for symptoms for the rest of your life, with annual or more frequent checkups as well as regular self-examinations.

Even a brief delay in making the diagnosis can be tragic. Caught early, testicular cancer can be treated successfully and you can enjoy a full life.

274. *What can be done to prevent impotence after a man has surgery for prostate cancer?*

After age 50, prostate cancer is among the most common cancers in men. About 36 out of every 100,000 men develop prostate cancer every year. It occurs much more frequently as we age. Half of those with prostate cancer are 70 or older, yet very few are under 50.

Many males in the older group are less concerned about erections than they were at a younger age. However, each patient is different. When possible during treatments involving the prostate, every effort is made not to interfere with the parts of the body vital to erections.

Nevertheless, difficulty with erections occurs in about 40 percent of men with prostate cancer even before they receive any treatment. In many of these men, the impotence is due to other chronic illnesses, not the cancer.

Advances in treating prostate cancer are encouraging. Basically, doctors use radiation and surgery. The prostate gland, seminal vesicles and part of the urinary bladder usually are removed during surgery. This often, but not always, causes impotence.

However, there have been important advances in radiation therapy, and it may not cause impotence. But I must point out that one scientific study revealed that smokers were far more likely to develop impotence following radiation for prostate cancer than were those who do not smoke.

In one particular form of radiation treatment, called brachytherapy, a radioactive source is placed in close proximity to the cancer. It delivers only a low dosage to the surrounding normal tissues, but an extremely high one to the cancer. Results have suggested that brachytherapy prevents impotence in a great majority of men who are treated with it, yet some experts question its long-term effectiveness against certain types of cancer.

275. ***There may be some money exchanged as the result of your answer, so I hope you will look it up to be sure. One of the guys on my bowling team claims he had three testicles, and that his doctor insisted that one of them be removed. The rest of us think that he just had a tumor or something like that. Is it possible to have more than the normal two testicles?***

Let me reassure you that I check all my answers, but this answer was double-checked, since there's so much at stake. Pay up, fellows, the story is completely possible. The condition is called polyorchidism, and it has been a medical curiosity for centuries. Ancient literature credited such men with supervirility and super sexual abilities. But those were just legends!

Actually, most additional lumps or bumps in the scrotal sac are either tumors or cysts, but there are many documented cases that prove more than two testicles are possible. The most common cases have three glands, but there have been reports of as many as five testicles.

Usually the "extra" testicle is on the left side. The patient usually has no symptoms, other than that of a mass. A biopsy, which obtains a piece of tissue for examination under a microscope, is the only sure way to make a diagnosis.

Since these extra glands are not in a normal anatomical position, they may become twisted (torsion), which creates a surgical emergency. As this is a frequent complication, and since these glands frequently turn into malignant tumors, many physicians recommend they be removed surgically before problems occur.

10.

The Special Concerns of Aging

Grow old along with me.
The best is yet to be.
The last of life for which
the first was made.

ROBERT BROWNING
English poet (1812–89)

Growing older can be a fulfilling time, an age when you know what you want out of life but haven't stopped going out and getting it; an age when you have fond memories of the past and still time to make many more happy memories.

Unfortunately, old age is the subject of so many myths that many people fear aging. We live in a society that practices *ageism*, prejudice against people on account of age. Advertisements make us believe that only young people enjoy themselves, are sexual, or have energy. Old people, according to commercials, are tired, feeble, confused, silly and prone to indigestion, constipation, denture stains, arthritis and bladder incontinence. Even more unfortunately, there is a grain of truth in these myths. Although aging is not a disease, getting older means more aches, pains and other changes for your body. Your vision may weaken, your hearing may be less acute, your knees and other joints may start predicting the weather, and you may slow down a bit. Very few people age without one or two physical problems, but the good news is that very few people get all of them.

Answers from the Family Doctor (Questions 276-305)

To my older readers, remember you are not alone. The percentage of the American population that is over 65 is growing as more people live longer. At the turn of the century only 4 percent of our people lived past age 65. Now, more than 12 percent of the population is older than that and 40 years from now, it will be more like 20 percent. Even more important, today's statistics indicate that a 65-year-old man can expect to live another 13 years, while a woman of the same age has about 18 years to enjoy. Yet, though there is no special frontier at the age of 65, no special anatomical or physiological changes that occur, age 65 continues to mark the passage into what is socially recognized as "old age." It is this age around which Social Security and Medicare benefits revolve, when annuity payments begin and when retirement starts for many. Yet no biological laws demand that old age start here.

It is important to understand the aging process, just as it was important to understand what was happening to your body when you went through puberty. Aging is inevitable. It is impossible to stop the flow of time, and almost impossible to stop the effects of time's passage. There is only one known way to keep from aging and that is to die young. Aging, with all its problems, is preferable to that. With a positive outlook, you can make Robert Browning's words true for you: "The best is yet to be."

What is "aging" anyway? It would be easy to define aging as the effects of a long life, but it isn't that simple. We all know people like comedian George Burns, who is keeping a busy schedule of performances well into his 90s. Or producer George Abbott, who worked in the theater into his second century. Former New York Congressman Hamilton Fish Sr. remarried just a few months short of his 100th birthday. Yet Rita Hayworth died of Alzheimer's disease at age 68. Why do some people get old so young while others stay young so old? The nebulous answer is that we don't really know.

Heredity is to some extent a factor. Someone once said that the best way to live a long healthy life is to pick parents who lived to healthy old ages. While it is true that some of the infirmities of old age, such as impaired vision and hearing or arthritis, do run in families, there is more to aging than your family tree. Different people may age at different rates, but their problems will be similar. In any event, we don't get to pick our parents.

How well we take care of ourselves also can help us lead longer lives. People who smoke, are sedentary, overeat and drink generally do not live as long as people who do not smoke, keep their weight down and exercise regularly. Keeping active is the best advice most people will get on how to stay young for an extended period of time. Activity helps both the mind and body, since parts that are used regularly usually keep working. More people rust out than wear out.

There is no simple explanation of aging, although several theories exist. These theories basically fall into two camps. One set of theories says that aging is related to how fast we live — that is, how fast our heart beats, our lungs breathe and our metabolism works — and that outside events, such as exposure to chemicals and accidents, and plain wear and tear, cause damage to our cells that eventually accumulates and wears us out. The other set of theories is based on the idea that aging and death are programmed into us and are an essential part of our lives, like growth and adolescence. These two groups of theories overlap to a great extent, and both may be at least partly right. Both sets of theories rest on the fact that throughout our lives our bodies reproduce and replace the cells that are the building blocks of human flesh. The *genes*, which are contained in a chemical called *deoxyribonucleic acid* (DNA) in each cell's nucleus, tell the cell how to create proteins and other chemicals and when to reproduce.

Most cells in our bodies use the information in DNA to create replacements for themselves at regular intervals. Red and white blood cells are being replaced constantly, as are the cells of the skin and those that line the digestive systems. Other cells, most notably nerve cells in the brain and nervous system, are meant to last a lifetime. As they die off, they are not replaced, although the remaining nerve cells do work harder. As we age, however, DNA is damaged through wear and tear, like a document photocopied too many times. Although the body can repair DNA and does so regularly, it may be that the body slowly loses this ability, so replacement cells that are made are not as good as those made earlier in life. The chemical structures, especially those formed by proteins, that are made based on faulty DNA instructions may be faulty as well.

A protein called *collagen*, which is an important component in skin and connective tissue, becomes less pliable with age and loses its ability to stretch and relax. Some researchers say that unstable molecules called *free radicals*, which are produced normally during metabolism, cause damage to our bodies. This damage accumulates and eventually leads to breakdown of individual cells and organs. On the other hand, other researchers say that certain genes are switched off as we get older, in a predetermined pattern. They point out that different creatures have different life spans that cannot be extended past a certain point. Mice live much shorter lives than people do, but parrots live longer. These researchers note that the maximum human life span is probably in the range of 115 to 120 years. The oldest documented human life was 120 years, while longer life spans for certain groups of people, notably those living in the Republic of Georgia who are said to be in their 150s, are unsubstantiated.

It now seems clear that our immune systems change with age, becoming less able to protect against infections by bacteria and viruses, as well as by other foreign substances. This reduction in the body's defenses explains the increased frequency of cancer, immune disease and infectious disease as the years add up. It also underlines the importance of taking the actions we can control, to prevent that which is preventable, and the need to establish achievable health goals as we enter this stage of our lives.

While each of these theories may include some information that is correct, the present fact is that more people are living to old age than ever before. Research may not be able to extend life past a certain point, but it can help us make the years we do have better. The main goal of *gerontology*, the study of aging, is to allow more of us to age as well as we can with minimum disability. The problems that come with age follow certain patterns. Knowing the patterns, you can plan to avoid undesirable consequences by not giving the problems a chance to develop.

As long as you're going to age — and we all will — it's best to understand as much about it as you can. Then consider the actions you can take to make an extended life span enjoyable — years to expand your horizons and do all the wonderful things that everyone contemplates achieving when they're younger.

The advice available to the older person is so abundant that it could in all likelihood take the rest of your life to read and absorb, but all the best counsel can be reduced to three important fundamentals. They are: Exercise regularly, with due consideration to your physical ability; maintain an appropriate state of nutrition by eating a well-balanced, nutritionally sound diet; and preserve a positive mental attitude by remaining involved in intellectual pursuits. Individuals who follow such a simple regime, no matter their age, can feel better and enjoy life more than any 35-year-old who's working under stress, drinking too much, smoking and overeating, and allowing the weight to mount up while pursuing a sedentary, couch potato existence.

Change the word "exercise" to "activity" and you take the sting out of it for some people. Yet it conveys the same message and achieves the same rewards. Walking is sufficient. A good pace that doesn't tax the system is enough to maintain muscle strength and preserve the mobility of joints, while improving both the cardiac and pulmonary reserves. The secret is not overexertion but regularity: 25 to 30 minutes per session at least three times a week. Walking with two or three others transforms it into a desirable social event and helps keep motivation high. In addition, many seniors with an active athletic past, such as in tennis or golf, are able to continue the pursuit of their sport indefinitely.

Eating can be another social event, and the choice of nutritious foods is made ever easier by the new labeling information now required by the Food and Drug Administration. Checking content for excess salt, cholesterol and fat content, as well as caloric value of each portion, makes the scheduling of a nutritious diet a snap, even an interesting task that is but a small challenge to your calculating skills. Older folks don't require the same caloric intake as they did in younger years, and a declining sense of taste can be compensated for by launching adventures into the flavors of new spices, such as ginger, garlic, chili and curry. Planning and preparing the day's food can be fun, and even in institutional surroundings, the development of a "menu committee" can provide both challenge and satisfaction for the participant. The secret is to formulate a meal plan that is balanced and that assures an intake of all the basic nutrients, proteins, carbohydrates, fats, minerals and vitamins, while adhering to the principle of "moderation in all things."

A healthy mental attitude requires a persistent curiosity: the desire to learn more; to achieve new accomplishments; to explore new vistas. Crafts provide the opportunity to learn new manual skills, keeping fingers and hands busy and dextrous. Painting and sculpture offer new avenues of expression, and time becomes an asset instead of an encumbrance; moments for living instead of waiting. The older years become truly "the golden years."

Help is available for the American senior citizen from many sources. Principal among these are government agencies, the federal government, the Social Security system (including Medicare programs), the National Institutes of Health, and the offices of senators and congressmen. Many state governments have established commissions and divisions to deal with the special problems of the aging and provide some health services through Medicaid programs. County and local services also are available, and all of these resources can be found in the special pages of the local telephone directory — quite literally only a telephone call away. When all else fails, a visit to the social services department of a local hospital can put you on the right track.

Additional support can be found in many self-help and special interest organizations for seniors, such as the American Association of Retired Persons and the Gray Panthers. Their monthly publications list an array of available resources, with enough information to help senior citizens get assistance.

Questions and Answers

276. ***Though some friends think I'm too old, I want to start an aerobics class to get back into shape. However, I don't want to hurt myself, and I have never been known as athletic. Are there any precautions I should take to avoid unwanted and unneeded problems?***

First get a medical exam. Your doctor may want to do a cardiac stress test to make sure you won't jolt your heart. Then start slowly. I recommend low-impact aerobics to my older patients. Low-impact aerobics can give their bodies the same overall workout and cardiovascular conditioning as regular aerobics, but it doesn't put too much stress on their joints.

With high-impact aerobics, many people develop pain and swelling in the joints, which can aggravate arthritic conditions. Pain also may develop in the muscles and tendons, because of the pounding effect of all the jumping.

In low-impact aerobics, one foot is always on the ground. The dance steps usually involve stepping back and forth or side to side, while at the same time moving the arms and upper body. There are no jumping or bouncing steps.

The goal of aerobic exercise is to get your heart rate up to 60 to 80 percent of your maximum rate. To calculate your target heart rate, subtract your age from 220. This gives your maximum heart rate. Your target zone is 60 to 80 percent of that number. For example, a 45-year-old person's target heart rate zone is from 105 to 140 beats per minute. To gain full aerobic benefits, you must exercise at least 20 to 30 minutes each time. In addition, the exercise routine must be repeated at least three times a week.

Remember to do a cool-down period; just slow down your movements for several minutes to return your heart rate back to normal. Then stretch your muscles to avoid cramping. Take a moment to consider how great you feel and how much good you have done for yourself — and enjoy your day!

277. ***Why would a woman who virtually never took a hard drink in her life suddenly become an alcoholic? On a visit to my mother, we became aware of a change in her living habits, and we discovered a trash can***

full of empty bottles, mostly vodka, hidden in the basement. Her neighbors also have noted inexplicable actions that just don't fit. What is happening here, and how can we help?

There may be many explanations for changes of behavior in an older woman, but I will go along with your supposition, based on the unusual findings in the basement trash can.

Alcoholism in older people differs greatly from the disease we find in younger people. There is a classification of people who start drinking in later life called reactors, who use alcohol as a response to the stresses that accompany aging. It's more frequent in women than men, and about one-third of drinking problems of the elderly fall into this category.

These reactors do not obtain the high that young drinkers seek, but may have memory lapses, headaches and confusion as a reward for their alcohol intake. Their response to alcohol also is much stronger because of their age, changed physical makeup and changed physiology.

The most difficult part of diagnosis and treatment is recognizing that the problem is not simply a change due to aging but has an actual basis in the overuse of alcohol. Once you can get your mother to admit to the practice, she probably will do well with therapy. She may be reluctant to enter an institution for care, so remember persuasion is a better tactic than confrontation. Once in a counseling program, older people tend to be reliable about attending meetings and sessions.

You also may have to examine her current lifestyle and its implications as part of the cause of the problem. Changes in her living situation may be required. But with family support, careful attention to her personal needs and expectations and professional assistance, your mother's chances of beating this late-blooming problem are good.

278. ***I have just learned of another person with Alzheimer's disease, this time a member of our own family. I don't understand where this disease came from, for I surely never heard of it years ago. Could it be the result of an infection like AIDS, which is another disease that was not known when I was just a girl? Perhaps you could shed some light on this new epidemic.***

Your perceptions are correct. There are many more cases of Alzheimer's disease diagnosed today than in the past. Alzheimer's is one of the two illnesses that account for the largest number of dementia cases now seen. It's diagnosed in 50 to 60 percent of all dementia cases.

During the past century, this type of dementia was rare, as few people reached the age of 75. Today, in the United States, more than half the population attains the age of 75, and more than 25 percent live to the age of 85. That leads to the astonishing fact that at present, more than 2.6 million people have dementia in our country, a number that is expected to reach more than 4 million by the year 2000, and almost 9 million by 2040. That's as many as one in 30 Americans. Thus it is a developing problem with far-reaching implications for the future.

The cause of the disease is not yet fully understood, but present thinking does not include infection as one of the possibilities. The only well-established risk factor is age. There may be a genetic link, for a history of Alzheimer's in the family increases risk about fourfold.

Another link may be to aluminum, for it's found in brain cells of Alzheimer's patients in elevated amounts. But it's not clear whether the aluminum accumulates in cells that already are altered by the disease, or whether this substance is acting as a toxin that causes the illness.

Previous head trauma may be another risk factor, since statistics reveal that such injuries increase the possibility of Alzheimer's by 2.8 times. It's clear there is a real need for more research in this area if the increasing number of cases is to be reduced.

279. ***Although I have passed 75, I still wish to keep my health as perfect as possible. When I last visited my doctor, he told me that I was slightly anemic, but that testing for the cause was not necessary. Does this mean that my anemia is a part of getting old, and there's nothing to worry about?***

I wish I had an exact answer for your question, and I suspect that many physicians would, too. There is quite a bit of controversy about anemia in older people. Some researchers say there's evidence that anemia is a normal part of aging, and that the standards used to measure normal levels of hemoglobin in younger people should be reduced for evaluating older patients.

Other researchers say although anemia of some degree is very common in older people, it should not be considered as a part of the aging process. They believe that all causes of anemia should be carefully sought and proper treatment prescribed.

Anemia may be the result of many chronic diseases, as well as poor nutrition. However, intensive testing for specific causes in people with a low-grade anemia rarely provides a clear-cut answer that identifies a specific cause. I think your doctor knew that when he told you the tests were unnecessary.

We consider anemia to be low grade if the hemoglobin is just below 14 grams/deciliter (g/dL) for men and 12 g/dL for women. A person is at high risk if the level is below 12 g/dL for men and 10 g/dL for women.

Most often the anemia is not the result of a single factor but rather the effect of several components that combine to lower the hemoglobin. By correcting the diet, paying attention to iron metabolism and vitamin intake, and treating any chronic disease, the level of hemoglobin may be adjusted upward. Whether or not we can accurately lay the blame for your anemia on aging, your physician's reassuring "not to worry" statement was certainly in order.

280. *Is a case of acute appendicitis more dangerous to an older person? I always had the notion that only young people could develop this condition. Perhaps you can clarify this situation for me.*

Although acute appendicitis is primarily a disease of the young, it's not unusual in older people. The danger lies in delaying treatment (by mistaking the symptoms for those of other illnesses), since a ruptured appendix can lead to peritonitis, abscess and even death.

Time, say the experts, is a crucial factor in dealing with the disease because mortality rates are highest (especially in the elderly) when emergency surgery is required. Usually appendicitis follows a pattern: Pain begins at the navel and gradually moves to the lower right side of the abdomen. Nausea, vomiting, diarrhea, tenderness or low-grade fever normally follow.

With older folks, however, this course may not hold true. Other factors may hinder proper diagnosis. For instance, in 45 percent of cases, pain does not localize, and in older patients it's always less intense. Special problems, such as senility, fear or deafness, may make communication with the older patient difficult. And other conditions present at the time, such as heart disease, circulatory problems, diabetes and intestinal disorders like diverticulitis often mimic or mask the symptoms.

281. ***My father is a wonder. Without any doubt, he can predict the coming of bad weather, especially bad storms. He says he can feel it in his bones, and I've heard other people say the same thing. I no longer question this ability but would like to know how they manage to do this. Is it a psychic ability, or is there something special about their bones? Is there a medical answer to this question?***

Bad weather usually is preceded by a falling barometer, which indicates a lower barometric pressure. You have but to check your local TV weather reporter to verify that. Now assuming that your father isn't getting his "inside" information from the same weather report that you do, it may be that his joints are special. He may suffer from arthritis.

The pain that arthritics suffer on a daily basis often is increased when the atmospheric pressure drops. If the humidity is also on the rise, the ailing joint may give out a warning signal: an increase in the intensity of the usual pain and sensitivity. Some individuals are particularly aware of these changes, even when they are slight, and they can predict a change in the weather, most often from fine weather (high barometric pressure) to bad weather or an oncoming storm. When researchers asked people with arthritis to keep a daily record noting when their joint pain was more severe, the days of increased pain coincided with days of low barometric pressure.

I don't think it's totally clear why this happens. Arthritic joints are inflamed and often produce additional liquid that stays in the joint. The tissue in normal joints is able to reduce the amount of liquid in the joint to match the changing air pressure, while the arthritic joint maintains the fluid and the increased pressure. Since an inflamed joint is more sensitive anyway, it may be able to sense this additional pressure as well.

So you can believe your dad the next time he tells you that his bones are predicting bad weather. It's not an expression of psychic powers, but a physical sensation he's experiencing.

282. ***It seems as though we all sit around and complain about our stomachs much of the time. Why do elderly people have so many digestive disorders? Are some gastrointestinal problems more common to senior citizens?***

Elderly people suffer from digestive disorders because of many different factors. Although the gastrointestinal (GI) tract usually does not change greatly due to the aging process, there are influences other than aging that take their toll. Malnutrition, a reduction in exercise or a problem with any other part of the body may lead to digestive symptoms that range from abdominal pains to constipation to dysphagia (difficulty with swallowing).

The number of cases of cancer somewhere in the digestive system is very high among the elderly. Chromosomal instability is often the cause, but other factors include a diet low in fiber and high in carcinogens or a chronic inflammation of the lining of the stomach.

Diverticular disease also is common among the elderly. Here again, a low-fiber diet is one of the leading causes of this painful problem, in which pouches or sacs form in some part of the digestive tract. A low-fiber diet often causes constipation. This, in turn, increases the pressure in the colon that promotes the formation of these sacs. Ulcerations near the diverticula can cause colonic hemorrhage that complicates matters.

The incidence of gastric ulcers rises with age. In many cases, these ulcers are found in people who must take aspirin and other kinds of medications, as the elderly often do.

Diseases of the mouth and esophagus also are found more frequently among the elderly than among younger folk. Many of these problems can be prevented with regular teeth brushing, gum massage and flossing.

Gallbladder problems also develop in the elderly, because as individuals age their bile contains fewer acids that break down the substances that cause gallstones. But you can do more than talk about your digestion. A change in diet, a bit of exercise and a little prudence can work wonders.

283. ***We've been going out with a couple our age for years, ever since we both bought apartments in this community. Last night at dinner they announced that they've decided to go their separate ways and are filing for divorce. We're devastated and don't know how to react. It's as if someone died. What can we do for them? And how can we deal with our own feelings? Is there anything you can tell us that might help?***

It's hard to stand aside and watch as two close friends end their relationship. It's in many ways like losing a loved one. But just as in cases of grief after the passing of a friend, the first and probably the hardest thing you must do is to accept the fact. The least productive and most agonizing effort would be to try to intercede to change what two adults already have decided for themselves.

You do not have to make a choice between them. It's possible to maintain an ongoing friendship with each of them, as they begin to construct new lives. A great deal will depend upon the course of their divorce proceedings, which may be very destructive or, more happily, may leave them both emotionally and psychologically intact.

They may wish to continue to see you separately. That's fine, but be careful not to become trapped into sessions in which their personal anger against the former partner is being vented. It's a no-win position, so change the conversation to more neutral and happier subjects. If these meetings begin to fall into a repetitive pattern, it may be best to ease off the relationship for a while and let the wounds heal.

This is a good time for you and your spouse to open some lines of communication to discuss with each other your personal feelings about the couple. Don't become divided by taking sides, but try to develop a unified position that both of you can accept. These conversations may help you overcome your own grief or anger about your friends' divorce. It's quite possible that both of you are developing your own strong feelings, and it's very important that you share your feelings.

Just as their relationship has changed, your relationship with each of them must change. Trying to keep things as they were won't work, so strive to establish new common ground for a continuing friendship. While both of you may offer support to them during moments of great stress, don't overdo it and try to act as a replacement for the portions of their lives that they're losing. Sympathy and understanding are fine, but activities such as cooking for the divorced husband are not conducive to a healthy relationship between him and you.

While the first shock of their separation seems hard to bear now, another more dramatic incident may be in the future. As your friends seek to achieve new lives, they may decide that the best opportunities lie over the horizon and decide to leave. This may provoke another episode of pain, but even here you have some opportunities to act as friends who are considerate, caring and helpful. Assisting with the moves or accepting the responsibility of caring for precious possessions until your friends become settled can help greatly. Then you can look forward to the pleasure of visiting and corresponding, which at the very least will help you keep in touch with these people you seem to care for so much.

284. ***I have read this term several times but have never understood it. What is a "dowager's hump"? What causes it to form, and what do you have to do to get rid of it?***

When certain women grow older, past the age of menopause, they develop a curvature of the spine as a result of the bone condition called osteoporosis. As the deformity becomes more pronounced, it's called a dowager's hump. One of the definitions of dowager is "an elderly woman of wealth and dignity."

Osteoporosis is predominantly a disease of women. It's a generalized progressive reduction in bone mass that causes the bones to weaken. The spinal column supports our skeleton and provides us with a standing posture. It is composed of vertebrae piled one upon the other like a tower of building blocks. As the mineral content (calcium, among other minerals) in these bones diminishes, they begin to collapse slowly, with the front (anterior) end of each "block" becoming smaller. This changes the shape of the vertebra from a square into a triangular form. This creates the curve in the spinal column that we describe as a hump.

There is no cure for dowager's hump as yet. It may be prevented by an active, healthy premenopausal lifestyle that includes proper nutrition that supplies the calcium and other minerals needed to build strong bones. Once the process has begun, it may be halted by replacing the female hormones lost at menopause and using supplementary calcium.

While real cures are still being investigated, there seems little hope of discovering a medication that would reverse the process and reduce the hump. That would require a new growth process similar to the rejuvenation Ponce de Leon sought from the Fountain of Youth.

285. ***I'm in my 70s, and as I grow older I find myself less sure of my footing and have grown unsteady on my feet. I've been fighting off using a cane, probably because of pride, but I wonder if there isn't some other way to deal with this problem.***

I think your question touches many lives, and I'm happy to respond. As life spans get longer, we must dedicate attention to making those additional years productive and filled with happiness and fun. We're aware that things change as we grow older, and we do lose some strength. But it's probable that more strength is lost in older people than need be, simply because life slows down a bit and activity diminishes.

The loss of muscle strength is more noticeable in the legs than in the arms because we continue to use our upper members even while sitting. Therefore, if there are no other medical or neurological causes, the solution may lie in regaining some of the strength in the legs through proper exercise.

Just as exercise is effective in reducing the risk of heart attacks by increasing our cardiovascular fitness, an exercise program also may be designed to increase flexibility and muscle strength. A complete program includes training exercises that develop and maintain strength, low-impact aerobic exercises and some flexibility maneuvers as well. By using a complete program, you can regain the force necessary to walk with greater assurance and steadiness.

More and more programs are being developed just for people like you. A call to your local YMCA or to your physician may be the first step to getting your "steps" back in order and avoiding the need for a cane.

286. ***I guess my advancing age is the reason I'm losing the edge on some of my senses. The eyes are a bit worse; things don't smell as they once did; and now the hearing is going. It's such an important sense that I wonder if there's anything new to help people who lose their ability to hear.***

How right you are! The sad part is that we can lose some of our hearing acuity from so many causes. But there is good news. Thanks to advances in medicine, surgery and technology over the past 30 years, nearly everyone can improve their hearing.

The most significant advances have been for disorders of the middle ear. One of the most common problems is middle-ear effusion (a buildup of fluid), which typically has been treated with one or more drugs, including antihistamines, decongestants, steroids and antibiotics. Not all patients, however, respond to such treatment. Now, some of these patients, particularly those with chronic otitis media, can be treated surgically. The procedure involves inserting a ventilation tube into the ear to relieve symptoms as well as to prevent permanent ear damage until the eustachian tube can function completely.

Researchers also are beginning to make progress in managing problems of the inner ear. One of the most exciting and promising developments in this area is the cochlear implant. A small, self-contained device is placed surgically in the portion of the ear called the cochlea. The patient wears another device that transmits sound through electrical impulses to the implant. The use of this procedure generally is limited to those patients who once had normal hearing but are now totally deaf and cannot benefit from a conventional hearing aid. Although the procedure cannot restore normal or near-normal hearing, it can restore some degree of usable hearing.

Progress also has been made in the treatment of sensorineural hearing loss, which is caused by aging, genetics, infections and injuries (particularly loud noises). Currently, only limited medical and surgical treatments are available. However, improvements in technology have resulted in new high-fidelity hearing aids that can improve substantially the hearing of nearly all patients.

With all these new and exciting developments and the many causes of deafness or hearing loss it's important to have the right diagnosis for your particular problem, so the right remedy can be applied to help you.

287. ***Although it seems to be worse lately, I have had to use a laxative for most of my adult life to keep regular. However, I think it never has been as bad as it is now, and I wonder if my medicine isn't being made as strong as it used to. I'm sure there are many others who would like a word from you about caring for their constipation.***

Your question is one that is asked by many people; in fact, the word constipation comes from the Latin meaning "to crowd together." More than $250 million is spent each year in this country for laxatives, so there must be many people who feel they need help. But many people who use laxatives normally would have five to seven movements a week anyway, which is really all that is necessary to maintain health. However, as people grow older, their bodies do change in function. It becomes harder to move around (which helps the process of digestion), and new diets may fail to contain enough bulk.

When chronic and severe constipation is the complaint, a good medical evaluation is necessary to determine if there are any underlying medical problems that might yield to treatment. But many times changing to a diet that adds additional fiber and encourages you to drink six to eight glasses of fluid daily can help remedy the situation.

Add a bit of exercise, perhaps a long walk, to your daily schedule of activity, and you may achieve your goals. If your current laxative seems less than effective, then try choosing a bulk-forming preparation that contains materials that absorb water and form a larger mass that can stimulate the bowel's actions.

There are many types of laxatives and all have different actions on your system. Your physician is the best source of advice for your situation. However, I don't think that the manufacturer has reduced the amount of active ingredients in your current medication. It's just that you have been changing bit by bit over all these years, and your needs are now different.

288. *Is there any real way to ensure you'll live longer? I've seen some pills in health-food stores that claim to extend your life. Is it possible that they really work?*

I'm sorry to say that with all of the advanced technology we have, there is still no magic elixir that can provide us with a Fountain of Youth. Scientists have been studying gerontology (the study of what happens to the body during normal aging), but they haven't figured out how to slow or stop the aging process.

A large number of Americans are obsessed with youth and staying young. They allow quacks and manufacturers of useless products to make tens of millions of dollars every year. I'm not saying that all of these manufacturers are insincere and intentionally ripping people off, but there is nothing to prove that these products work. Some of the products you might have seen in health-food stores include Dismutase (SOD), Dehydroepiandrosterone (DHEA), and Gerovital-H3.

DHEA, a hormone produced in human beings by the adrenal gland, seems to help curb caloric intake. There have been no scientific studies on people to conclude DHEA supplements have life-extending effects.

Gerovital-H3 is marketed as a treatment for age-related bodily changes. A Romanian doctor reported this substance has helped laboratory rats live longer lives, but those results have not been found by other scientists studying the compound.

There really is no proven method of guaranteeing a longer life, but there are things you can do to help you live a healthier life and perhaps indirectly prolong life. The National Institutes of Health concluded that people who are slightly underweight live longest; other scientists disagree. Exercise, begun early in life, is believed to play an indirect role in life extension. Active people have fewer problems with their hearts and are generally healthier, but studies on athletes done by the National Institute on Aging have not found athletes to have longer lives than the general population.

Proper diet, exercise and a life lived within the rules of good health will make your existence a healthier and more enjoyable one, and it will prevent many diseases that can shorten your time here in this world. Still, it seems there really is only one way you can truly increase your longevity, and that is to choose parents with the right genes. Since that choice already has been made for you, you must make the effort to choose a lifestyle that provides you with the best possible chances for a long and happy life.

289. ***I hate the signs of aging that I can detect in others, and I'm most distressed by those same signs when I find them in myself. Now my husband keeps telling me that I'm losing my memory, and I'm not sure that he's wrong. What can I do about this problem?***

All of us experience moments of forgetfulness from time to time. A busy schedule, worrying over health problems and just plain "too much on our minds" can contribute to temporary lapses of memory. This is perfectly normal and nothing to be alarmed about. But if your memory loss becomes noticeable and troublesome, and you find yourself forgetting recent events (as do an estimated 3 million to 4 million Americans over age 60), it's time to see your doctor.

Some of the early signs of true memory loss that your doctor will be alert for are repeatedly forgetting things like keys, glasses and appointments, retelling stories or events in the same conversation, problems recalling new names and places, difficulty learning new facts or skills, and a progressive lack of interest in appearance and personal hygiene. He'll want to know if you have trouble getting out words "on the tip of your tongue," if your attention span is short and, most importantly, if you often forget things that happen from day to day.

The key words to remember are repeated and often. Occasional slips are inevitable in this hectic world; frequent memory loss is not, and it could signal some physical problem. Among the many possible causes are poor nutrition, diabetes, anemia, thyroid problems, depression and medications or combinations of medications you might be taking. Whatever the cause, the important thing to know is that it's treatable. Early diagnosis can definitely better the chances for improvement.

290. ***I was visiting my father in his new nursing home when I noticed that another patient on his floor was tied into her wheelchair with straps. Now I'm worried that they might treat my father this way. Do you know of any rules that govern the use of these measures in nursing homes?***

While such restraints were pretty common in nursing homes in the past, today they are considered a major no-no. Yes, there is legislation that deals with this issue in the Nursing Home Reform Act (contained in the Omnibus Budget Reconciliation Act), which Congress passed in 1987.

The use of physical restraints (and medications as well) was limited to treating medical symptoms, and the law specifically prohibits their use for the purposes of discipline or convenience. This act forms the basis of the guidelines used by state nursing home inspectors, and it's used by the Health Care Financing Administration, which regulates Medicare- and Medicaid-certified facilities. Since these regulations went into effect, the use of restraints and sedating drugs has been watched closely.

While there are restrictions in the use of these methods of controlling patient behavior, the patterns of behavior in some patients may tax the ingenuity of nursing home staffs. However, in many cases, restraining an agitated patient just makes the situation worse. When improperly applied, restraints can cause injury in the form of skin abrasions and ulcers.

However, there are times when a restraint such as you noticed may have a proper place in caring for these patients. That's when there's a question of safety. The situation that comes to mind first is safety during sleep. When bedrails are judged insufficient to prevent a patient from falling out of bed, restraints may be indicated. They're usually placed in such a manner as to allow the patient to move about with some freedom. In fact, all uses of restraints must be governed by concern for the patient's freedom, dignity and safety. They must be applied in a manner that is comfortable and improves the quality of the patient's life.

291. ***I have noticed that my doctor seems more concerned about all my medicines than in my younger days. He has even changed the dose on some medicines I have taken for years. Is there any reason for all this checking and changing?***

Older people use more medicines than younger people, and they also are much more susceptible to drug reactions and interactions. Most drug studies are conducted on young and middle-aged people, so drug problems are not always identified quickly in older people. For this reason and several others, caution is important.

As we age, our bodies change. These changes affect the way drugs are absorbed and used in our bodies. For instance, the older adult has a slower blood flow to the kidneys. This changes the rate a drug is excreted from the body. If the drug stays in the body for a longer period of time than expected, the dosage should be altered in order to avoid overloading the body with the drug.

Distribution of the drug in the body's tissues may be altered in older people when blood flow slows down. The older body typically has more fat than muscle, so fat-soluble drugs are not distributed as they would be in younger people.

Older people are usually more sensitive to anti-coagulants, narcotics and anti-hypertensive drugs. Barbiturates may create more sedation than usual or may cause agitation. Antihistamines, including those found in over the counter preparations, may create more drowsiness.

Older individuals also may have more chronic health problems that can interfere with the actions of drugs, as well as medicines previously prescribed. Health problems become more complex, and this may require taking several different drugs prescribed by different doctors.

The most important piece of advice I can give you is this: Whenever a medication is prescribed, be sure your doctor knows about every other medicine you're taking, whether by prescription from another physician or something purchased over-the-counter at your pharmacy. This will permit a careful choice of your new medicine and help avoid drug interaction problems.

292. ***When we look around our retirement community, it's apparent that women must be stronger than men somehow, for there are many more women here than men. Yet all the men were hard workers, and most of them were big, strong men. Is there a medical explanation for why women outlive their husbands so often?***

Your observation that more women survive their husbands than vice versa is correct, and your community is not the only one in which that is true. Over the age of 65, the ratio of widows to widowers is about four to one. Despite the fact that more boy babies are born, about 106 boys to 100 girls, by age 75, there are three women to every two men left living.

To try to find the reasons for this, we must look at three factors: differences in the makeup of the genes carried by men and women, the influence of hormones during life, and the types of lifestyles and environments with which men and women live.

To date, studies of the molecular makeup of genes have failed to reveal any differences to account for the advantage in life span that women seem to possess. Research is ongoing in this area, for it still seems likely that part of the answer may lie in the genes.

Since male and female hormones differ, research into the part they play in the metabolism of cholesterol and the resulting development of atherosclerosis and heart disease will be potentially more productive. The reduced probability of developing coronary artery disease in women is certainly part of their longevity.

Smoking was once a factor. Lung cancer was thought to be a man's disease, until women in large numbers took up this habit. As many as seven years of the difference in life expectancy may have been lost by men due to the effects of tobacco. Work-related accidents, deaths due to car accidents, suicide and homicide all take a greater toll on males as compared to females, so that more women survive the years prior to retirement.

However, as age progresses, the gap diminishes. By age 85, the life expectancy of women is but one year longer than that of men. Hopefully, new knowledge about heart disease prevention and smoking cessation will continue to narrow the differences in life expectancy between men and women.

293. ***I'm a long time past my last period, and as a widow, my sexually active days have passed. That is why I'm just a bit put out by my physician's insistence that a pelvic examination be part of my physical checkup. It is not a procedure that I liked much when I was younger and felt it was necessary, but now that I'm past all that I feel it's a waste of time. Don't you agree?***

I'm afraid you're not going to like what I have to say. Though I fully understand your point of view, the fact is there are still many afflictions that may yet affect this area, and you're placing a large obstacle in the path of their diagnoses.

Many conditions are age-related — not the least important of which is genital cancer, which is more common in the older age group and can be diagnosed readily during the pelvic exam. There are still infections, though not necessarily sexually transmitted, that may occur.

You're preventing their early diagnosis, and thus early cure, when you omit the pelvic examination from your regular physical. I'm not advocating that you be examined each time you visit your physician, but certainly it's wise to consider this procedure during a once-a-year annual checkup.

It's also during this exam that problems that may lead to incontinence can be observed, and this exam offers an opportunity to discuss other intimate conditions with your physician. I don't believe his insistence is anything more than a meritorious and professional concern for your well-being and health.

294. ***When Dad died three years ago, my mother decided to stay in her home of many years rather than come live with any of us. Now we know she is lonely, depressed and has few friends to visit, yet she is determined to stay put. In the old days, we had a family dog that Mom adored. Do you think she's too old (age 72) to start again with a new pet that might offer her some companionship?***

All things being equal, if your mother's physical condition is about average for a woman her age, and if she has ample vision and hearing, I think a new pet to offer her companionship and love is a super idea. It may be the motivation needed to put her back on track and help fight off her understandable depression.

The secret is in the proper selection of the pet. A medium-sized dog that requires regular outings is the best choice. This will motivate your mother to take walks, which would benefit her health as well. A big dog might be too strong. Try to adopt an alert dog that is already house-trained, but not too frisky.

Your solution may well put an excellent idea into the minds of many, but before selecting a pet make sure your mother approves of the plan.

295. ***I have a question of a rather delicate nature that I find difficult to bring up with my own physician. Though not an old man by today's standards, I find my sexual ability declining. I know my wife would appreciate more attention, but I don't know what to do about my situation. I'm hoping you may be able to provide me with some advice.***

I'm always disheartened when someone feels restrained in discussing an intimate problem with his or her physician. It means that the relationship is faulty at a time when it is most needed to help with a problem that is not easy to correct. While I'm happy to offer you some insight, I truly hope that you will continue your search for a solution with the consultation and advice that only a personal family physician can offer.

Your problem is not a rare one, and impotence is one of the most common forms of sexual dysfunction. In one form or another, it may be a problem for more than 20 million American men.

Impotence can be either a physical or a mental problem. One of the most easily remedied causes of impotence stems from the unwanted side effects of many prescription medications. Anti-anxiety, anti-depressant and anti-psychotic medications, sedatives, some blood pressure medications, as well as medication used for stomach ulcers and epilepsy must be included in the long list of prescription medications that may be causing your situation. Review any medication you're now on with your physician, since changing or altering dosages may lead to a remedy. Of course, alcohol, illegal drugs — marijuana, cocaine, amphetamines, narcotics — and even nicotine all can be culprits.

The presence of an erection while sleeping (nocturnal penile tumescence) is an indication that the patient is physically capable of a normal erection, and it may be discovered by using one of a number of home monitors that are now available. You're also entitled to a complete physical examination and laboratory work-up to help determine the reasons for your problem.

Impotence has many causes, and it is not a condition that is either all black or all white. Many new effective techniques and treatments now exist, but you will discover which is best for you only by confiding your problem to your doctor.

296. ***Mother came to live with us recently. In the past four months she has had four bad spills. We're quite concerned and would like some tips on preventing additional accidents. Can you help?***

Since falls are a major medical health problem for the elderly, prevention is obviously very important. However, before preventive measures can be taken, it's important to determine the causes of these repeated spills, which aren't always easy to diagnose. Most patients who fall repeatedly attribute their falls to tripping, but this is rarely the case. There can be environmental, physical or psychological factors that contribute to these accidental "spills." A doctor needs to investigate many possibilities before an appropriate evaluation can be made.

Since the home is the most common site for accidents, home hazards should be considered. Slippery floors, loose or torn rugs and poor lighting are all dangerous. Safety measures such as providing handy light switches and good illumination should be taken. Installing handrails for the toilet, bath and stairways, and making floors, bathtubs and carpets nonslip are good precautions as well. Be sure to show Mother the changes you've made and explain that their use can help prevent these accidents.

When physical causes are suspected, doctors will perform a complete physical exam as well as investigate cardiac and neurologic concerns. They also should probe the patient's medical history to determine if she's taking any medications that possibly can be linked to the problem.

Impaired vision or hearing, stiff joints, weak muscles and impaired gait are other factors that may contribute to a fall. To pinpoint potential problems, the patient should be questioned about palpitations, pain, dizziness and shortness of breath. If such factors are present, simple tests, such as monitoring cardiac rhythms, can provide the needed clues. Balancing exercises may help patients with vertigo, and some patients may benefit from sleeping with the head raised or by resting in a sitting position for a few minutes before they stand or walk.

Many elderly people who fall have multiple problems. Without knowing your mother's particular medical history, it's difficult to offer you more specific advice. I suggest you talk things over with her, encourage her to talk about any problems that may not be readily noticeable and suggest she get a complete physical exam. Her falls may not have any serious underlying complications, but there's no harm in seeking a professional consultation.

297. ***I have an adorable and lovable grandfather. He is not only warm and caring, but alert and interesting. Every time he drops something, slips or forgets where he has placed his glasses, he mumbles, "I guess I'm getting senile." I wish there were something I could do to prevent that disease from striking him. Can you help?***

Have I got good news for you! There is no such disease as "senility," and it's not a "must" condition for those who are getting older.

Surely, there are some changes in the way an older person thinks, just as there are physical changes that occur with age. But according to a 1980 report from a task force sponsored by the National Institute on Aging, "Normal aging ... does not include gross intellectual impairment, confusion, depression, hallucinations or delusions. Such symptoms are due to disease and indicate the need for diagnosis and treatment."

To be sure, there are incurable diseases that strike the elderly, such as Alzheimer's disease, which causes mental impairment. But there are some 100 reversible conditions that mimic this disorder, and they can be treated effectively.

Although medical research is working on many of the problems of aging, it may well be that your grandfather may never need them. The best methods of avoiding the problems of aging are to maintain an active life that involves both body and mind, pay careful attention to a balanced diet, and carry out a well-conceived plan for physical fitness. Regular, brisk walks are as useful and beneficial to older people as regular training programs are to athletes. While all these suggestions may help, my guess is that your visits with your grandfather may well be the best preventive medicine available.

298. ***I often read magazine articles that offer advice about sex to older men. They are of little use to me, for as I advance in age and pass my menopause, I could use some information, too. How about giving us older gals some help and advice?***

I'm truly pleased to answer your question. Actually, I get more letters from older women about this subject than I do from the fellows.

An older woman can indeed have a wonderful, healthy sex life after menopause. Despite some physical changes, an older woman's sexual response cycle usually remains in good working order. Orgasms still can be achieved, although in some cases, the intensity and duration may be slightly less than in premenopausal women.

The physical changes that might hamper sexual activity include atrophy of parts of the vagina, which increases the risk of trauma, infection and vaginitis. The pH factor rises and necessary secretions diminish. Elasticity is lessened in the vaginal wall, and the cervix shrinks. However, most women are still very capable of achieving sexual pleasure and should consider it a healthy part of their lives.

Aging ovaries produce less estrogen than they used to, and many doctors recommend estrogen replacement therapy. In many cases, the added estrogen helps relieve or reduce hot flushes, atrophy of the genitals and osteoporosis. The therapy also may promote a sense of well-being. There are some possible negative side effects though, so every patient must discuss the benefits and risks with her doctor before estrogen is prescribed.

Another factor that may impede the sex life of an older woman includes the availability of an acceptable partner. Because women statistically live longer than men, many elderly women are either widowed or their husbands are seriously ill or disabled. The woman herself may have non-sexual physical ailments, such as arthritis, neuromuscular disease or osteoporosis, which can impair sexuality.

The older woman may sink into depression because of her own or her partner's physical ailments and lose interest in activities that are pleasurable, such as sex. It's important for both older women and men to continue to develop hobbies, interests, friendships and loving relationships, so that their self-worth remains high and their interest in their own sexuality will be maintained.

299. ***As a young girl, I took a great deal of pride in the smoothness and softness of my skin. There is no greater reminder that the years have passed than when I look at my skin now and see all the changes that have occurred. What makes skin age so, and is there any way to prevent it?***

Why skin ages is still pretty much of a mystery, although recent research has revealed some definite answers. It's believed that a natural aging system is set in motion at birth and later is compounded by the wear and tear of everyday life, as well as by environmental damage. As we all know, too much exposure to the sun's ultraviolet rays damages the skin and accelerates the aging process.

However, there are more subtle factors that influence the skin's aging process. Within the dermis (the skin layer just beneath the surface layer) are the cells that form the elastic tissue of the skin. In time, their elasticity deteriorates and causes wrinkling.

Pigment cells also deplete with age. Since these cells act as a protective barrier to sunlight, their loss increases susceptibility to sun damage. Immune cells, known as Langerhans cells, are reduced by nearly half their number over time, which weakens the skin and makes it more prone to certain skin cancers. As we grow older, the connection between the top two layers of skin becomes weaker, which permits those hateful wrinkles to develop.

With all this knowledge, I'm sorry to report that, at present, there is no known remedy for the skin aging process. Avoiding intense sun exposure is the best advice dermatologists can offer, since moisturizers and estrogen-containing creams have shown no long-lasting positive results. However, a prescription acne product developed a number of years ago has a subtle rejuvenating effect on the skin — it can erase and flatten some of the wrinkles. You might wish to ask your doctor about this.

300. *My dad, who is 75, has a number of skin growths. Should he just leave them because of his advanced age, or should he seek some medical treatment?*

Well, a dermatologist friend of mine says it's never too late to treat skin growths. In older people, she thinks it's very important, from an emotional standpoint. Some growths are badges of age that she feels people don't always wear proudly. So, by all means take your dad to a doctor.

The typical growths found in the elderly are small, discolored skin tags in which malignant transformation is rare and treatment is relatively simple. Removal usually is accomplished through scraping, freezing or acid treatments. Liver spots, which are another type of skin growth, frequently go untreated and are waved off as a sign of aging. But there is no need for this, since they are simple to treat and respond to bleaching or liquid nitrogen peels.

The more serious growths are cancers, and they must be treated. Basal cell carcinoma, which is found most often on the head, neck or upper trunk, is a slowly advancing cancer that is easy to remove through cryosurgery. Squamous cell carcinoma that develops as a solitary nodule sometimes necessitates deeper procedures, as does malignant melanoma.

Let your father be treated for these growths, either for his ego or for his life.

301. *Some time ago, my wife and I moved to this retirement facility so that we would have more of a social life than was possible before. However, ever since we arrived, I have been unable to sleep well, and get only a few hours a night. Will this loss of sleep cause me any harm?*

It's not how many hours of sleep you get, nor even whether the sleep is light or interrupted, that is important, but rather how well you have rested. If you still feel perky in the morning, no matter what pattern your sleep took, you're fine and no harm will occur.

With advancing age and a change in your home environment, you have some very understandable reasons for a change in the amount and type of sleep you're experiencing. As we grow older, our need for sleep changes. We spend more time awake in bed than before, and have less light and deep sleep, but our bodies function just as well.

You might consider a number of things that could make your sleep habits change. These include various medications: blood pressure pills, cortisonelike medications, and various anti-depressants and antihistamines. You might wish to discuss these with your doctor.

Then, too, aches and pains, the need to visit the bathroom, irregular heartbeats, difficulty in breathing, outside noises you have yet to become accustomed to, and even your wife's snoring (does she?) all can contribute to breaking up a night's rest. Are you napping more during the day? If so, that, too, can contribute to making your night's sleep less satisfying.

Try a few of these suggestions, in addition to correcting any of the situations I have outlined above:

- While you should establish a regular routine for retiring and rising, it may help to stay up a bit longer and participate in some relaxing activity.
- Stay away from stimulants like coffee or tea in the evening.
- If you suffer from a condition that causes a chronic pain, ask your doctor to help you change the schedule of pain medication, so that you take one before retiring.

Answers from the Family Doctor (Questions 276-305)

Review your problem with your physician, who should have some insight about you and may have just the remedy you need.

302. ***I'm a senior citizen now living in a retirement home. I don't like this living among so many people who are deteriorating in body and mind, although there also are many fine, intelligent people. I know I will not always be able to take care of myself. Would I have been better if I had moved into a smaller place? I like peace and quiet, good books and knowing what is going on in the world. Please give me your opinion, and I thank you.***

After a lifetime of living in quarters of your own choosing and making, it's hard to adjust to the group living of a retirement community. This is a time when one wishes for quiet calm, when all the adjustments needed to live a lifetime of happiness, sadness, triumphs and defeats have been mastered. When all one wishes for are simpler pleasures, the need to adapt one more time may seem a difficult task.

Still, I'm sure you can achieve it with little effort if you develop the proper perspectives and attitudes. Many people choose a home based upon convenience for relatives, location or costs, without the necessary information that lets them choose the right environment for their lifestyle. It isn't too late for you to search for another location, but the effort necessary to assure yourself that the people and surroundings meet your needs may require help from your friends and family. If you do find such a facility, then your choice seems clear.

However, you might consider the possibilities that exist in your present location. Are there other people who share your views? Who read as you do? Are they seeking someone to share their ideas with and to discuss their points of view? The odds are that you'd have a better chance of finding such people in a larger place, with more candidates to choose from. Is there a social worker, nurse or administrator to help you with your search?

With your obvious alertness, you might want to start a book club or a discussion group to share the new experiences gained through reading. Perhaps by turning your eyes and spirit outward rather than retreating into solitude, you can convert your present surroundings into a new world of friendship and happiness, and find new paths of enjoyment.

303. ***My doctor says my stomach is atrophying. I'm horrified. I have no idea what this means, nor how dangerous it is. Could you please explain, without frightening me further?***

Atrophic gastritis (atrophy of the stomach) is a common condition in older people. In most of them, it causes little or no problem. The condition is characterized by inflammation and atrophy (which means "to waste away" or "fail to grow") of the lining of the stomach, not the stomach as a whole. The inflammation is accompanied by a shortage of hydrochloric acid, which is one of the acids the stomach secretes to digest food, as the amount of acid-producing tissue is reduced. The symptoms for atrophic gastritis include indigestion, a feeling of fullness in the stomach after small meals, weight loss, hives and wheezing.

Because gastric acid protects the intestinal system in addition to digesting food, atrophic gastritis is sometimes complicated by intestinal infections. People with atrophic gastritis are more likely to pick up bacterial and viral intestinal infections, such as traveler's diarrhea. In some cases, atrophic gastritis can be accompanied by nutritional deficiencies, such as pernicious anemia or a lack of calcium. Pernicious anemia, if present, is treated with vitamin B-12 shots and iron supplements.

Atrophic gastritis was once thought to be a risk factor for stomach cancer, but recent studies have shown this not to be so. However, carcinoid tumors of the stomach, which are not malignant, may be associated with atrophic gastritis. Your physician probably will examine your stomach through an endoscope at regular intervals to check for these growths and to keep an eye (literally) on your condition.

304. ***I'm 70 years old, and with the passing years I seem to be losing a bit of my hearing. Many people who are my age seem to be in the same boat. Is a "tin ear" something we just have to accept as part of getting older?***

Recent studies show that about one in three Americans 65 years of age or older — including former President Reagan — experiences some sort of hearing impairment (defined here as deafness in one or both ears, or any other trouble hearing).

The statistics are quite revealing. In men from the ages of 65 to 74, almost 30 percent report some hearing loss. Women seem to be better off, as only 17.5 percent in this age group have difficulty. About 13 percent of males 65 to 74 reported deafness in one or both ears, compared with 8 percent of the women. And about 8 percent of both sexes said they use a hearing aid.

In people over 85, the percentages of individuals with partial or complete deafness becomes somewhat greater. So, you're not alone. I'll just shout a bit louder when addressing answers to my older readers!

305. ***I had to laugh when I walked behind our group of women on our daily walk. We're between the ages of 71 and 83, and it was just like a group of ducks were waddling down the avenue. We all seem to have the same peculiar walk, yet none of us is particularly ill. Is this a natural result of aging? We would like very much to know.***

I doubt that anyone is comparing you to ducks. Just look around you. You will find all kinds of peculiar gaits, as people hustle to and fro.

But your observations are correct. We do change the way we get about as we age. Our steps become smaller and more cautious, and we place our feet a bit wider apart for balance. A stooped posture and a diminished arm swing along with a bent position of the knees and hips complete the picture. It's more difficult to start to walk, and it's harder to turn easily. The fact is, it's generally called a "senile gait," but you don't have to be senile to walk this way.

Although doctors are not sure of the exact cause, it probably is produced by a number of factors that come on with normal aging, including changes in the brain and the central nervous system as well as in the nerves that go out to all parts of the body. Other changes in bones, muscles and joints exert an influence as well. Except for an added risk of falling, it's generally a mild condition and not disabling.

Walking is great exercise, so keep on with your walks. And don't worry about the way you look, but be more careful to avoid tripping. That way you may enjoy all the benefits of your daily exercise with none of the risks.

11.

Pregnancy, Childbirth and Parenting

Some wonder that children
should be given to young mothers.
But what instruction does
the babe bring to the mother!
She learns patience, self-control, endurance.
Her very arm grows strong so that she holds
the dear burden longer than the father can.
The coarsest father gains a new impulse
to labor from the moment of his baby's birth.
Every stroke he strikes is for his child.
New social aims, and new moral motives
come vaguely up to him.

THOMAS WENTWORTH HIGGINSON
American Unitarian clergyman
and abolitionist (1823–1911)

Pregnancy, according to an encyclopedic definition, "is a normal physiologic process, which begins with conception, follows through development and growth of the fetus and delivery, and ends with a return to a fully normal state approximately six weeks after birth." But that's just the beginning, and a world of details accompanies the miracle of birth. Let's explore some of them.

Pregnancy causes modifications in the manner in which the mother's body functions to permit the fetus to grow and develop. For the fetus, pregnancy is a time of dependency on the mother for nutrition, and so it shares in all the hazards to which the mother may be exposed, an excellent argument for good prenatal care for both mother and baby-to-be. Although pregnancy proceeds normally for most women, others may have complications that can lead to unfavorable outcomes for both mother and baby. Careful supervision often can avert the more tragic consequences.

The average time of *gestation*, from conception to delivery, is 266 days, but calculating this time is usually difficult in actual situations. Therefore a time of 280 days (40 weeks) is generally used to calculate the due date, or expected date of delivery. For this calculation, the date of the last menstrual flow preceding conception is used, rather than the day of conception. It assumes that ovulation takes place 14 days after the menses, which is average for most women.

The gestation (from the Latin *gestos*, which means to bear) period is further divided into *trimesters*, roughly about 13 weeks, or three months, for each trimester. This provides a convenient and useful framework that can be used for measuring the progress of the pregnancy, and certain events can be described as reference points in each of these periods.

The first trimester starts for the mother with the end of her menses. This is due to changing patterns of hormones, as the developing *placenta* produces high levels of *HCG* (human chorionic gonadotropin). It is this hormone that activates the reaction in the home pregnancy tests, which are now so accurate that women no longer have to await a doctor's visit for confirmation of the good news. It's also during the first trimester that some of the common discomforts of pregnancy occur. Fatigue is a very common complaint, and it may start early in this period of time. Nausea and vomiting may start at about the eighth week. Sore breasts or tingling are the results of hormonal stimulation of the breasts to prepare them for their role in the infant's nutrition. Urination also is more frequent as the enlarging uterus begins to occupy some of the internal space usually taken by the bladder.

By the end of the first trimester, almost all of the recognizable organs have developed in the fetus. The heart begins to beat at about the fourth week, although it cannot be heard during the early examinations. At about the eighth week, all the toes and fingers are recognizable, as are the mouth, face and eyes. The reproductive systems are already distinguishable as either male or female.

During the second trimester, the mother's waistline continues to expand. The additional pressure from the enlarging uterus on the intestines can cause constipation. Occasionally the uterus may contract (called *Braxton-Hicks contractions*), but these contractions subside spontaneously after a few moments, and they're considered a normal part of the pregnancy. Under hormonal influence, more and more of the mother's blood flow is diverted to the growing uterus, placenta and fetus, with the result that the mother can experience moments of lightheadedness. In some cases, these may even advance to episodes of fainting. This has no ill effect upon either the mother or the baby, though the experience may be a disturbing one. While heartburn is also an increasing discomfort during the second 13-week period, usually this trimester is more comfortable for the expectant mother than the first one was and the next one will be.

This second trimester sees a thin-walled skin develop on the fetus, bone marrow begins its functioning, blood is formed, and the organs of the body start to work. As the trimester advances, the bones begin to harden, scalp hair begins to appear, and some fat develops in the subcutaneous layer of the skin. The fetus, which began its first small movements earlier, now can be felt by the mother at about the 20th week. This event often is called the *quickening*, and some say that this moment represents the exact middle of the pregnancy. A birth date prediction calculated at 20 weeks from this point is often quite close to the mark.

As the woman enters her third or last trimester, the level of discomfort increases, with headaches and the development of varicose veins and hemorrhoids (which are really varicose veins of the rectum and anus). The uterus is now so high in the abdomen that it restricts the motion of the diaphragm a bit, causing some shortness of breath. In the last weeks, insomnia is common.

It's during the third trimester that the fetus gains most of its weight. The ear cartilages develop, the nails grow over the tips of the fingers and, in the male, the testes descend into the scrotum. Investigations of the *in utero* fetus reveal that it has begun a pattern of behavior that closely approximates the cycle of wakefulness and sleep that is seen in the newborn baby.

When the last days are reached and the fetus' head drops, there is increased discomfort in the area of the pelvis. False labor, or uterine contractions that do not result in the dilatation of the cervix, can cause an unnecessary trip to the hospital or birthing facility, often in the middle of the night.

Today's unborn infant doesn't get to spend its nine months in the womb with the same privacy as those of a generation ago. Modern technology offers a number of procedures that permit the physician to keep a close "eye" on development and growth. In addition to checking the mother's weight, the apparent growth in size of the uterus and the sounds of the fetal heart as heard through the stethoscope, a physician may employ other methods to gain important information about the fetus:

- *Amniocentesis* collects a sample of the fluid that surrounds the fetus in the uterus, from which cells can be obtained that reveal the chromosomal makeup of the fetus.
- *Chorionic villi sampling* (CVS) can be performed in the ninth or tenth week. It examines a small bit of tissue taken from the placenta, which sustains the fetus, for chromosomal abnormalities at this early stage of pregnancy.
- A procedure known as *cordocentesis* draws blood from the umbilical cord while still within the uterus by using ultrasound images to guide the needle, and it obtains a specimen that can provide information about the chemistry of the blood.
- *Electronic fetal monitoring* provides tracings of the heartbeat and fetal movement, and shows the baby's response to external stimuli. This evaluation can be started at about the 28th week of pregnancy and has become a commonplace procedure.
- *Ultrasound* produces images that are used to evaluate the growth of the internal organs of the fetus, fetal movement, lung actions, the amount of amniotic fluid present and the condition of the placenta. It also may be used to determine the sex of the infant before birth. Many baby picture albums now include these images as "the baby's first photo."

Thus the unborn approaches the important day of birth with a chart full of documented information that can help provide safe passage when the time comes.

Labor and delivery begin with the onset of regular contractions. Advance notice of this event may be found with the discovery of a "bloody show," which is blood-tinged mucus that, in reality, is the plug that had been located in the cervix until the first stirs of labor released it.

Labor itself is divided into three parts. The first begins with uterine contractions and continues until the cervix dilates fully to about 10 centimeters (four inches). This may take anywhere from two to 24 hours, or sometimes even longer. The second stage begins with a completely dilated cervix and continues until the baby is born. This stage lasts less than two minutes for most women. The mother experiences a bearing-down sensation and an intense desire to "push." By contracting the muscles of the abdomen, she adds additional force to the action of the uterine muscles, and the baby is pushed from the uterus through the vagina to the waiting world. After the birth, the third stage of labor continues until the placenta (the afterbirth) passes out of the vagina, which takes place about 10 to 20 minutes later.

General anesthesia seldom is needed or used during a normal birth these days, and pain can be controlled by the judicious use of regional anesthesia and some medication. Natural childbirth is accomplished by many parents after proper training, which reduces the fear and muscle tensions that result from the anticipated pain and allows a birth that is less traumatic and certainly less painful for many women.

With the arrival of a newborn baby, life changes for the family. It matters little whether this is the first child or the latest of many, whether the family consists of a single parent, or an extended family with grandparents hovering in the background. There is the constant need to support the new life, provide appropriate nutrition and comfort, and deal with the mysteries of the developing personality and mind. But help is available in many forms: the physician, the advice of neighbors and friends, the past experiences of the grandparents, and the ever-present *Baby and Child Care* books by Dr. Benjamin Spock, which have helped to raise more than one generation.

And whether you refer to Spock or some other authoritative text, knowing the milestones that mark the normal progress in the development of a child can be most valuable. Understanding that a newborn can breathe only through its nose (which makes it essential to keep these passages clear), or that tears don't form until 1 to 3 months of age may help the parents monitor the baby's health. As the weight increases from 140 to 200 grams (averaging 5 to 7 ounces) a week during the first six months, and growth continues about 2.5 centimeters (1 inch) a month during the first half-year, strength increases and the baby becomes more mobile. By 6 or 7 months old, definite likes and dislikes for certain foods are dramatically displayed. Teeth show up at 5 to 7 months. By 6 months, sitting up is pretty well managed; at 8 months crawling starts; and by 11 months, the baby may be standing with help and moving around the room on the way to walking independently. By the first birthday, the baby will have tripled its birth weight, grown 25 to 30 centimeters (10 to 12 inches) and will be babbling with sounds that seem almost like real words. Mind you, these ages are all just averages, and every baby deserves to make its own mark, in its own good time. And every child deserves regular well-baby checkups, so that the parent can remain informed and so that remedies can be applied when progress is too slow.

Raising children in a changing world is a never-ending challenge, and it's a process that requires never-ending study. During the school years, membership in the parent-teacher association provides an excellent opportunity to tap into the knowledge and experience provided by the teachers that share your child's day with you. And school officials can be the introduction to resources you may need and not know how to find.

Preparing a child for a stable future place in society may be beyond our powers to imagine today. Awareness of the problems that can beset our offspring, and the determination to do something about them, are timeless strategies. It is merely a question of applying the advice in a timely fashion.

And so the first prenatal photograph is soon joined by a succession of constantly changing portraits that document the progression from newborn to baby to toddler to child to adolescent to young adult and on and on. Too fast? Then stop now and take this moment to smell the roses and enjoy your children, however old they may be.

Questions and Answers

306. ***I'm having a lot of trouble disciplining my asthmatic daughter. Every time she is punished, she begins wheezing. I'm afraid she'll have a full-blown attack, so I let her get away with what she's done. Does the stress of punishment actually bring on asthma attacks? What can I do? My other children get jealous because Nancy gets away with so much.***

It's true that any extremely frustrating, frightening or upsetting situation may trigger some wheezing in an asthmatic child. But discipline is essential for any child. Start by having a good heart-to-heart chat with Nancy. Explain that you love her, but that everyone, including children, must live by certain rules. When we don't, we must accept the consequences.

Many asthmatic children suffer from added emotional problems. They may be afraid of dying. They often suffer from feelings of inferiority because they can't compete in some activities or because of repeated absences from school. These emotional problems may lead to depression.

If you can't regain control of the discipline problem, I strongly suggest seeing a psychologist or a social worker to help you and Nancy. Also, check to make sure that your daughter is taking her medication when she is being corrected. Some children purposely skip medication while "grounded," knowing full well it'll spur symptoms. It's their way of getting back at concerned parents.

307. ***My mother believes in giving a baby something solid to eat just before bedtime, as a means of getting the child to sleep through the night. My physician never heard of this and pooh-poohs the whole idea. Do you think that I would be hurting my 3-month-old baby if I tried this feeding solution?***

I doubt that you would be doing any serious damage to your child's health by offering a feeding before bedtime, but I guess I come down on the side of your physician. (The American Academy of Pediatrics Committee on Nutrition advises holding off on solid food until the baby reaches the age of 4 to 6 months.)

Over the years, there have been many reports that such a feeding — usually a cereal prepared with either breast milk or formula — could encourage an infant to sleep from four to six hours.

However, when the idea was put to a scientifically conducted test at the Cleveland Clinic Foundation Pediatric Primary Care Center, an analysis of the results failed to demonstrate any difference between children who were fed before bedtime and those who were not. Researchers concluded that a child's ability to sleep through the night was a developmental and adaptive process that occurred regardless of diet composition.

308. ***My young teen-age son is having a terrible time because he's developing breasts. He refuses to take gym at school, because he does not wish to disrobe and have the other boys make fun of him. We're more concerned that this may be the sign of a serious disease. Can you help us?***

Although you do not mention your son's age in your letter, I'm willing to wager he is 13 or 14, which is a time of puberty when almost 40 percent of normal boys undergo some degree of breast development. It may not be as evident in others as in the case of your son, but it can be discovered by careful palpation during the course of a physical examination.

While the reasons for this growth are not clear, it probably results from a temporary imbalance between the male and female hormones that normally exist in all of us. The medical term applied to this diagnosis is pubertal gynecomastia, and it is a totally benign condition. Usually it will resolve itself within a few months, although in rare cases it can take longer.

Since gynecomastia has many causes, and in view of your son's problem at school, he's entitled to a complete physical and history to verify my impressions. Your family doctor can explain the condition to him and offer the reassurance that I believe will be forthcoming. With this reassurance and new understanding, your son will be able to deal with his inner fears. Perhaps a note from the doctor can relieve your son of gym classes until the situation returns to normal.

309. ***My mother and I are developing a dangerous generation gap concerning the hazards of breast-feeding to a baby's developing teeth. She has a whole list of abnormalities that she claims are due to the effort my baby seems to be putting out during feedings. Can this really cause crooked teeth later on for my baby, or am I developing maternal anxieties unnecessarily?***

Put your worries aside and let your mother read this. My authority is no less than the Academy of General Dentistry, which is all for breast-feeding and the nutritional and psychological benefits it provides newborns and infants. Now the academy feels there may be definite advantages to tooth development as well.

A study conducted by the Johns Hopkins School of Public Health reviewed the dental histories of more than 9,000 children to see if their teeth were crooked and to check their history of breast-feeding. Their study indicates that children who were either bottle-fed or breast-fed for less than a year had a 40 percent greater chance of misaligned teeth than babies who were breast-fed for a year or more.

It seems that during breast-feeding, babies develop stronger mouth muscles when they work at suckling, as your child does. The results are proper growth and alignment of teeth. As this benefit and other advantages of this natural nutrition become more and more apparent, the number of mothers breast-feeding their babies has increased to 56 percent, from a low of 25 percent in 1970.

It's time your mother caught up with you and the millions of mothers who are providing their babies with the best nutrition possible — mother's milk.

310. *My baby has colic. I feel if I hear her cry one more time, I'll be judged an unfit mother through neglect. I'm at my wit's end. What can I do?*

Let me tell you the story of one of my patients. I think it will help, and I'll change her name and enough details to maintain her privacy.

Donna came into my office a while back. That bundle of joy in her arms was causing her incredible anxiety and stress. Donna and her husband were on the verge of separation, ready for divorce court. They both had been joyous during Donna's pregnancy, planning their new baby's whole life for the first 18 years, which included its scholarship to Harvard.

Then reality loomed its ugly head. This new life demanded their constant and undivided attention. Perhaps no moment in mankind's history on Earth is as forceful as when parents realize that their infant is totally and completely dependent.

Donna was 32 and had given up a career in advertising to stay home with her baby. But motherhood was a harsh taskmaster, and there were no immediate rewards in terms of paychecks and promotions. Her visit was not a routine well-baby one. She complained that the baby had prolonged periods of crying for no apparent reason. During these times, she had looked for all the obvious causes. Was the baby hungry? Wet? Did she want to be held? Nothing seemed to work.

The onset of colic varies, but usually occurs between two and three weeks of age. It's marked by rhythmic attacks of screaming without known cause. Each attack can last for several hours and can't always be distinguished from the ordinary daily periods of crying common in infancy. Usually the distinguishing factor is the length of the attack. So a diagnosis of colic occurs by ruling out other possibilities.

Many theories have been posed as to the cause of colic: food allergy, immaturity of the gastrointestinal tract, progesterone deficiency, improper feeding techniques, emotional factors. The truth is that the medical field isn't quite sure, and it attacks the problem using many different therapies.

I'm sure that you, like Donna, have tried the obvious remedies. Talk to your pediatrician about a formula change or a pharmacologic approach (using some sort of medication). Both these methods are hit-or-miss, however. Do follow these maxims:

- Create an emotionally stable environment for your baby.
- Never overstimulate her in the evening near bedtime.
- A pacifier may help to calm her and satisfy her need for non-nutritive sucking.
- Improve your feeding techniques by holding her at a 45-degree angle while sucking and taking constant breaks to burp her.
- If you're bottle-feeding, make sure the nipple hole is neither too big nor too small and the formula neither too hot nor too cold.
- If you're breast-feeding, consult your physician about omitting allergenic foods from your diet.
- A swing, a rocking chair, a clock or a mobile also might help to calm her.

If all else fails, remember that the baby will outgrow colic around 10 to 12 weeks of age, so hang in there for the duration. Colic won't hurt your baby. It's not your fault she has it. Make sure that you plan periods away from your baby, alone, with friends or with your husband. These periods away are as important to your baby as the loving care and attention that you shower on her.

Donna made it, and I'm sure you will, too.

311. *Would you answer a simple question for a mother with a need for some information? Please explain what causes diaper rash.*

More than 60 percent of babies between 4 and 15 months experience an occasional rash in the diaper area. The symptoms may vary from a mild redness to painful open sores that extend into the folds of the thigh.

In the past, diaper rash was blamed on such factors as teething, diet and ammonia in the urine. But experts now say that diaper rash may be caused by too much moisture, as well as by the wearing-away of the skin's protective barrier from continual contact with urine and stool. Wetness starts the process by removing the skin's natural oils. Moist, unprotected skin is damaged easily by the constant rubbing action of the diaper, which possibly leads to a stubborn long-lasting yeast infection.

To prevent this, doctors advise prompt care of the diaper area, especially after a bowel movement. Avoid excessive cleansing with soap and disposable wipes, which can dry and irritate the skin. If a rash still develops, despite every effort, a bland ointment containing zinc oxide may be of some help.

312. ***Can you please tell me if I should feed a child who is having a sudden bout of severe diarrhea? Some friends say yes, but my mother says no. I'm getting conflicting advice on this question and would be grateful for your advice. What do you say?***

Acute diarrhea in a small child is not the same relatively benign discomfort as it is for an adult. Infants and small children with diarrhea can become dehydrated extremely quickly and may die. It's always been the standard treatment to withhold solid food from a baby with diarrhea and give him or her only water or a rehydration fluid for the first 24 to 48 hours.

However, recent evidence points to the value of giving babies some lactose-free formula after they've already received some fluids. Babies who received a soy-based infant formula (not one with milk in it, which can cause further diarrhea) had diarrhea for a shorter period of time than did babies treated with just water and rehydration fluid. Because of this finding, it might be a good idea to start a baby on some formula early in the course of his or her illness.

Rehydration fluid is water with important nutrients like potassium added. It's sold in pharmacies under the name Pedialyte. Your doctor also can tell you how to make your own rehydration fluid and how to use it. I'm sure your own doctor has some ideas about this, and it would be wise to ask him or her about this subject and follow the advice.

313. ***My 8-year-old son complains about being dizzy. What causes a child to be dizzy? Can it be dangerous? I know I could deal with the problem if I had some idea of what I was dealing with.***

Dizziness in children can have a number of different causes, ranging from a psychological disorder to a brain tumor. Don't ever ignore dizziness in a child; it may indicate a serious underlying problem that needs treatment.

You also should be aware of dizziness in a child who's too young to have the vocabulary to describe the sensation he's experiencing. A child may describe dizziness as a spinning feeling, or he may indicate that he's feeling unsteady or lightheaded.

Watch, too, for other symptoms that may accompany dizziness. Does the child suffer from nausea, vomiting, faintness, pallor or headache? Does he black out or lose consciousness? Is the dizziness brought on by rapid movement of the head? How long does the dizziness occur, and how frequently? Is your child able to play or to carry out normal activities despite feeling dizzy?

If dizziness occurs in your child, ask your physician about it. He will need to take a complete history, and he'll ask you and your child a number of questions to try to pinpoint the cause of the dizziness.

In addition, a thorough physical exam will help rule out a number of possible causes. Lab tests (which look for blood abnormalities, diabetes, etc.) and even a CT scan (computerized tomography) will help in the diagnosis. In particular, your doctor will be interested in any ear or neurologic disorders, which often have dizziness as a symptom. For instance, any obstruction, such as impacted ear wax, in the auditory canal could result in dizziness.

Chronic ear infections or previous ear surgery could be the culprit. Your doctor will want to know if your child suffers from any kind of hearing loss, tinnitus (ringing in the ears), pain or feeling of fullness in his ears (in one ear or two).

Other possible causes of dizziness include:

- Medications such as aspirin, antihistamines, phenytoin and barbiturates (used to treat epilepsy and other seizure disorders).
- Injury to the head, neck or spine.
- Infections such as meningitis, encephalitis or brain abscess.
- Disorders such as diabetes, low blood sugar, high or low blood pressure, or hypothyroidism.
- Diseases of the blood such as anemia or leukemia.
- Diseases of the central nervous system such as multiple sclerosis.
- Lead, arsenic or alcohol poisoning.
- Thiamine or niacin deficiency.
- Meniere's disease (although it's more common in adults).
- Migraine headaches.
- Seizure disorders such as epilepsy.

Dizziness also can indicate benign paroxysmal vertigo of childhood, which is a fairly harmless and common childhood disorder characterized by recurrent attacks of dizziness that last a few seconds to a few minutes. During an attack, the patient may have nausea, vomiting and appear pale with a constant involuntary movement of the eyeballs. This disorder usually disappears after six months to a year, and it rarely occurs after the age of 6.

As you can see, this is not a simple question with an easy answer. I sense the urgency in your words and emphasize that you should get your child to the doctor as soon as you can. Hopefully, the answers in your case will be simple and without serious consequences.

314. ***My older sister has just gone through the frightening experience of an ectopic pregnancy. She is fine now, and the doctor says she will be able to have another pregnancy soon. I found it difficult to understand just what happened, and I am anxious about myself. I, too, want to have a baby and want to know if my sister's experience may mean I will someday have to face the same problem. Could you explain ectopic pregnancies, so that I can know what to do?***

While still relatively uncommon, the number of ectopic pregnancies more than doubled between 1970 and 1980. They increased again during this past decade and now account for approximately 1.5 percent of all pregnancies. However, ectopic pregnancies are most important, because they're responsible for about 13 percent of pregnancy-related deaths.

The word ectopic comes from the Greek *ektopos*, which means displaced. The term graphically describes the condition, for an ectopic pregnancy is one in which the pregnancy develops outside of the normal position in the uterus. About 98 percent of ectopic pregnancy cases occur in one of the Fallopian tubes, which are the long tubular passages that run from the ovaries to the uterus. Three symptoms are characteristic of a tubal pregnancy: abdominal pain, absence of a normal menstrual period, and vaginal bleeding beginning after the missed period. An examination will show tenderness in the area and frequently the presence of a mass. Although this may resemble appendicitis or acute salpingitis (infection of the Fallopian tubes), a positive pregnancy test is often the confirmation that helps make the diagnosis.

Some conditions make an ectopic pregnancy more likely to occur.

They include salpingitis, endometriosis, a previous ectopic pregnancy in one of the tubes, or surgery on the Fallopian tubes, which includes a previous tubal sterilization. When such a pregnancy occurs, it must be removed surgically by removing all of the Fallopian tube or the portion of the tube in which the pregnancy is located.

Since none of these factors involves an inherited trait, it's most improbable that your desire for children will be impeded by the same obstacles that were overcome by your sister.

315. ***With the due date of my first baby fast approaching, it seems that all my girlfriends' conversations now turn to the "cut" the doctor may make during the birthing. Can you tell me the scientific name for it and explain its use? Does it cause a lot of pain?***

When a delivery can be helped by providing a bit more room for the baby's head to pass through, a physician may elect to perform an episiotomy. The term is from the Greek word *epision*, which describes the pubic region. It's through this area that an incision is made.

There are several advantages to the procedure. It can allow a quicker and easier birth, and it can reduce pressure on the baby's head. Since the forces pushing the baby through the birth canal are powerful enough to stretch and tear vaginal tissues, making a clean surgical incision at the appropriate moment prevents the complications that torn tissue can provoke. With everything else that is going on at that moment, many women are unaware that the cut has been made.

After the birth, the incision is repaired by suturing, like any other surgical incision, and is permitted to heal. While the swelling and pain pass in a few days to a week, the area may remain tender for a month or so. Total healing usually is complete in about six weeks.

The mainstay of care is hygiene. The area must be kept clean and free from any possible contaminating elements that can cause irritation or infection. Your own physician will guide you through this period and counsel you about resuming normal activities and relations.

316. ***This is the third time in as many months that my 4-year-old son has had a seizure during an illness with high fever. What am I doing wrong? Is there any chance that he will have some permanent damage?***

Up to 5 percent of children may experience a febrile seizure or convulsion (febrile means fever) by age 5. This major side effect scares the dickens out of most parents. However, a convulsion also can be a symptom of a more serious condition, such as a brain infection.

Febrile seizures can be either simple (a single seizure) or complex (more than one, or one that lasts longer than 15 minutes). Most febrile seizures last less than five minutes and are associated with fevers above 102 degrees Fahrenheit. Removing excess blankets and other coverings may help cool the child a bit and can help prevent seizures. Usually, children who have febrile seizures are better by the time they see the physician. Aside from the doctor giving acetaminophen to the child to reduce the fever, there is no treatment.

Your child has had repeated febrile seizures, so he should be followed more closely. Up to 40 percent of children who have one febrile seizure will have another one during a fever, usually within a year. Your physician may discuss the advisability of your child taking anti-convulsant medications until age 5 or so to prevent future episodes.

Only 2 percent of children who have febrile seizures develop epilepsy and another 1 percent have nonepileptic seizures. Occasionally, children are found to have mental retardation, coordination problems, or sensory or perceptual abnormalities after febrile seizures. But these problems probably existed before the seizure and are noted only because the child undergoes testing afterward.

317. ***Do you know what the thinking was in giving a number as the name of a disease? I'm referring to "Fifth disease," which is a recent addition to my daughter's medical history. Where did the name come from?***

You're a bit confused, but it's easy to straighten out. Normally diseases have names that describe the condition or bear the name of the discoverer. However, in the case of children's diseases, there are five of them that have similar rashes. Four received names. They are German measles, measles, scarlet fever and roseola (once known as Filatov-Dukes disease or Fourth disease). When the fifth childhood rash was discovered, it simply was named Fifth disease (it's also known as Erythema Infectiosum).

Fifth disease affects school-age children worldwide, with infants and adults affected only infrequently. A low-grade fever accompanies the infection, which characteristically produces a rash that gives the child a "slapped-cheek" appearance. This rash is usually itchy, and it becomes worse if the child is bathed in warm water, becomes upset or rubs the skin. The rash fades after about 11 days. No treatment is required, and complications are rare. This childhood disease is considered to be a very mild one. Compared to some of the jawbreaking names we give diseases, I think Fifth disease is a simple one to remember.

318. ***There have been three separate occasions when my son returned from playing with his friends and he was flushed and feverish. I don't mean just hot and sweaty, but actually had a temperature of over 100 degrees, which I took with an oral thermometer. My doctor advised me just to watch him, and, of course, it went away without any medication. However, I'm still worried and hope that you might be able to offer some explanation.***

You sound very much like a normal, caring mother, for many parents worry about elevated temperatures when they occur in their children. In this case, however, I doubt that there is cause for concern.

There is really no such thing as a "normal" temperature. Even in normal individuals, it may vary as much as two to three degrees in a 24-hour period, with the lowest reading being found during sleep and the highest temperature recorded during the late afternoon.

When fever is noted after a healthy workout or period of play, it is not a cause for concern, especially when it comes down in a short time, without medication. In this case, it is considered a normal variation in the constantly changing level of body temperature.

It may interest you to learn that the so-called "normal" body temperature of 98.6 degrees Fahrenheit was determined by averaging the levels found in just a few individuals in a study conducted in the 19th century. Most doctors today therefore do not react too strongly to brief variations from this level. And that is good advice for you as well.

Any serious conditions usually produce fevers that are both higher and sustained over a longer period of time. It's generally conceded that a rectal temperature over 101 degrees F (38.3 degrees Celsius) is abnormal.

319. ***My daughter, now 11 years old, has complained constantly over the past several months about pains in her legs. I have taken her to the doctor,***

who gave her a complete examination including X-rays and blood tests, but he could find nothing. He finally described the problem as "growing pains." Is there any treatment for this, or may I hope that it will disappear by itself as she grows older?

It appears as though your doctor has given this problem the attention it deserves, because the diagnosis of "growing pains" is made only when the other possible reasons for the complaint have been investigated and no evidence of any other causes for pain can be found. The term is used for a condition of benign, recurrent limb pain in young children and probably has nothing to do with the actual physical process of growing up.

The pains may come on at any time but seem to occur most frequently in the evening or at night. Usually they are located in the thighs or calves, and the pains leave after an hour or two. The children are otherwise healthy, and the laboratory tests, as well as X-rays, are always normal.

Frequently there is a history of similar experiences during childhood in other members of the family. Some experts in pediatric development believe that growing pains may be due to the emotional growth of the child, and warn that evidence of emotional disturbances may be common.

You must continue to support your daughter in an understanding and open manner, continue to watch her closely, and react if other symptoms appear. The most likely course is that the complaints and pains all will disappear in time with no lasting health effects. Use a lot of love and a little patience. They are great medicines for any situation in growing children.

320.

My baby is 5 months old. I started losing a lot of my hair when he was 4 months old. My doctor says that this was because of hormones, and that the hair loss will stop in six to 18 months. Would you please explain why this happens? Is this a common problem with women who have had babies, and is there anything I can do now to stop it?

You're experiencing a problem with the improbable name of telogen effluvium, which is seen commonly in women after childbirth. The good news is that "this too will pass."

Hair growth occurs in a cyclical pattern, with active growth (anagen phase) continuing for two to six years. A brief period of regression (catagen phase) then occurs during which a club (stubby) hair is produced instead of the normal long hair you're now wishing for. Then a rest period of about three months takes place (telogen phase).

When reactivation occurs, the club hair falls out (telogen effluvium), and new hair growth, and a new cycle, begin. Normally about 85 percent of scalp hairs are in the anagen phase, while the remaining 15 percent are resting.

Hair shedding may follow any type of body stress, such as surgery, high fever, crash diets, acute blood loss, the use of certain drugs and after giving birth. But as your doctor correctly advised you, new growth will take place soon and your hair will return to normal.

There really is nothing you need do now, for the process will run its course. There are no means of stopping it once it has begun. You can best help yourself by using this new understanding to reduce the stress and anxiety that you're naturally experiencing at this time and turn your energies to your baby.

321. *Since there are many apparent changes in a woman's body during pregnancy, I wondered if her heart also might be affected by the pregnancy. Does the mother's heart change while she is pregnant?*

It most certainly does. During normal pregnancy, labor and delivery, a good many changes take place. This provides physicians with a special opportunity for observing important cardiac adjustments during a temporary state of high stress.

To begin with, the heart rate increases as much as 15 beats per minute above nonpregnant levels, with the most significant increases occurring before the eighth week of pregnancy. Blood pressure either can increase or decrease, depending on the woman's age and whether she's had previous pregnancies. Blood pressure levels appear to increase with advancing age and decrease if previous pregnancies existed.

In addition, cardiac output (the amount of blood the heart pumps out) at rest increases during pregnancy, from 30 to 50 percent above normal, and peaks at the end of the second trimester. It is believed that the increased heart rate and increased stroke volume (which is amount of blood that is pumped out with each heartbeat) are responsible for this change in cardiac output.

The resistance to blood flow in the arteries of the body decreases during pregnancy. Together with the increased cardiac output, blood flow to various organ systems is altered as well. Uterine and kidney blood flow markedly increase, as does blood flow to breasts, skin, limbs and mucous membranes.

One of the most significant changes, however, involves the left ventricle, or lower left chamber, of the heart, which pumps oxygenated blood out through the aorta to all the tissues of the body. Left ventricular volume and chamber size gradually increase throughout pregnancy, which results in the enlargement of the heart's cavities and wall mass. This enlargement contributes to the increased cardiac output. However, despite the dimensional changes, the heart's function remains normal.

Within five weeks after delivery, all blood flow and structural and functional changes are back to pre-pregnancy values. This indicates that the heart is a remarkably adaptive organ that can respond to the changing demands placed upon it by the needs of a pregnancy. Physicians are hopeful that these findings will one day lead to insights concerning possible treatment for problems of an ailing heart and the need for it to adjust to stress.

322. *My kid just doesn't seem to listen to anything I say and certainly can't sit still long enough to have a talk. Even my neighbors are beginning to make comments. One friend thinks that I'm dealing with a child who has a condition that has the word "hyperactive" in it. I need some advice and information. Can you help, please?*

I certainly can offer you a few bits and pieces of advice that may help. But this is a condition in which the child must be observed and examined by a physician in order to get a clear understanding of the problem to make a correct diagnosis.

I believe your friend is referring to a condition known as attention-deficit hyperactivity disorder (ADHD). It is a neurological condition that causes a child to be easily distracted from the task at hand, inattentive, impulsive and hyperactive, when compared to other children of the same age.

In some cases, particularly with girls, the hyperactivity is less pronounced or less noticeable. With or without hyperactivity, this condition may affect from 2 to 10 percent of all children, and hyperactive behavior is the most common problem now being referred to child guidance clinics in the United States. The diagnosis will depend upon the presence or absence of certain behavior patterns, and the severity will be judged by the effect on the child's ability to function.

There are 14 behavioral criteria listed for ADHD, and at least eight of them must be present for six or more months to make the diagnosis. Here are but a few for you to use in your own preliminary evaluation of your child:

1. Often fidgets with hands and feet, or squirms in seat.

2. Has difficulty remaining seated when required to do so.

3. Is easily distracted by things happening outside the immediate area.

4. Has difficulty awaiting turns in games or group situations.

As you can see, it is not a simple task to arrive at the correct diagnosis, which is a must if an effective therapeutic plan is to be fashioned. Prescription medications are one route that is available to you, but this is a problem in which the solution is neither instantaneous nor complete.

You should proceed step by step through a complete evaluation, while gathering all the information and resources that you may need to help you cope effectively. Your ability to help your child is most important in the outcome of any treatment.

323. *Is it possible that my 9-year-old youngster can have hypertension? He was found to have high blood pressure on a recent physical. I thought this was a condition only of the elderly. If children do have it, can my son be treated?*

Hypertension can occur in children. When it does, the cases generally are mild and, frequently, are found in families with histories of hypertension plus excess body weight.

Treatment usually begins with the physician taking your child's medical history, giving a thorough physical examination and obtaining an understanding of the family's medical history. Such information enables a doctor to determine whether your youngster suffers from some other disorder or from secondary hypertension. The latter is much more common in children than in adults.

Secondary hypertension is caused by, or is associated with, a variety of diseases, such as kidney, central nervous system, endocrine and/or vascular disorders. When such diseases are cured — by a course of therapy under your doctor's supervision — the child's high blood pressure usually returns to normal. Doctors have observed that secondary hypertension usually occurs in their youngest patients with the highest blood pressures.

Because of today's readily available blood pressure measurements, mild hypertension is being discovered in children much more frequently than before. When doctors treat it, their goal is to reduce blood pressure without producing side effects that could interfere with your youngster's normal growth and development.

Mild or borderline high blood pressure usually is treated by diet modification for weight control and an exercise program. Your child's physician may prescribe anti-hypertensive drugs to prevent possible damage to blood vessels and/or other organs. Usually very small dosages are given and, if necessary, are increased slowly. Once weight control and increased exercise become routine, the goal is to reduce and, it is hoped, withdraw medication if your child's blood pressure remains in an acceptable range.

324. *My mother called the condition a "lazy eye." But when I took my baby to the doctor, he diagnosed it as "amblyopia." There seems to be a lot of treatment involved, and I would like to know more about this problem, Will you please answer this very important question for me?*

Amblyopia is decreased or poor vision in an eye that has no detectable damage in either the eye or the visual pathway. The eye doesn't develop normal sight during early childhood, usually because the child experiences double vision from a turned-eye condition and so blocks out (suppresses) the image falling on the turned eye to avoid seeing double. The eye then becomes "lazy" from not being used. Vision is now poor in that eye, and the eye is considered to be amblyopic. This also occurs when one eye is out of focus with the other because of a stronger degree of nearsightedness, farsightedness or astigmatism.

Children should be checked at 6 months, certainly before age 3, so the doctor can diagnose and treat the condition while the child is still young. Once the visual system is completely developed, vision in the eye cannot be restored. Remember that the condition can go undetected, because the child is not aware that he is seeing out of only one good eye. A careful eye examination will reveal vision problems as well as any eye disease, such as a cataract, that can lead to amblyopia.

Treatment for amblyopia involves forcing the child to use the weaker eye. The stronger eye may be patched, glasses may be prescribed to correct errors in focusing, and surgery or exercises may be recommended to correct misaligned eyes. Early detection and prompt treatment can prevent the blindness that can develop from amblyopia.

325.

After much testing by our doctor, the youngest of our three children, age 6, is thought to have mononucleosis. It seems the first test results were not too clear, but now our doctor seems convinced. We were wondering if this is a rare thing, and what we should do to protect our other children? How long does the infection last, and is there any special medication that should be given? Thank you for any help you can give.

Cases of infectious mononucleosis (IM) are not as uncommon as once thought. Because the test used to diagnose the infection, called the heterophile antibody test, may not show the same results in children — especially very young children — as it does in adolescents and adults, IM was believed to be rare in these youngsters. However, newer and more sensitive tests that can reveal the presence of the Epstein-Barr virus, which causes the disease, now enable physicians to make the diagnosis more readily.

Sometimes it takes many days or even weeks to see the full pattern of the disease in children. Usually there are a fever and fatigue, with enlarged glands in the throat and neck. Both the spleen and liver may become enlarged. Skin rashes and abdominal pain are seen more commonly in the younger patients than in older ones.

The infection does not seem to be too contagious even among other family members. Adults rarely develop the infection, probably because they're already immune due to a prior contact that failed to develop symptoms. Even older brothers and sisters can escape the clinical disease in many families.

There are no specific medications for treating IM, but rest and reduced activity are usually the mainstay of the supportive therapy that is necessary. Although the illness may linger for some weeks or months, it's almost always self-limiting, which means it will disappear over time.

326. ***What can you tell me about the relationship of pregnancy and diabetes? My daughter is expecting my first grandchild and has been told she has "sugar." This is something new, for she never had this condition before. Can you please explain what is going on?***

Some women who get pregnant get diabetes, but this type of diabetes, called gestational diabetes, usually goes away when the baby is delivered. The physical changes of pregnancy cause the diabetes in these women.

Women who get gestational diabetes usually have at least one of these characteristics:

- They have had a previous stillbirth.
- They have had babies that weigh more than 4.1 kilograms (9 pounds).
- They have had babies with birth defects.
- They have a family history of diabetes.
- They have had obstetric complications, such as high blood pressure.
- They have had gestational diabetes with a previous pregnancy.

Of course it is also possible that even when none of these characteristics are present, the condition will still develop.

It is especially important for a woman with this type of diabetes, or any form of this disease, to get early prenatal care. The doctor will require a thorough history to spot any of the risk factors and test and treat your daughter accordingly. Uncontrolled diabetes is not healthy for the baby or the mother. It can cause birth defects and death for the baby if it is not fully treated. The good news is that proper treatment can prevent such tragedies.

Of course, a woman who had diabetes before she became pregnant will not be "cured" by the delivery of her baby — she still will be diabetic afterward. Since there is no history of this disease in your daughter, it is likely that her sugar problem will disappear after the birth of your grandchild.

327. ***I'm having the hardest time getting my young son off to school each day. He will use any excuse not to go. One of the teachers called this a "school phobia" and suggested that I seek some counseling and help for my child. What do you think? Does this phobia really exist?***

I think many experts agree that there is a condition called school phobia, and that it may be more common than once thought. However, in many cases, it is more truly a fear of leaving home than a horror of being in school.

Actually, many of these children want to attend their classes, but they suffer from the effects of a separation anxiety and wish not to leave the protection of their home and parents. Some fear their mothers will desert them when they are away at school, and they will put up quite a battle when the moment to leave arrives, clinging to the mother, crying and screaming. Many develop complaints of headache, dizziness, abdominal pains, nausea and vomiting, all of which resolve themselves quite rapidly when they are permitted to stay at home.

To be sure, some events at school, such as a school bully or an overcritical teacher, may aid the development of the problem, as will a fear of certain subjects. Most of these children have an average or superior intelligence, and the problem occurs in families of all social, ethnic, religious and economic classes.

Do not confuse school phobia with truancy, which is when the child leaves home without any problem, but does not attend school and roams the streets with others who also are "taking the day off." These youngsters are frequently poor students, and their parents are unaware of the absence. School phobia is a complex problem in many cases. Seeking professional help is well advised.

328. ***I break out into a cold sweat every time my 4-year-old son starts wondering where babies come from. I have doubts that I know enough about educating youngsters of his age about reproduction and sex, yet I feel there must be an answer both to his question and to my problem. I wish you could take over for me. What do I do?***

If the answer that you are not alone will help you to relax, then be assured there are many other parents in this same boat. The hardest part is overcoming your own doubts and feelings of inadequacy but, fear not, you can manage quite well if you stay calm and follow a few important tips: Stay cool, stay accessible to your youngster and stay simple; don't panic when such questions arise, but listen carefully.

You may be making more out of the question than Junior is intending. When your reaction shows that you don't find such discussions difficult, you will remain the first person the child asks for such information, an important position you don't ever want to abandon. Once the intent of the question is understood, answer as fully but as simply as possible. Don't launch into that complete lecture you have been rehearsing for this moment, because it is just not necessary. There will be time enough for that in the future, if you don't lose the child's thread of curiosity that promotes the questioning at this time.

You're just at the beginning now, with plenty of time to read up on the advice from the experts and to become prepared to continue such conversations throughout the emotional, social and sexual development of your offspring. Explaining reproduction and sex is only part of your responsibility to guide your child through the trials of growing up and to teach the ethical principles and values that motivate your own life.

329. *My daughter recently went for a routine prenatal checkup. She was told she had a urinary tract infection and was given medication to clear it up. She had no signs of the infection. Was it really necessary to take this medicine while she's pregnant? Is it safe?*

Many pregnant women experience urinary tract infections (UTIs) with symptoms that they can't detect. Urinary tract infections are the most common infections experienced by women, and they are the most common complication of pregnancy.

Pregnant women who are diagnosed as having a UTI should most definitely follow the prescribed regimen. Usually with asymptomatic bacteriuria (the presence of germs in urine, but without symptoms), the course of treatment lasts five to seven days. If this type of UTI is left untreated, it can progress into a more serious complication. The more dangerous situation, called pyelonephritis, usually requires hospitalization. This infection can result in premature labor and endotoxic shock.

It is, therefore, very important to take UTIs seriously and adhere to the doctor's advice, especially during pregnancy. Once the infection is cleared up, careful monitoring should be continued throughout the rest of the pregnancy, because UTIs often recur.

330.

My 8-year-old son has occasional episodes of shivering that are frightening. His head and arms tremble out of control for no apparent reason. I have taken him to several doctors, and epilepsy has been ruled out. The doctors say what my son has been having are "shuddering attacks" and they aren't dangerous. What do you think?

It sounds like the doctors have made a good diagnosis. Shuddering or shivering episodes are common in children, and many young people pass through this experience at one time or another to some degree. You can be reassured that this disorder appears to be benign and nonthreatening. These bouts usually involve rapid shuddering tremors, primarily of the head and arms, so that your son's case appears typical. These attacks are different from common shivering, because they last longer and occur more often.

Testing done with an electroencephalograph and videotape monitoring can confirm that the incidents are nonepileptic in nature. They actually are associated with abnormal posturing of the arms.

Parents of children with shuddering attacks also may have a history of similar episodes. There is no treatment for this disorder. Since the attacks apparently do not cause any real damage, medications are not indicated. It would seem that you have little to fear here, and that time will put everything in order.

331.

It feels like a war, and I'm losing. There is seemingly nothing I can do to get my 2-year-old son toilet-trained, despite all my efforts. He is a bright child, and all of his playmates are well on the road to control, but we're getting nowhere. What is a mother to do?

Your frustrations are showing, so sit down for a moment, take a deep breath and let's talk. Most authorities agree that if you've been trying for several months and your child reaches the age of 2½ without successfully achieving training, you may assume that he's resisting in a conscious way. And you haven't reached that age limit yet.

However, it's time to change strategy. By now he knows what you want, and he's capable of performing, but he will fight your efforts unless you turn the responsibility over to him. There should be no more scheduled sessions just sitting, no more frequent questions or reminders. Reminders are just another form of parental pressure. One last discussion will tell him that "peepee" and "dooty" are his to deal with and that you know he doesn't need your help.

By withdrawing attention from the bathroom battle, his need for attention can be met only when his performance merits it. Of course, you must stick by your guns, but offer positive reinforcement freely — small rewards like building blocks or pennies may do it. Create a visual aid, like a poster or calendar, and mark it boldly for every victory, while you heap on the praise.

Even sitting on the potty chair counts, for once that routine is established, he's on his way. Don't stand around while he is on the chair, let him come to you with his success story. Once you have informed him about wet or soiled clothing, have him help you clean them. Having him rinse a soiled garment in the toilet bowl will keep him aware of his duties and help motivate him to avoid this unpleasantness.

Accidents will happen, but avoid any harsh criticism or punishment. Do not embarrass him, as it is counterproductive. And don't be embarrassed yourself. Discuss strategies with the parents of your son's playmates. Let them know what your situation is and what rules are governing your actions, so they can use the same guidelines when your child is visiting with them. They may have developed routines that could be helpful for you, so discuss toilet training openly.

Once you have all your ducks in a row, you may be pleasantly surprised at the speed of your child's progress.

332. *My daughter has a newborn baby that she is nursing. She believes that this is enough protection against another pregnancy, which would be most difficult at this time. Is my daughter safe now, or is it still possible for her to become pregnant while nursing a baby?*

The long-held belief that the process of nursing a newborn is a safeguard against another pregnancy may not be the absolute truth that some people think it is. It makes sense that nature would provide a mechanism that allows a mother to devote all her attention to a baby. This may lend some support to those women who tell of their lack of fertility during this period, but there is more to the story.

It is clear that fewer pregnancies occur immediately after childbirth in nursing (lactating) mothers than in mothers who do not nurse. The period of relative infertility lasts only six weeks in nonnursing mothers. In nursing mothers, the presence of a hormone (prolactin) that is stimulated by the baby's sucking can suppress the action of the hormones that promote ovulation for a prolonged period.

However, this protection seems to last only as long as nursing continues uninterrupted. While total breast-feeding provides protection against another pregnancy, any schedule that reduces regular nursing can lower the amount of prolactin in the blood, allowing ovulation and a possible pregnancy to occur.

One of the overlooked reductions in nursing is the elimination of the night feeding. This allows a period of eight to 10 hours to pass without the sucking stimulus, and the levels of prolactin may return to normal. Thus the protection your daughter seeks depends upon maintaining a nursing timetable that most families find unacceptable, as it disrupts the sleep and rest necessary to keep up with daily activities.

333. ***Could you please help the parents of a teething baby? Our adorable daughter has turned cranky and difficult to deal with. This is our first baby, and perhaps we're still a bit inexperienced. Any help you can give us would be very much appreciated.***

I'm probably opening Pandora's box in trying to answer this question for you and will be rewarded with a flood of mail that tells me I am all wrong, but here it goes anyway. Your baby's irritability is the result of the swollen and painful gums that accompany the natural process of teething.

Usually babies drool more and want to chew and suck a lot more to help reduce the discomfort and tenderness. You can help by massaging the gums lightly with a finger, when time is available. Try to give your daughter something cool to suck on, like a teething ring that has been kept in the refrigerator for a while.

There are some over-the-counter medications available, but I would check with your own doctor for his approval before using one. I don't approve of using a drop of whiskey for this indication, though I have heard of it. A hard biscuit or cookie can provide the child with something to chew away on. In certain circles, mothers swear by stale bagels as the perfect solution to the problem.

334.

Our 6-year-old son still sucks his thumb in spite of our pleas to act more mature. My mother suggests an old-fashioned solution of painting his thumb with a bitter liquid, but this sounds terribly antiquated to me. What do you think?

A study conducted at the Johns Hopkins University School of Medicine in Baltimore suggests that your mother's time-honored solution may still be applicable in our modern day and age.

Seven thumb- or finger-sucking children who were otherwise emotionally and developmentally normal had their offending thumb or finger coated with a bitter-tasting, commercially available solution after waking and before bedtime. All the children quickly stopped the offending habit. They did not resume it even when their parents ceased applying the liquid after five continuous days of nonsucking had passed.

As long as there is no underlying emotional reason for your child's thumb sucking, your mother's solution, while a bitter pill to swallow, is effective.

335.

As my pregnancy advances (I'm now in my seventh month), I find my back pain is increasing. I'm sure I'm not the first person with this problem, but I haven't really been able to find any decent solutions. I want to stay away from pills, but it is getting to the point where the discomfort is more than annoying. Do you have a suggestion or two that might help me get some relief?

I doubt that there are many women who escape the problem of low back pain occurring at some time during their pregnancy. A simple side view is enough to reveal that your center of gravity is changing, moving upward and forward, as the baby grows larger. This puts more strain on your back muscles as you strive to walk erect against the weight.

Assuming that the pain is not the result of an old condition that existed before your pregnancy and is not caused by such things as a urinary infection, or aggravated by excessive weight gain, there are a few measures you can take to reduce the discomfort. And I agree with you, forgo any unnecessary medication during this time.

The first assignment is to take a good survey of the tasks that cause the greatest pain and seek to alter the way you approach them. When seated, if your knees are lower than your hips, you can be putting extra pressure on your back by tilting your pelvis forward. Try placing a book or block of wood on the floor to rest your feet on, and place a small cushion or folded towel under your thighs to help elevate your knees a bit higher. Standing is better than sitting, so try to keep erect when possible.

Avoid jobs that require you to bend over, and raise your work surfaces to a more comfortable level. If you must lift something, keep the load as close to your body as you can.

Exercises can be a big help in strengthening your aching muscles, and your obstetrician can advise you about the best ones for you. There are times when a relaxing massage can loosen those tight muscles and provide just the right prescription for the relief you need.

12.

Feeling Fit: The Role of Nutrition and Exercise in a Healthy Lifestyle

Moderation resembles temperance.
We are not so unwilling to eat more,
As afraid of doing ourselves harm by it.

François, Duc de la Rochefoucauld
French courtier and
moralist (1630–80)

I don't know of any word that has taken a greater beating in recent popular literature than the word ***nutrition***. My big deluxe unabridged dictionary yields the following explanation: "a nourishing, or being nourished, especially the series of processes by which an organism takes in and assimilates food for promoting growth and replacing worn or injured tissues." I doubt that this truly expresses the thoughts that go through the mind of a diner at an expensive restaurant when presented with the bill of fare.

It might, though, if he or she were a nutritionist, a scientist working to discover the intrinsic elements in food and the nutritional needs for human growth. Or a dietitian, who translates nutritional facts into diets that maintain normal health and correct nutritional deficiencies.

The foods consumed by humans must contain adequate amounts of 40 to 50 highly important substances, in addition to water and oxygen. The body starts with these essentials and creates the thousands of substances required for life and physical activity. Commencing with the basic building blocks contained in food, substances with complex structures are constructed, many with more complicated formulas than in the original food.

The amount of energy contained in food is measured in *calories*, which are a bit different from the calorie measurement used in physics to calculate heat. Since the amounts of ordinary calories burned in human metabolism are quite large, it was decided to use a "large calorie" or kilocalorie when speaking in metabolic or nutritional terms. The food calorie is thus 1,000 ordinary calories, and all nutritional information uses this convention. Another convention used in nutritional mathematics is that 1 gram of pure protein yields 4 calories, 1 gram of fat is equal to 9 calories, and 1 gram of pure carbohydrate provides 4 calories.

For a food to supply calories for energy, it must have three basic atoms in its molecular makeup: *carbon*, *hydrogen* and *oxygen*. These atoms form the basic structure of both carbohydrates and fats. Protein contains *nitrogen* and *sulfur* in addition, and so it plays a different role in the body's metabolism.

Protein is the very essence of life, for no life forms exist without protein as a fundamental part of their structure. In turn, protein is made up of simpler components known as *amino acids*. There are 22 distinct amino acids in the body's proteins, of which only 13 can be synthesized by the body. The other nine must be brought into the body in the foods we eat, and it is these nine that are called the *essential amino acids*. A protein that contains all the essential amino acids is called a *complete protein*, and animal proteins are complete proteins. Meat, milk, cheese and eggs are all foods that are rich in complete proteins. By contrast, plant proteins are not complete proteins, however, it is possible to combine incomplete plant proteins in a manner that provides the body with all the essential proteins.

Proteins are necessary for the production of new tissue and the repair of older ones. All of the hormones and enzymes in the body are made of proteins, and the agents of defense, called the *antibodies*, also are made of proteins. When the body's reserves of carbohydrates and fats are gone, proteins can provide the energy necessary for the body to continue to function. Yet for all its vital importance, the most widespread nutritional deficiency worldwide is insufficient protein intake. Because of this lack, whole populations suffer from lowered resistance to disease and infections, and from shortened, unproductive lives.

Carbohydrates are the most abundant and least expensive source of energy from food. Dietary carbohydrates can be divided into two groups:

sugars and *starches*. The most basic carbohydrates are simple sugars (*monosaccharides*), such as *fructose* and *glucose*. Link two simple sugars together, such as one glucose and one fructose, and a *disaccharide* is formed. *Sucrose*, or ordinary table sugar, is the most well-known form of this type of carbohydrate. Combine several simple sugars together and the result is a *complex carbohydrate*, known as starch in plants and *glycogen* in humans. Starches are found in grains, beans, nuts, potatoes and root vegetables. When the starches, or complex carbohydrates, enter the body as food, the body's digestive process breaks them down into the simple sugars, uses what it needs for energy, and stores the excess carbohydrates as glycogen, primarily in the liver.

Fats are the most concentrated source of energy. The basic structure of a fat starts with a number of carbon atoms linked together, called a *glycerol*. Carbon atoms can bond with either hydrogen or oxygen atoms to complete the structure of a fatty acid. When three fatty acids are attached to the framework, a *triglyceride* is formed. When no hydrogen atoms are missing from the makeup of a fatty acid, it is called *saturated*. Most animal fats are high in saturated fatty acids, as are some plant oils, with coconut and palm oils being good examples. When a single pair of hydrogen atoms is missing from the structure of a fatty acid, it is called *mono unsaturated*. Olive oil contains a large percentage of this type of fatty acid. When two or more pairs of hydrogen atoms are missing from the fabric of the fatty acid, it is *polyunsaturated*. Vegetable oils such as sunflower and safflower oils, as well as fish oils, are composed mainly of polyunsaturated fats.

As a general rule, the less liquid a fat is at room temperature, the more saturated it is. And since cholesterol is synthesized in the body from saturated fatty acids, they are the ones to avoid. Cholesterol blood levels of more than 200 milligrams per 100 milliliters of serum have been linked to increased risks of heart disease, high blood pressure and stroke. Thus, most authorities now agree that a maximum of 30 percent of the daily intake of calories should be from fat, with the major portion coming from unsaturated fats.

Recently, the importance of *fiber* in the diet has been widely proclaimed. Known as roughage or bulk in days past, fiber comes only from plant sources: vegetables, fruits and grains; there is no fiber embodied in animal products. Fiber has no calories, but it provides the stimulus that makes saliva flow (from chewing) and promotes regularity. More recent research indicates that fiber may be useful in reducing blood cholesterol, improving the control of blood sugar in diabetes and reducing the incidence of cancer of the colon. While most Americans eat only about 11 grams of fiber a day, current thinking places the recommended intake between 20 and 35 grams a day.

Vitamins, which were discovered in 1912, were considered to be "an amine necessary for life," thus "vitamin." Vitamin B-1 was the first to have its chemical structure identified. Today there are 13 vitamins recognized: nine water-soluble (the B complex group and vitamin C) and four fat-soluble (vitamins A, D, E and K). Fat-soluble vitamins are present in the fats of the foods we eat and are absorbed into the body with these foods. The fat-soluble vitamins are then stored in body fats. Though vitamins provide no calories to the body and are needed in only comparatively small quantities, they are essential for normal metabolism of the other nutrients in the diet. When sufficient vitamins are not included in the diet, vitamin deficiency diseases, such as scurvy, beriberi, pellagra and rickets, develop and are present in a world where starvation and food deprivation still exist. Recent research in the field of vitamins indicates that there is still much to learn about the action of vitamins in the body, and that the function of the *anti-oxidants* (vitamin C, vitamin E and beta-carotene or pro-vitamin A) also may serve to prevent disease and cellular deterioration.

In addition to vitamins, the body requires a number of inorganic elements called *minerals* to complete its biochemical functions. The *macrominerals*, which are required in larger quantities, include calcium, phosphorous and magnesium. In addition, sodium, potassium and chloride also are needed, particularly since sodium can be neither manufactured nor stored in the body. The *trace minerals* are not needed in any great quantity, but they too serve vital functions in the complex chemical processes that sustain life. Included as trace minerals are iron, zinc, selenium and iodine, for which recommended daily allowances (RDAs) have been established by the Food and Drug Administration, as well as copper, chromium, manganese and molybdenum for which there are no RDAs.

While the term vitamin has been around for quite a while, exercise as a health-promoting activity has appeared relatively recently in the medical literature of the world. Until just a few decades ago, the normal daily life of most people involved a good deal of physical labor, which burned the calories, kept the muscles toned and tuned, and vitalized both the cardiac and respiratory reserves. But with the advent of office-based occupations, television and many leisure pursuits requiring little more effort than sitting in a chair, the need for physical activity has been translated into a recreational undertaking.

Activity (or motion) results from the contractions of muscles, and it demands energy. The energy comes from burning the sugars in the body, which is a process that always requires some oxygen. If the level of the exercise is not intense or is of short duration, the body's reserves of sugar (as glycogen) and the normal amount of oxygen circulating in the bloodstream suffice to keep up the action. Such an activity is classified as *anaerobic* (more correctly, without additional air). But as the intensity increases or is prolonged, the body will draw fuel from glycogen reserves, fats and proteins, and it will require additional oxygen; thus the activity becomes an *aerobic* exercise. The heart beats faster, increasing the amount of blood pumped by the heart (cardiac output) and increasing the blood pressure in the arterial system. To provide the additional oxygen needed, the rate of breathing increases. As more and more calories are burned by the hard-working muscles, heat is produced, as much as 10 to 20 times the normal amount, so that the mechanisms of the body that regulate heat become active. The sweat glands produce perspiration, and as the sweat evaporates from the skin, it helps to cool the blood.

The benefits of regular exercise are many and cannot be overemphasized. In addition to the physical benefits to the cardiovascular and respiratory systems and the increase in muscle strength, exercise helps bones to develop and remain strong. The levels of both blood pressure and cholesterol can be reduced toward normal in cases where they are elevated. And there are psychological benefits as well, since exercise can be used to reduce stress and is thought to promote a feeling of well-being. While not exactly the Fountain of Youth that Ponce de Leon sought, regular exercise has been shown to retard or postpone some of the consequences of aging. Its advantages for the older citizen include the maintenance of muscle tone, mobility of the joints and flexibility of the tendons and ligaments. Reducing the risk of heart attack and preserving the power and muscle force that make getting about a lot easier are even more important when the years add up. These results may be achieved by simply walking at a brisk or moderate pace for 25 minutes or more, three times a week.

For the millions of Americans who are currently more than 9 kilograms (20 pounds) over the normal weight for their height and age, exercise provides the greatest boon. When it just isn't possible to restrict the amount of food we eat or to change the eating habits of a lifetime, the answer to the weight problem may lie in changing the pattern of activity by just a bit. It is generally accepted that burning 3,500 calories more than are taken in by eating leads to the loss of 0.45 kilograms (one pound). Thus, if you walk 30 to 40 minutes a day (in addition to your present level of activity) and don't increase your food intake over your current diet, a weight loss of seven to 10 kilograms (15 to 20 pounds) is possible in just a year's time. And that kind of weight loss stays off, for the change in activity level becomes a permanent part of the day's activities. Of course, different rates of walking and different body weights change these average numbers a bit, but the fundamentals still hold. It is that first step that is the hardest, and the one that most people fail to take.

I began this chapter with a quote that serves well to conclude this book. It calls for moderation as a guiding principle upon which to base actions. Of all the health hints that are contained herein, none is more important. It is when belief is placed in concepts that advocate excess, such as too much exercise, or too little food, or too much weight lost in too little time, that health slips through our outstretched hands. When programs that promise totally "unbelievable" results are accepted as being true, our financial health disappears with equal haste. The secure road to health depends upon three important actions you can initiate and control yourself: 1) Ask the questions that obtain for you the answers you need to understand the problem. 2) Become firmly convinced that the solution lies in taking the proper actions. 3) Once the path is clear, follow through consistently and continually until the goal is achieved.

Moderation is the pathway to good health
When its principles are applied moderately;
invoking neither guilt nor shame, and understanding
that a brief, limited voyage to 'excess' can provide the spice
that makes the diet palatable.

ALLAN H. BRUCKHEIM, M.D.
American physician, author, lecturer (1928-)

Questions and Answers

336. ***We are striving to follow all the rules of healthy living, but they seem to change as fast as a politician's promises. It is hard to keep up. We are striving for a low-cholesterol diet and, as such, eat eggs only once a week. However, now my husband devours pancakes instead, and I worry that this may not be too healthy, either. What's your word on this breakfast food? We use a prepared mix, if that will help you answer.***

I think that flapjacks form a fine food around which to build a nutritious breakfast. Using a mix is just fine, for it provides you with all the nutritional information you need to make the correct choice right on the package.

Most mixes are low in cholesterol, provided no eggs or whole milk are required to complete the batter. Mixes range in fat content from a low of 2 grams to a high of 12 grams in one case. However, many contain large amounts of salt, ranging from 230 milligrams to a high of 880 milligrams.

The average serving of three or four 4-inch pancakes will provide from 180 to 300 calories, until you add the toppings. That's when both the calories and cholesterol can begin to add up, unless you maintain your vigil and read labels. A tablespoon of butter or margarine adds 100 calories and 12 grams of fat. Consider "lite" syrups or fruit preserves instead. Then enjoy!

337. ***While we were preparing a barbecue for some guests, one friend told me that we all were being exposed to cancer by eating the food I had cooked. Though I tried to pass it off as just another tall tale, she usually knows about things like this and I began to wonder. Can you put my mind to rest on this one, or perhaps explain what she was referring to?***

While, to many people's thinking, all the data isn't in on this subject, some studies conducted by the National Cancer Institute link cancer in animals to foods cooked at very high temperatures.

While stove cooking may be done at more moderate levels, a blazing barbecue may reach 350 degrees Fahrenheit and sometimes much above. During such high-heat cooking, a group of chemicals is produced in the food; these are called HAAs (for heterocyclic aromatic amines). These chemicals can damage the DNA in laboratory test bacteria and therefore are identified as mutagens, for the changed DNA produces new strains of mutated bacteria. The theory states that these types of mutations might lead to cancer in humans over time.

Another potential danger is the result of fat dripping on the hot coals. This produces a smoke that contains smoky hydrocarbons (polynuclear aromatic hydrocarbons), which are deposited on the surface of the food you are preparing and also have been suspected of being carcinogenic.

These tips will help you cut down on the amount of these chemicals in barbecue-grilled food:

- Use cuts of meat and chicken with all possible fat removed.
- Use cooler-burning fuels, like ordinary charcoal, real hickory wood or maple, rather than mesquite, which burns at a higher temperature.

- Place the food 5 inches or more above the coals to reduce the chance of charring, for the blackened meat contains the largest amounts of the undesirable chemicals.
- Precook your foods by microwaving, boiling or poaching before a final pass on the grill. This is another way to reduce the production of hydrocarbons or HAAs.

When all is said and done, though, if you ignore these few tips your risks are considered to be few, unless you're on a regular daily diet of barbecued meats and poultry.

338. ***I'm seeking information about a type of food poisoning called "bottled poison." I know it is very serious, because my brother-in-law almost died from this condition. I have looked in all the books in our small library but can find nothing written about this. Can you provide me with any information to help us understand what happened?***

My first thought was that this was a case of poisoning from illegally produced whiskey, "moonlighter's hootch" or moonshine. Such liquor has been known to produce serious problems that might be considered food poisoning.

However, I felt that you would have understood that situation, and therefore you had been mistaken about the real name of the condition. So, using my computer word search, I entered the word bottle and found the term botulism nearby. I believe this condition fits the circumstances you described.

Botulism is indeed a most serious type of food poisoning. It's capable of causing death if the amount of poison in the food is great enough. The poison, or toxin, is produced by an organism called Clostridium botulinum. It is the most potent bacterial poison known. The organism is found in the soil and in sea water. It forms spores that can contaminate food that is improperly processed or cooked. The spores can resist low cooking temperatures, then produce active organisms, which in turn produce the toxins that taint the food.

The toxin affects the nerves of the peripheral nervous system. Symptoms of botulism include double vision, dry mouth, nausea, vomiting and a progressive paralysis. The paralysis starts with muscles in the face and then travels down the body, affecting the arms, chest muscles and finally the legs.

Treatment includes induced vomiting — if the poisoned food was eaten recently — gastric irrigation and laxatives. Antitoxins may be used within 24 hours after the start of symptoms, but they have some serious side effects. These antitoxins are considered for use in only the most severe cases, which also require hospitalization in an intensive care setting.

339. ***I have had it with all my jock colleagues who brag about their exercise programs. This exercise fad is just bunk — why should I bother?***

Sounds like you need some information. There's abundant evidence that exercise arms you with protection against heart disease, diabetes, hypertension, obesity and many stress-related conditions.

Several studies have compared the incidence of heart disease in active and sedentary people. One such study looked at postal delivery people and postal clerks, and it found significantly less fatal and nonfatal heart disease in those who deliver mail. Another study showed that physical training increases the body's sensitivity to insulin, which shows a positive role in preventing and managing maturity-onset diabetes (non-insulin dependent).

There currently is no evidence that exercise lowers cholesterol levels, but endurance exercise increases high-density lipoproteins, or "good" cholesterol, in the blood.

You sound like someone who doesn't enjoy exercise. People like you can increase their physical activity in small ways that will add up to some significant health benefits. Instead of looking for a parking place close to work, park in the far corner of the lot. Take the stairs instead of the elevator. The extra steps will do you some good.

If you don't like exercise, find a way to get involved in some physical activity that you find comfortable. It pays off in improved health.

340. ***One of my friends is always on a diet. And she's always handing out information on how to lose weight. This week's big tip is to remove all bread from your diet. Does this make any sense? I love bread and would rather eat that than anything else, but I also have a weight problem.***

Actually, I love a good piece of bread as well, so your question was one I had to answer for myself. Truly, bread takes a bad rap in most cases, for the average slice of bread is only 60 to 90 calories. And you easily can include a slice or two in any sensible diet.

However, there are lots of types of bread, and you will have to do some label reading to know just where you are. Some light breads, which contain 35 to 40 calories, are merely thinner slices, so compare equal weights per portion when evaluating both the caloric and nutritional content of your food.

Bread can be a very good source of fiber, minerals and vitamins. A slice of bread that will help both weight control and good nutrition will contain from 2 to 3 grams of fiber per slice.

The secret in establishing a healthy diet that will keep your weight down is to control portion size rather than to change foods. It's almost as hard to eat foods you don't like as to give up those that you love. So eat your bread, but in moderation and after you have carefully checked the labels for content.

341. ***My boss is trying to lose weight, but I think he's on the wrong track. He gobbles down a quick lunch, then spends the rest of his lunch hour "speed walking." He thinks this helps to burn off the calories he has just consumed. I was taught that exercise after eating was dangerous. Is my boss in some type of danger? He really is too good to lose.***

Well then, let's see if we can keep him fit without any undue risks. Your lesson in the dangers of eating first then exercising probably came from similar admonitions — such as no swimming after eating — that I received as a lad. And they still hold true.

As the process of digestion starts, foods are broken down into the fatty acids, amino acids and simple sugars used by the body. Large amounts of blood are sent to the abdomen, where the intestines are located, to aid digestion and absorption. Since active muscles demand increased blood flow, exercise can pull the blood away from its digestive functions, which results in distress, cramps and indigestion.

While a bloated or full feeling that results from gorging on a feast can be relieved by low level exercise like walking, your boss' actions will not help him accomplish his weight-loss objective. However, reversing the pattern might.

Vigorous exercise before a meal can raise the metabolic rate at which calories are burned. This rate remains elevated even when the exercise stops, and this "afterburn" can help in weight control. In addition, exercise also may decrease appetite and help your boss resist the temptations of overeating. The exercise also will burn the stored reserves of glycogen (the body's ready source of energy), and the new food carbohydrates will be used to replenish this glycogen rather than being converted to fat.

So here is a health tip for your boss (and other readers): Use exercise before meals as an appetite suppressant, and restrict after-meal exercise to a slow walk, which aids digestion.

342. ***Now that my confidence in all the over-the-counter cold remedies has been shaken by recent television news reports, I suppose you will tell me that chicken soup is no good either. I have had to put up with my mother-in-law's stories for years about how effective this home remedy is. But I'm asking you for more scientific analysis of the idea. In straight talk now, is chicken soup really any good for treating the cold, and would you take it if you had a bad cold?***

I suppose I should include something about chicken soup to respond to the many questions that are submitted about the "broth that heals," but I resist displaying my biases so openly. Yes, if (and when) I get a cold, chicken soup heads the menu. There are a lot of fairly simple reasons and one or two scientific ones.

Surely you know how important liquids are in treating a cold. Chicken soup can add to the volume, along with the juices and tea that most people consume. When made in traditional fashion, with carrots, onions, celery, parsley, garlic and other spices, chicken soup contains a good amount of vitamin A and the B vitamins niacin and riboflavin. When your stomach is fragile because of the effects of the cold, chicken soup provides a soothing way to get the calories and minerals your body needs to fight the virus.

From a more scientific point of view, there isn't too much in the way of laboratory or even clinical tests of the theory. More than 15 years ago, some physicians at Mount Sinai Medical Center in Miami Beach, Florida, compared the effects of chicken soup with that of hot water and cold water. Both hot water and chicken soup were found to speed up the disappearance of virus-filled mucus from the respiratory tract. Chemical analysis showed that homemade chicken soup contains chemicals that are similar to medications that can thin mucous secretions, which provides quicker relief from coughing and sneezing.

Don't lose faith. A tradition that has lasted this long must have something going for it. As the old punch line goes, "It may not help, but it couldn't hurt."

343. ***Please write something about the eating sickness that is causing my daughter to shrink away before my eyes. Tell her it could affect her heart. Please help an anxious mother deal with this problem.***

Anorexia nervosa is a serious illness. Fifteen percent of all anorexia sufferers die, which makes it the deadliest of all psychiatric disorders.

Sudden deaths among anorectics often are due to the serious damage that the disorder causes to the heart.

Researchers have known for a long time that anorectics have abnormal heart rhythms, including heart rates that are too fast, too slow or lack the proper rhythm. Their hearts also are shrunken in size.

It always had been thought that when the body is starved, the heart and brain are spared at the expense of other parts of the body. But an anorectic's heart appears to lose more weight and size proportionately than the rest of the body. The size of the heart's left ventricle in anorectics is especially reduced. Bulimia — eating and then vomiting — also can cause heart problems due to chemical imbalances in the body.

Because of these heart changes, anorectics cannot exercise as long as normal during exercise stress tests. Their heart rates and blood pressures do not respond normally to the extra effort of exercise as a healthy person's would. It is still not known whether the heart returns to normal after the patient regains her weight or whether these changes are permanent. Some studies have shown that the heart does increase in size as weight is gained.

Your daughter needs professional treatment. Even a mother's concern may not be enough to get her on the right path. This warning should be clear enough to help make her seek medical care.

344. ***I'm home now after my first heart attack. My doctor said it was a moderate one. My family has presented me with all sorts of books on health, diet, exercise. It looks like a life's work to get through them all. Before I start, I want to know if changing my diet and some of these other things have been proven to prevent another attack. Along with my natural anxiety about the future is a skeptical attitude about so-called health cures.***

You're right! It is a "life's work" — *your* life. Trying to learn how to restructure your lifestyle after a heart attack may be overwhelming when you're swamped by all the books you have collected. So let's take it more slowly and look at a few basics.

Don't confuse good nutrition, sensible exercise and removing stress from daily living as being a quack "health cure." Heart attacks result from damage to the arteries that bring nourishing blood flow to the muscles of the heart. When they become clogged by obstacles loaded with fats (atheromatous plaques), blood flow is either cut off or diminished. The muscles no longer can function and they die from lack of nourishment. No amount of dieting or exercise is going to bring those muscle cells back to life. But the goal now is to get the maximum out of your remaining heart muscles and to prevent recurrence of the same problems that led to your first attack.

Reduce the amounts of fats in your diet and increase fiber, fruits and vegetables, and you can reduce the size of those obstructions in your heart's blood vessels. Start a cardiac rehabilitation exercise program, and you can get the most from your healed but scarred heart. Lose some weight, if need be, and reduce the workload on your body. Reduce the stress factors in your life, and "get a load off your mind."

I wish I could provide specific proof with absolute affirmation that, in your case, all these things will work as predicted. No one can do that. But the odds are very much in your favor. This is evidenced by literally hundreds of scientific reports. Should you choose not to accept these new challenges, it would be equal to putting your life back on the block. Check with your own physician, who knows your story, and accept the recommendations that can bring you reasonable expectations that another attack will not occur.

345. ***Ever since my husband read that the Chinese have fewer medical problems than we do, it has been one Chinese restaurant after another. I like the food well enough, but it is getting just a bit boring. Are we doing anything positive for our health that makes choosing this one cuisine a reasonable option? Do you think the diet in China is the basis for their better health statistics?***

Your husband's reading is correct enough. It seems that Americans do suffer more from "diseases of affluence" than the citizens of China.

For example, only four out of 100,000 men die from heart disease in China, while 67 out of 100,000 American men succumb to the ravages of heart disease. Breast cancer is five times more frequent in American women, and American women run eight times the risk for cervical cancer than their Chinese counterparts. And the statistics on both colon cancer and diabetes reveal that the Chinese diet is apparently more healthful than ours.

It is not the quantity of food, as the Chinese eat more, both in ounces and calories, than we do, but they consume far less fat and much less animal protein. The major meal in China is rice with vegetables, occasionally with meat, fish or poultry added for flavor and variety.

But that is the diet as served in China, not your local Chinese restaurant, where most of the food is prepared by frying, which adds fat to the diet that does not form part of the menu in China. Add to that the sodium in the soy sauce, the great reliance on beef, pork, chicken and seafood rich in cholesterol (shrimp and lobster) and sauces made with sugar, fat or oil and cornstarch, and we're no longer discussing the healthy cuisine as eaten in China.

You can get back to some of the elements that make "authentic" Chinese cooking so beneficial. Start with a simple soup to reduce your appetite and satisfy you with smaller portions. Make rice the main component of the meal, with just a bit of vegetables and meat to add flavor and variety. Use chopsticks while eating, because they slow you down to permit that full feeling to develop and you leave most of the heavy sauces back on the plate.

346. ***Please compare two men who are exercising. One is walking and finishes 3 miles in one hour. The other covers the same course by running at 6 miles an hour. Who is burning the most calories? Do both exercise periods yield the same health benefits? I'm sure there must be a formula for all of this.***

Great question! Even though math is not one of my strong points, there are some simple formulas to help. For the purposes of a valid comparison, I chose to make both men the same age, 45 years old, both weigh 175 pounds, and both are 5 feet 10 inches tall. That's pretty average.

The walker covers the course at 3 miles per hour and burns 278 calories. Not bad. The runner, at 6 miles per hour, covers the same course in 30 minutes and burns ... 278 calories. The runner's only advantage is that he finishes faster.

However, since the slow walker had a longer sustained period of exercise, it's probable that he burned more fat than the runner did, since we start burning calories from fat only after sustained exercise of 20 minutes or more. Since his pulse rate was elevated for a longer period of time, he most probably improved his cardiovascular reserves. That means he strengthened his heart a bit, which probably had a positive effect on any elevated blood pressure and gave a boost to his immune system.

These answers are easy to explain. Since the formula for caloric burn from exercise depends upon distance, sex, age, height and weight, the results are the same for both men in this example. If you wish to include the other benefits of exercise in a calculation of health benefits, time plays an important role. Thus the person who exercises for longer periods of time or works out more frequently will show the greatest gains.

All of this may be quite pleasing to you if you are the slower man in the example, as I suspect you are. I know it gives me a measure of satisfaction as the younger guys fly past me on the track, yet are long gone by the time I have finished. For I know, as you now know, that it is indeed the turtle who often wins the race, for health, that is. If you doubt me, check out the life expectancy of a turtle versus a hare.

347. ***My physician suggested I follow the seven simple guidelines to a healthy diet, which I said I would do. But he never told me what they were, and I didn't ask. Do you know what they are?***

Of course, and I am happy to pass them on to you and my other readers:

1. Eat a variety of foods. Include fruits and vegetables, whole cereals, lean meats, poultry, fish, peas, beans and low-fat dairy products.
2. Maintain a desirable weight.
3. Avoid too much saturated fat and cholesterol.
4. Eat foods with adequate starch and fiber.
5. Avoid too much sugar.
6. Avoid too much sodium.
7. If you drink alcoholic beverages, do so only in moderation.

These guidelines may sound easy, and they are. Your health will profit immeasurably if you follow them.

348. ***I was astounded when my son told me he's now a vegetarian and is avoiding all types of meats. He assures me that this is a healthy diet and by staying on this diet he never will have a problem with high cholesterol. Maybe so, but what about other risks? Can you please offer me some insight into the safety of such diets?***

There are many types of vegetarian diets, and they vary considerably in the nutrients they might lack. Many reasons are given by those who choose these diets: religion, a belief that eating animals is immoral, cost, or that some people just enjoy the flavor and variety a vegetarian diet offers.

Some vegetarian diets include dairy foods, eggs, chicken and fish, but no other animal flesh (semi-vegetarian). Others include milk but no animal flesh or eggs (lacto-vegetarian), and the pure vegetarian diet excludes animal foods of any type (vegan).

Depending upon the extent of his restrictions, your son's diet may provoke deficiencies in vitamin B-12, vitamin D and calcium. Some deficiencies in the micronutrients — iron, copper and zinc — also are possible. Animal flesh, eggs and milk contain the eight essential amino acids the human body requires to fulfill the total protein requirements for complete nutrition.

These amino acids are also available in a plant-based diet, but it takes a variety of grains, legumes, seeds and vegetables to provide all eight in the needed quantities. But the list of products is long: black-eyed peas, soybeans, peanuts, lentils, sprouts, peas, rice, wheat, corn, rye, oats, millet, barley, buckwheat and all the beans (kidney, lima, navy, etc.), as well as all the nuts, vegetables and fruits. These can be mixed and enough included in the diet to obtain all the necessary nutrition.

Vegetarians are aware of these needs and usually show great diligence in studying the essentials of healthy nutrition, and display great ingenuity in obtaining all the essentials.

349.

My wife insists there is a chemical in wine that can produce a cancer. She says everybody knows about this, even the FDA, but that no one is doing anything to protect us. Could you please look into this and let us know where we stand?

It wasn't hard to discover the answer to your question, for a great many people do know about it, and a great deal is being done. To start with, the chemical in question is called urethane, which is a natural product of the fermentation process in which yeast turns fruit juice into wine. It's known also as ethyl carbamate, and it's not a product of any new technology.

Some amounts of urethane are present in many alcoholic beverages. The amounts differ significantly in quantity from one alcoholic product to another and even between bottles of the same variety or brand.

Both the Food and Drug Administration and the Bureau of Alcohol, Tobacco and Firearms have sampled some of the products on the market. Imported fruit brandies had the highest levels, with about 1,200 parts per billion (ppb), sake was next with about 300 ppb, and then bourbon with 150 ppb. Ordinary grape table wines only have about 13 ppb, but dessert wines can contain up to 115 ppb.

The problem is that no one knows just how much risk these amounts represent, for the studies being conducted at the FDA's request by the National Toxicology Program are not yet completed.

However, no one is waiting around. Led by the Distilled Spirits Council of the United States, the American Association of Vintners and the Wine Institute the industry is pursuing strategies calculated to lower the quantities of urethane in all alcoholic beverages. These strategies include changes in wine growing (lowering the amount of fertilizers used), using a new type of yeast in the fermentation process, and making modifications in the manufacturing plants and processes. Recent tests have shown marked reductions in the urethane contained in recently processed alcoholic beverages.

In general, domestic products contain less urethane than imported brands. For now, there seems little for the moderate consumer of spirits to be concerned about, but prudence would seem to dictate limiting the consumption of products containing high levels of urethane, such as fruit brandies.

350. ***For the past two years, I participated in an aerobics class at least three times a week. I now feel fit, trim and happy. Unfortunately, I have been transferred to another office, in another town, with a schedule that just doesn't permit me to continue my current level of activity. How long will my present state of fitness last?***

Not too long if you stop your training program completely. Fitness can be measured in terms of endurance, the ability of your heart to function as measured by its ability to beat (or maximal heart rate), as well as other criteria, all of which begin to decline rapidly during the first 12 days after you stop exercising. They continue to retreat from the high levels you achieved after that, but in a more gradual fashion. This reduction in fitness is called detraining. If you value your hard-won gains, you may wish to take these words of advice:

Although you always can retrain to get back to your highest level of fitness, the road will not be as long nor as difficult if you manage to fit even a little exercise into your new schedule. Make your sessions more intense, a bit faster or more energetic than your usual session. A shorter period of time then can provide almost the same benefits as a longer session. Try for two sessions a week if you can't make it to three, or even just once a week if that is all you can manage.

Any exercise you do now will reduce the time needed to get back into high gear when you start your program again, and any activity now will slow down the detraining effect. And that includes running upstairs on a regular basis instead of using elevators and walking instead of taking public transportation.

You still will be better off than those who have never trained, even after three months, but continuing complete inactivity eventually will put you back to square one.

351. ***My boyfriend is on a new health kick, and this time it is yogurt. Every conversation seems to turn to the marvels of this food (boring!). Can you please discuss this, so that I can set him straight and put a stop to his endless lectures on "long life through yogurt"?***

Ever since bacteriologist Elie Metchnikoff credited yogurt for the long lives of yogurt-eating Russians living in the Caucasus Mountains, the legend has grown, supported by innumerable articles in health magazines and journals. From a strictly scientific point of view, there are some interesting nutritional points that can be offered.

Yogurt is made from milk and contains many of the nutritional benefits of this liquid food. It is converted into yogurt by the action of two bacteria, Lactobacillus bulgaricus and Streptococcus thermophilus, through a process known as lactic acid fermentation.

Depending on the techniques used in bringing the final product to the market, the bacteria still might be found alive and active in the yogurt or might not be present, destroyed by heat treatment after culturing.

While different yogurts contain different amounts of nutrients, all contain substantial amounts of protein, calcium and lactose. Different categories of yogurt — whole milk, low-fat and nonfat yogurts — contain varying amounts of fat, from a high of 7 grams per serving to the nonfat low of 1 gram or less per serving. Caloric values per serving also vary depending upon the amount of added sugar contained in many of the fruit-flavored varieties.

Current research is looking at the live bacteria variety and the lactic acid they produce. It seems that these bacteria do survive the digestive process and may have a role in reducing blood cholesterol levels and the incidence of intestinal tumors.

It may not be the road to long life, but the nutritional value of yogurt in a balanced diet cannot be disputed. This may not turn off your boyfriend's lectures, but at least now you have a bit more knowledge about the subject.

352. ***Do you have any tips on how to reduce sodium in my diet? It's taken some effort to make up my mind to do it, because I love salt so, but now's the time. I have been told that this is an important health consideration.***

I sure do have some good tips, and they're easy to do. If you're concerned about sodium, you're probably already keeping the salt shaker in a hard-to-reach place in your kitchen. If you're still using salt in cooking or at the table, gradually reduce its use until you've stopped.

The next thing to do is to learn the foods that are high in sodium, and some of these may surprise you. Read labels on prepared, canned and frozen foods. Foods that are low in calories and fats still can be high in sodium. Examples are cottage cheese, milk and tuna. Generally, canned vegetables are higher in sodium than frozen ones. Bacon, ham, olives, luncheon meat and canned soups are generally high in sodium.

Know that softened water is high in sodium, as are many over-the-counter drugs. You may be getting unwelcome and unnecessary sodium in antacids, mouthwashes, antibiotics, cough medicines and laxatives. Your pharmacist can help you evaluate the sodium content of any medicine you're taking.

Sodium is measured in milligrams, and a "no-added-salt diet" usually means you should limit your sodium to 4 grams per day, which is 4,000 milligrams.

353. ***My husband and I take our daily vitamins quite faithfully. But we do have our differences in technique. Hubbie takes his vitamins before his meals, while I was taught to take them after my meals. Would you please straighten us out and tell us who is right? I also would like to know if it is better to take them in the morning or in the evening.***

According to most experts, the proper time to take vitamins is at mealtime, along with your food. In this way, vitamins are absorbed along with the rest of your food, and they provide you with the greatest benefit. Mealtime is considered to span from a few minutes before a meal to up to a half-hour afterward. By that standard, you're both right, and I like things that way.

However, some authorities are more specific and maintain that the very best time for your vitamins is immediately after eating. So perhaps you're more right than your husband. But they all agree that it is best to spread out your vitamins over the day, by taking some after each meal. This will provide the highest level of vitamins in the body's system over the longest period of time. If it is not possible to take some after each meal — either because your dosage is not that high or because you're just not home during the day — divide the quantity you take into two doses, one for the morning, the other with the evening meal.

Finally, if you must take all your vitamins all at once, then it is best to take them after your largest meal of the day, which for most people is dinner — most commonly the evening meal.

To be complete, I also must inform you that at least one reference provides the advice that oil-soluble vitamins should be taken before meals and water-soluble vitamins should be taken afterward. That's pretty difficult to do if you are taking a "one a day" multivitamin preparation.

Now that we have worked our way through all this information, here's my final word: Just take them! — your husband as he wishes, and you as you wish. And may you both take them together for many years to come.

354. ***The new buzzword going around is "yo-yo" dieting. If I understand the articles in the paper, you might be better off if you stayed fat. It sure would save a lot of guilt and probably considerable money, too. Still I find it hard to believe that fat is better than thin, so I hope you will try to explain what all the frenzy is about.***

The wave of articles in the press and stories on television were inspired by the results of a study published in the *New England Journal of Medicine*. It was based upon findings in the ongoing evaluation of adult residents, ages 30 to 62 years, of Framingham, Massachusetts. The study was started in 1948 and is collecting health statistics over the lifetimes of these individuals.

A review of the health records of 3,130 participants revealed that individuals whose weight fluctuated frequently over a period of 32 years had a greater risk of coronary artery heart disease than those individuals whose weight remained relatively stable.

An additional conclusion was that the more the weight changed, the greater the risk of coronary artery heart disease. That doesn't mean individuals who are substantially overweight won't achieve a better health profile by shedding those excess pounds. It translates into recommendations for safer, slower weight loss maintained through good eating and exercise habits.

355. *I've taken some medical advice and am now on a diet. But I get terribly upset and frustrated because there are days I actually gain weight. My scale shows as much as a 2- or 3-pound gain even on days I have been most careful. What's a gal to do?*

Probably the best answer to this frequently asked question is to weigh yourself only once each week. That allows the ups and downs in your daily weight to average out, and you can gain a better sense of your progress.

It isn't fat that is causing the changes to occur, but retained water. Certain liquids, such as coffee, actually act as diuretics, which help your kidneys pump out extra fluid and cause the weight to drop. Foods that contain extra salt, for example Oriental foods with soy sauce and Italian foods with a great deal of commercially prepared tomato sauce, can add several pounds overnight.

If you consume from 3,000 to 3,500 fewer calories than you burn in a given period of time, you can expect a real loss of about 1 pound by the end of that period. Add on extra exercise, which burns 350 to 550 calories per hour depending upon intensity, and you can lose even more. It may seem slow, but it's safer, and with the newly acquired health habits, the pounds will remain off over the long haul.

356. *Do you know anything about a new diet to prevent cancer that requires you to eat lots of veggies and fruits? I'm especially interested in knowing how much is enough. It seems to me that you have to eat tons of these foods to get any benefit. Please explain.*

The new diet is part of a program called "5 a Day for Better Health," sponsored by the National Cancer Institute (which represents the government) and the Produce for Better Health Foundation (which represents the fruit and vegetable industry).

Research has shown that a diet rich in fiber, low in fat and containing lots of fruits and vegetables can have a significant impact on lowering your risk of cancer. This educational program seeks to bring you these benefits.

You don't need "tons," but the daily servings required can be made up of five (or as many as nine) choices from the following servings: one medium fruit, three-quarters cup of 100 percent juice, a half-cup of vegetables or fruits, one cup of raw leafy vegetables, and one-quarter cup of dried fruits.

You can pick and choose as you wish. Currently, most Americans eat only about three servings of these foods a day.

For more information, you can contact the Office of Cancer Communications, National Cancer Institute (NCI), Bethesda, Maryland 20892, or call the Cancer Information Center at 1-800-422-6237.

357. *An article in the paper stated that doctors now think triglycerides are more important than cholesterol in predicting your chances of suffering a heart attack. Why then would a doctor still take a blood test for cholesterol? Shouldn't he be using the triglyceride test instead?*

Though triglycerides have taken on a new importance in evaluating the risks of heart attacks, relying on a single test with absolute numbers is a trap we all can fall into. No single factor is an absolute predictor of future events, and no numbers are absolutes.

When dealing with cholesterol and triglycerides, it's probably more useful to consider them as part of a total picture of the fats that circulate within the bloodstream. The values found on tests for lipoproteins can be useful tools when looked at in a comprehensive manner. Thus the current thinking is to use cholesterol tests for screening, but to order the more complete lipid profile, which includes triglyceride levels, for a more realistic evaluation when the situation warrants it.

A full profile includes tests for cholesterol, triglycerides, high-density lipoproteins (HDL) and low-density lipoproteins (LDL). These tests indicate the level of each chemical in the bloodstream and also permit the cross-comparison of HDL and LDL, also known as the HDL/LDL ratio. A physician can use these findings along with an assessment of the patient's history and physical examination to determine just what treatment, if any, is needed.

For example, a borderline-high triglyceride coupled with an acceptable LDL value may require treatment in an individual whose family history includes close family members who have had coronary heart disease. Others with the same test findings but no family history risk factors might not require treatment. That leaves me with a realistic but somewhat unsatisfying answer to your question: "It all depends."

You should have a full evaluation of your personal risk factors before tests are ordered. Then it's not the results of the tests alone that will determine your need for treatment, but the entire medical picture. And for that, I recommend a full discussion with your own physician.

358. ***My doctor is treating me for a moderate elevation in my blood pressure. I'm determined to comply with all his suggestions, but his latest request for me to give up my morning coffee is a bit hard to take. Do you have any information that might help me convince him to rethink this new restriction? I do love that first cup in the morning.***

The medical literature really is divided on this one, with as many studies showing coffee as a risk factor in circulatory system problems as there are articles that say that coffee is safe. I believe it depends upon two factors: How much coffee you drink each day, and how long you have been drinking coffee.

For the most part, no risk is seen when the quantity of coffee is below four cups a day; some articles put that number at less than six cups. If you are talking about only one or two cups with breakfast, I can find no evidence that this amount would create a problem. In addition, the reaction to coffee that increases blood pressure seems to be present only in people who have not developed a tolerance to caffeine.

It may be that the best way to fulfill both your desire and the instructions of your physician is to switch to a decaffeinated brand. At any rate, an open discussion with your doctor is in order. This subject is not as black or "with milk" as it would seem.

359. ***When I checked the amount of calories that men and women lose when exercising, I found some numbers that puzzle me. Even when a man and a woman weigh the same, the man loses weight faster because he burns more calories for each hour of activity. It isn't fair! I don't understand why this is true. Could you please shed some light on this situation? I would be most grateful.***

Your calorie scale is correct even if it is unusual, for most tables used in calculating caloric burn and weight loss fail to indicate the differences between the sexes.

Men and women have different metabolic rates, even when their ages, weights and activities are the same. And the metabolic rate runs about 10 percent lower in women than men.

An average-sized woman in her 30s who lives a lifestyle that is fairly active will burn about 2,400 calories a day. An average man with a similar build and lifestyle will use about 3,000 calories per day. This difference also is reflected in the calculations for the various intensities of exercise programs. In every case, when using total body weight in figuring caloric burn, a woman is at a disadvantage.

The basis of this difference lies in the proportion of muscle that makes up the total weight of the individual. A man's body is made up of about 45 percent muscle tissue, compared with only 36 percent for a woman. Many factors might change the exact percentages, but these are close enough for this explanation.

The fact remains that muscles use the greatest amount of the body's energy. So the more muscle mass present, the greater the number of calories burned. For some scientific analyses, a researcher may choose to calculate the lean mass of the body when calculating the amount of energy used, and this can overcome the anatomical difference.

Since you must burn about 3,000 to 3,500 calories more than you eat to lose a pound of weight, the scientific method actually doesn't help when you are checking the scales. However, adding some muscle-building exercises to a pure aerobic program will add more muscle mass to your frame and eventually burn more calories for you.

360. ***At parties at some of my friends' homes, one of the appetizers served is steak tartare, which consists of raw ground beef with onions and other ingredients. I have read that raw beef could cause some serious infections, the names of which I forgot. So far I have refrained from partaking of this dish. Your comments would be appreciated.***

Keep your resolve strong and continue to refrain from sampling these "gourmet" appetizers. Recent outbreaks of food-borne illnesses in some Western states have heightened our appreciation of the risks involved when food is improperly handled and prepared.

In those cases, the infecting organism was a rare form of E. coli, but since it is destroyed by proper cooking the lesson is clear: Don't eat raw ground beef. That opinion is shared by the experts at the National Live Stock & Meat Board. It may cause a bit of consternation in your social circles and my French chef friends will object, but steak tartare should be served "medium" cooked, when an internal temperature of 160 degrees Fahrenheit is attained or when the center is light gray and the juices run clear.

Here are some other tips to keep your hamburgers nutritious and safe:

- Refrigerate or freeze meat immediately after purchasing.
- Never defrost frozen meat at room temperature on the counter top or in warm water. The proper technique is to defrost frozen meat in the refrigerator for 15 to 24 hours.

- Keep your kitchen work areas and cooking utensils clean, and wash your hands thoroughly in hot, soapy water before starting to prepare meals.
- Cook ground beef as soon as possible after thawing, and then cook it without interruption until it is ready to eat. Partial cooking may encourage bacterial growth.
- Do not leave hot foods out of refrigeration for more than two hours. Instead, refrigerate leftovers promptly, dividing large quantities into smaller portions to allow them to cool more rapidly.

Following these tips will reduce the chances of bacteria getting a foothold in your meat products, and thus prevent the production of the toxins that may cause serious illness — and even death.

361. ***I have seen exercise touted as being of benefit for many situations and diseases, particularly in preventing heart problems. But what can you tell me about exercise and diabetes? Do I run a chance of more risks than benefits from starting to get out and around a jogging track now? I am 53, and have had diabetes for just two years.***

I must answer your question from an "it depends" perspective, for much relies upon you and your history. If you have Type II diabetes (non-insulin dependent), exercise can help increase the effectiveness of the insulin you produce in your body and can help control your sugar levels.

Exercise also can be a valuable aid in reducing weight, an important consideration in a diabetic. Some people with a family history of diabetes, and thus an increased risk for developing the condition, can prevent its evolution and avoid it completely.

Individuals with Type I diabetes (insulin-dependent) may be able to lower the amounts of insulin needed to control their levels of blood glucose. All of that is provided, in addition to the benefits to heart, lungs and muscles you already know about.

If you're taking insulin, your dosage and schedule may have to be modified as you change the amount of energy you use for your activities. Regular home blood monitoring, both before and after exercise, and frequent consultations with your physician can provide you with the information to calculate any changes you may require.

You state you've recently been afflicted with this condition, so the possibility of long-term complications of diabetes in your case seems remote. However, in others, these require some serious consideration. The presence of some complications, such as those that may occur to nerves and blood vessels, would place restrictions on an exercise program. Aerobic exercise, jogging or walking is better than resistance exercise, such as weight lifting.

Starting a directed exercise program now during the early stages of your diabetes may win important benefits for you in the long run. Check with your physician to be sure you start out on the right foot.

362. ***I have been reading a lot about some new vitamins called "anti-oxidants," but no one has explained what they do in words an ordinary person can understand. Is the subject so complicated that nobody knows what they are talking about?***

The recent discoveries about this hitherto unsuspected action of some vitamins has captured the attention and imagination of many nutritional writers. They are not "new" vitamins, but in truth old friends.

Because anti-oxidants are complicated, usually only a few words explaining their actions are contained in articles that tell you how much good they might do for you. I'll try to explain anti-oxidants as simply as possible, even though some of my more learned colleagues may catch me taking a shortcut or two for the sake of clarity.

All atoms contain a nucleus and electrons that circulate around it. Atoms connect to each other to form molecules by sharing or exchanging their electrons. For example, water is formed by three atoms: two hydrogen and one oxygen (H_2O). The electrons they share are locked into a stable compound that is difficult to break down.

However, in some compounds there is a free radical, which is an electron that is not held firmly in the compound, so it is "free" to break away and attach to another compound or body tissue. You can liken it to hydrogen peroxide (H_2O_2), which contains one more oxygen atom than water does. When this common preparation is used to help clean wounds, the extra oxygen readily bubbles up as the liquid comes in contact with the wound.

Consider those bubbles of oxygen to be very similar to the free radicals in the body. When they combine with normal tissues, they oxidize some of the chemicals that form the tissue — a little like oxygen turning iron to rust (or iron oxide). And just as rust does not possess the strength of iron, oxidized tissues lose their strength or their ability to function as they are damaged by the oxidation process.

Free radicals are formed as the result of everyday metabolism, as the body converts foods to useful chemical molecules that it requires for energy and rebuilding. But free radicals also are formed by tissue damage (for example, from excess sunlight), cigarette smoke, toxic substances in the environment and radiation. The body possesses a number of defenses against free radicals, but they may be overwhelmed in times of stress or as we grow older and anti-oxidant enzyme activity decreases.

Enter our newly discovered champions, vitamins that can capture these free radicals before they attach to vital tissues, reducing the damage they do. Among the most studied vitamins are beta-carotene (a form of vitamin A), vitamin E and vitamin C. Though all are classified as anti-oxidants, each works in a slightly different way to eliminate the free radicals produced by chemical reactions in the body. Thus a combination of anti-oxidants can provide the protection that a single vitamin is unable to deliver.

Some conditions in which the symptoms may be lessened or prevented by anti-oxidants include cataracts, rheumatoid arthritis, cancers and heart disease. Anti-oxidants also may help to preserve the vitality of human sperm. The delight in this story is that good nutrition may be a method of preventing disease, and that is the best medicine of all.

363. ***I'm 28 years old and teach aerobics three or four times a week. My weight is about 128 pounds. The problem is reducing another 10 to 15 pounds. Even though I'm not overweight, I just don't feel physically fit. I do not overeat, and I watch my fat consumption, but nothing seems to help. I have battled my weight all my life, and it would be nice to finally win. Any advice or help would be greatly appreciated.***

Without a height measurement, it's hard to evaluate your situation. I probably would agree with you that you do not seem to be overweight. You would have to be 20 percent over your normal body weight to be considered obese. And that weight should be in excess fat tissue rather than in muscle tissue for it to be significant.

While regular aerobics does not tend to develop your muscles excessively, it would be interesting to know whether some of your body weight is due to your frequent workouts. While you claim you're not overeating, keeping a diary of everything you eat and converting it to calories might reveal that even for a person of your age, height and physical activity, you're still consuming too many calories for there to be a noticeable weight loss over time.

But my medical sensitivities are alerted by your statement that you "just don't feel fit." I would want to check out a few possibilities to be sure that both your physical functions and mental state are all functioning as they should. A thyroid problem can be at the base of your problem. And work and living situations can make a person feel less than fit without any physical basis.

Too many times a medical situation that is relatively easy to correct is lost in a poorly defined complaint, such as yours. I don't think your answer lies in another diet, but in an overall evaluation of your physical, emotional and social situation.

364. ***I often shop for food with a girlfriend, and we're both very conscious of the new trends for healthy cuisine. I always look for cholesterol content in prepared foods. I was about to purchase a package with a "cholesterol-free" label when she saw that it contained coconut oil and said it was loaded with fats. How can that be? I thought these labels were supposed to be a source of reliable information.***

While cholesterol is an important factor in your choice of foods, it's found only in animal products, such as meat, butter and eggs. But saturated fats, which can be found in vegetable products such as coconut and palm oils among others, also can increase the cholesterol content of your blood, even when you haven't eaten any cholesterol in your food.

This is because the body can create cholesterol from other fats, so you must be careful to avoid high-fat foods (especially saturated fats). While labels are generally pretty truthful, the law that regulates their wording and nutritional information is now in place. Until it is enforced by the Food and Drug Administration, be wary of labels that proclaim "Low Cholesterol" or "No Cholesterol" without noting whether the foods are rich in other fats.

365. ***I'm to have an exercise cardiogram, but I really don't know what that means or how it is done. Would you please explain?***

An exercise cardiogram is a test that checks to see how well your heart functions during exercise, rather than at rest. It's also called a stress test, since it shows how your heart responds to exertion.

An exercise electrocardiogram (EECG) can show abnormalities of the heart that a regular ECG won't, and it's helpful in evaluating people who have symptoms of heart disease or a past heart attack. The test is also part of the checkup for older people who are considering starting an exercise program.

During an exercise ECG, you're wired to the ECG machine while you walk on a treadmill or pedal on a stationary bicycle. The speed of the treadmill or the resistance of the bike is increased gradually so that you're exercising more strenuously.

Don't eat or smoke for two hours before the test. Wear loose pants or shorts and sneakers. Women should wear a comfortable support bra, a loose front-buttoning blouse, and they should avoid wearing a girdle or one-piece undergarment. The test usually takes about 30 minutes. It may take some time to analyze the findings, but then you can be sure that your exercise program will do you more good than harm.

366. ***My boyfriend is on the heavy side, but he thinks dieting is for women. He eats everything in sight. When we go to the movies, he gets a huge container of popcorn and tells me that it has no calories. He sometimes eats two! Can you tell us the truth about the calorie content of this common snack?***

Well, there is popcorn, and then there is popcorn. Popcorn prepared fat-free in a hot-air popper contains about 35 calories per cup, not bad for an evening's snacking.

Movie houses, for the most part, use hot oils in preparing their concoction, which jumps the calorie count up to more than 50 calories a cup. A small container of popcorn sold over most snack counters contains six cups, so you consume about 300 calories if you eat it plain. With a shot or two of that butter-flavored topping (it isn't real butter, you know), the calorie count zooms to about 650 calories.

Now, I don't know about your movie house, but I have seen some containers that contain 10 or even 18 cups of flavored popcorn, for which the calorie price is more than 2,000 calories. Surely he doesn't eat two of those!

For comparison, you might wish to consider that many weight-reduction diets provide only 1,000 calories for a whole day's meals. But those are contained in a well-balanced diet, not merely popcorn.

367. ***My wife pesters me to get more exercise as the prescription to cure all ills. I do walk when I can and get my heart to race a bit faster. I suspect that is what all exercise is for, anyway. Can you comment on this for me please?***

There is more to it, indeed, much more! Perhaps some explanations of the types of exercise will help.

There are several types of exercise, and a good exercise program should give you some of each kind each week. The goals of exercise are to strengthen muscles, improve cardiovascular health, increase joint flexibility and, in some cases, to burn calories and help in a weight-reduction program.

Aerobic exercise is any continuous vigorous exercise. As you exercise aerobically, your lungs do more work with less effort, your heart becomes stronger, and your endurance improves. Running, cycling, swimming and brisk walking are all aerobic exercises. To get the most from an aerobic exercise program, exercise continuously without rest periods for 20 to 30 minutes at least three times a week.

Anaerobic exercises — tennis, handball, running sprints — involve a short burst of activity, followed by a recovery period. They put a sudden high demand on the heart and lungs.

Strength-building exercises can be isometric or isotonic. Isometric exercises build strength by pitting one group of muscles against another or against something unyielding. Isometrics no longer are recommended, because the lack of movement can result in joint stiffening. This type of exercise also increases pressure in the chest and may cause dizziness or fainting.

Isotonic exercises build strength by having muscles move weight through a full range of motion. These exercises help maintain muscle mass, body proportions and good posture. Weight lifting is isotonic exercise, as are push-ups, pull-ups and sit-ups, when the weight of the body is being lifted or moved.

368. ***Could you please explain about fiber? It seems all the magazines tell how good it is but fail to explain just what it is. How much of this material is enough in your diet? I've had my share of overdoing a good thing, and I don't want to do that with this.***

In recent years, fiber has been described as the preventive element in food that may affect the development of many diseases, from cancer of the colon to atherosclerosis. The most widely accepted definition of fiber is that it is the portion of food, mostly from plants, that cannot be broken down by intestinal enzymes, and therefore passes through the small intestine and colon undigested.

Experts also agree that dietary fiber is important because it increases the bulk of the stool and makes it softer by absorbing water as it passes through the colon. This speeds up the process of eliminating organic wastes and toxins from the intestinal tract, possibly reducing the length of time the intestinal wall is exposed to poisonous substances.

The desirable daily fiber intake in the United States is approximately 25 to 50 grams a day, with 30 grams considered an optimum daily portion. Good sources are fruits, vegetables, nuts and whole grains, especially wheat bran.

Too much fiber, though, can have negative effects, because it can reduce the absorption of minerals, nitrogen and fat. And increasing the amount of fiber in your diet too rapidly, in your words "overdoing it," may lead to excessive gas, diarrhea and cramps. However, by slowly adding fiber-containing food to your diet over a period of time, you can gain all of its benefits with none of the annoying side effects.

369. ***Because of all the statements made, which incidentally seem to change daily, I'm totally confused about the role my diet may have in preventing cancer. Can you make any sense out of the endless numbers and "facts" that are printed or reported on television each day?***

The topic of health and disease prevention is one that most Americans seem to be very interested in, and the news media is just trying to keep up with all the latest developments published in medical journals each week. It's hard to report on all of this material and to separate those statistics that apply only to a few cases from those that are generally accepted by many researchers and clinicians.

Most doctors recommend reducing the percentages of calories obtained from fats in the diet. A reduction from 40 percent to 30 percent, for example, may provide protection from breast, colon, ovarian and endometrial cancer. Some experts would like to see that percentage pushed even lower, to about 20 percent of total caloric intake. This could reduce the risk of breast and colon cancer by as much as 80 percent. To accomplish this, you're going to have to learn the fat content of various foods and keep careful count.

Fiber is another big item in the news these days. Fiber may decrease the chances of colon cancer by increasing the bulk of stools, diluting possible cancer-producing material in the stool and decreasing the time they stay in contact with the cells lining the colon. Fiber is present in cereals, whole grain breads, fruits and vegetables.

Calcium also is recommended, not only as a measure to prevent osteoporosis but also to reduce the chances of colon cancer. Daily intake of 1,200 milligrams of calcium is recommended. Other dietary items, such as smoked, charred and nitrite-cured foods, have been linked with cancer in some studies. Stomach cancer also has been associated with long-term use of pickled and salted foods.

If cancer prevention is really your goal, there are two other items to be mentioned, although they do not deal specifically with food. They are exercise and smoking. Individuals with active occupations seem to have a lower risk of both breast and colon cancer. The use of tobacco can be linked to about 30 percent of all cancer deaths, and it has been associated with cancer of the lung, pancreas, bladder, kidney and possibly the cervix. Lung cancer is now the biggest killer of women (21 percent), even more lethal than breast cancer (18 percent).

In summary, if you want to prevent that which might be preventable, choose a healthy diet of foods low in fat and high in fiber, keep your weight down, exercise regularly and stay away from tobacco.

370.

I keep hearing about how good "complex carbohydrates" are for a healthy diet. But I'm not sure I know just what these carbohydrates are. Do they mean sugars or starches? I thought they were fattening and something to be avoided. Would you please clarify this situation for me?

Complex carbohydrates are made of long strands of simple sugars, but that is where their resemblance to sugar ends. This food classification includes starches as well as three types of fiber — cellulose, hemicellulose and gums. All are derived from plants. Starches are found in cereals, breads, pastas, barley, rice and vegetables such as potatoes, corn, peas and beans.

Since starches yield only four calories per gram (versus nine calories per gram for fat), they are great for dieters. Just leave off the fatty toppings and you're on the way to a healthy, calorie-conscious diet. Research has shown that people who eat a diet with lots of complex carbohydrates become full more quickly, and so unconsciously they decrease their intake of calories.

The Body's Systems

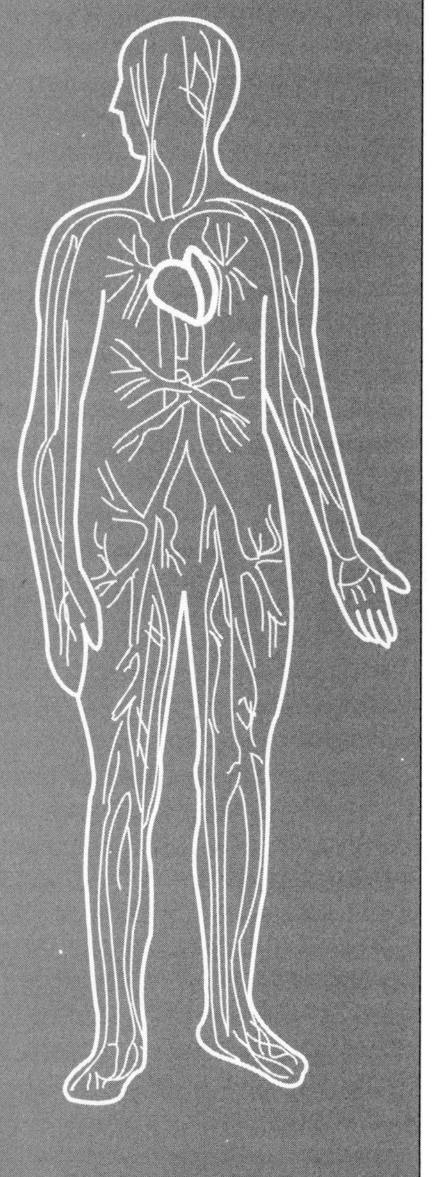

The Circulatory System

Whether we're consciously aware of the minute-by-minute efforts of our hearts or not, this single, relatively small organ controls our lives. More than once a second, it beats and pumps blood through our bodies, giving vital oxygen to the tissues and keeping us alive. At a typical rate of 72 beats per minute, the heart will beat 104,000 times in an average day in adults, and even more than that in children.

For many other body systems, there is duplication of the main organ, which provides two kidneys, two lungs or two eyes to the body, so that if one fails the other can take over the vital functions and do all the work necessary to keep us alive and well. But each of us has only one heart, so it pays to keep this important organ in the best possible working order.

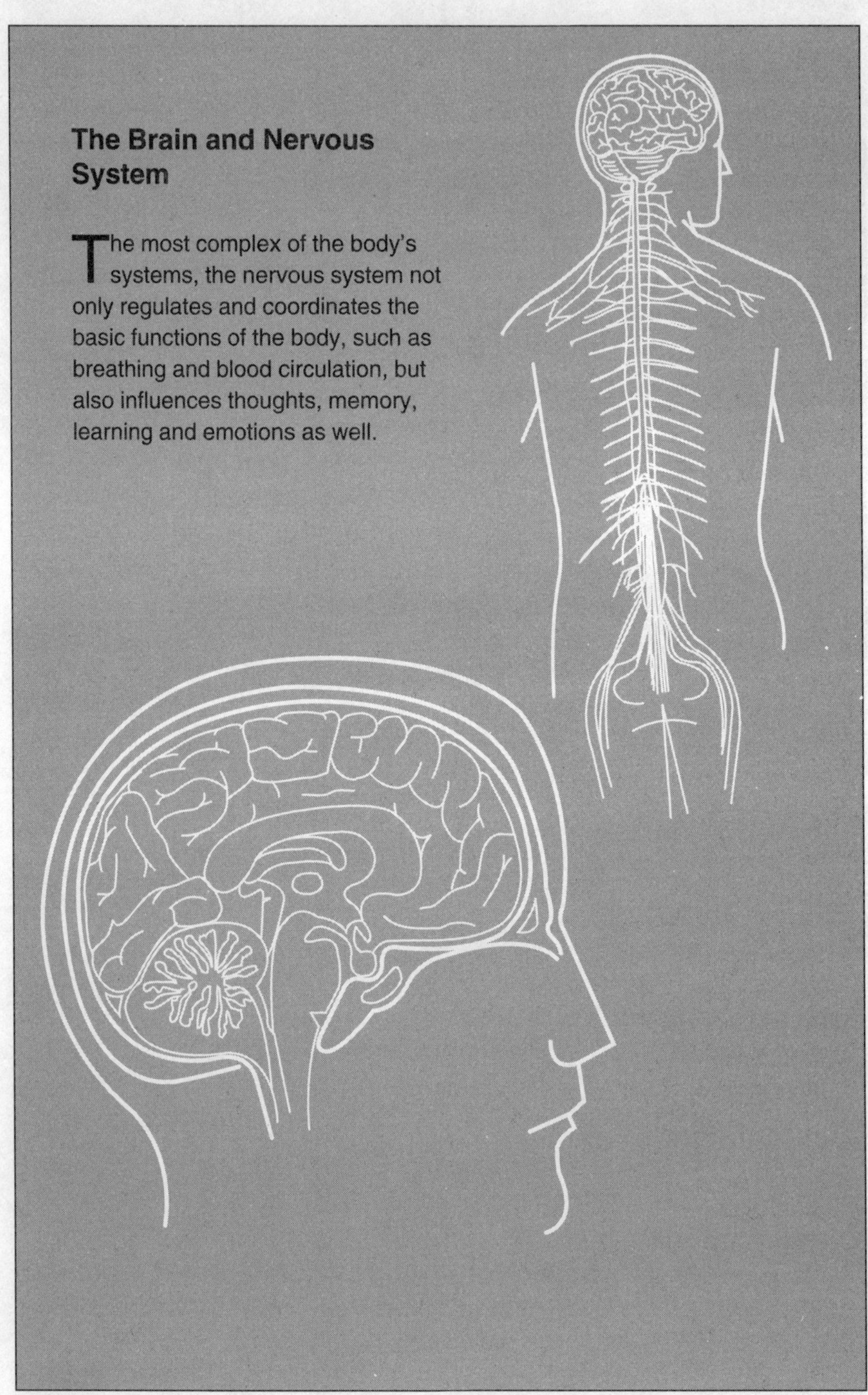

The Brain and Nervous System

The most complex of the body's systems, the nervous system not only regulates and coordinates the basic functions of the body, such as breathing and blood circulation, but also influences thoughts, memory, learning and emotions as well.

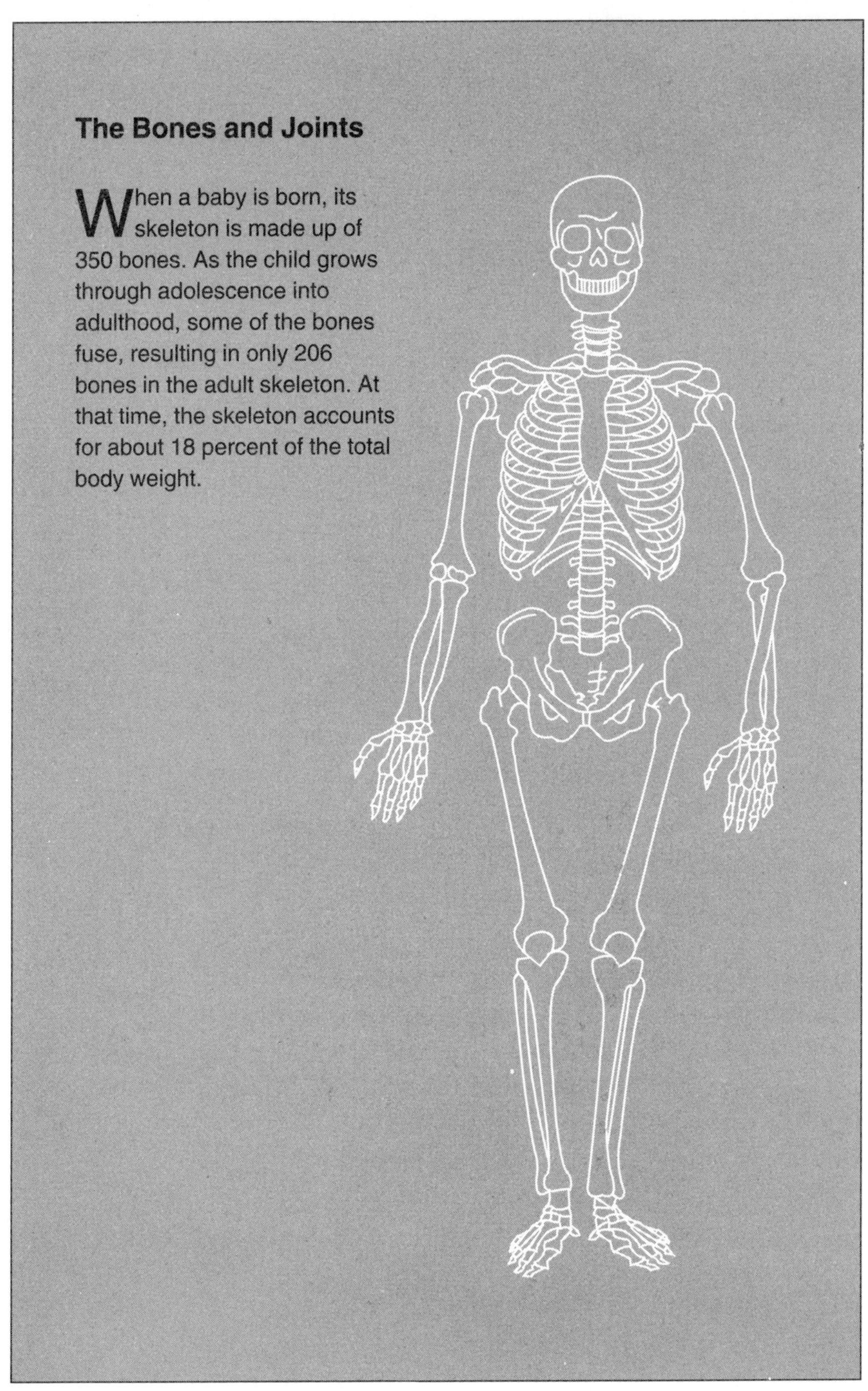

The Bones and Joints

When a baby is born, its skeleton is made up of 350 bones. As the child grows through adolescence into adulthood, some of the bones fuse, resulting in only 206 bones in the adult skeleton. At that time, the skeleton accounts for about 18 percent of the total body weight.

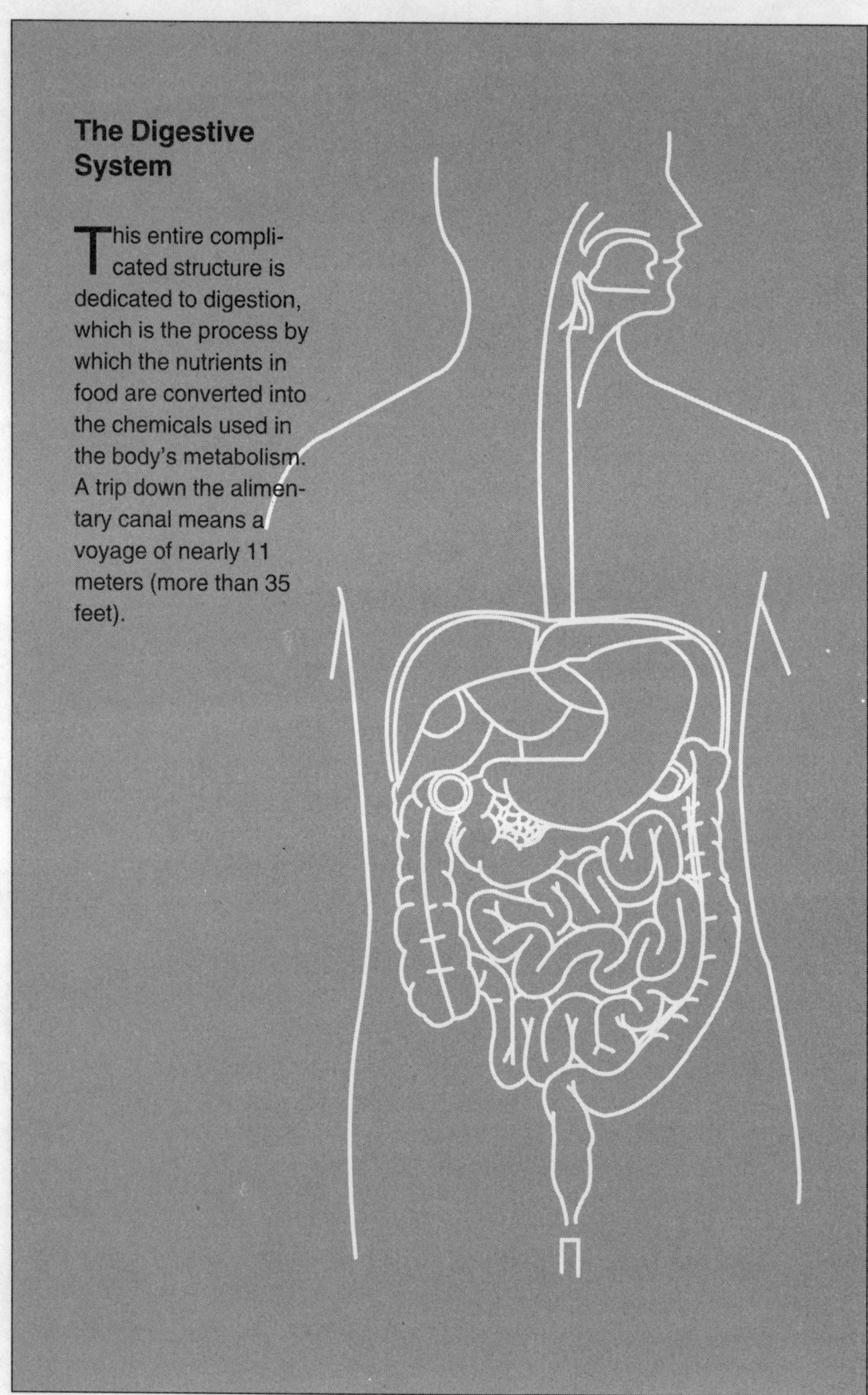

The Digestive System

This entire complicated structure is dedicated to digestion, which is the process by which the nutrients in food are converted into the chemicals used in the body's metabolism. A trip down the alimentary canal means a voyage of nearly 11 meters (more than 35 feet).

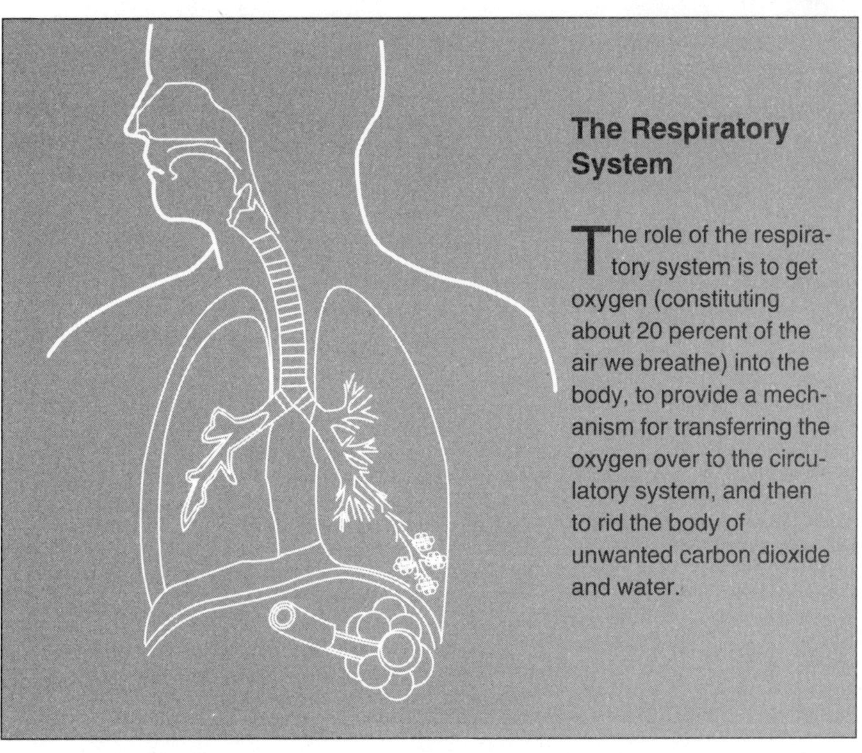

The Respiratory System

The role of the respiratory system is to get oxygen (constituting about 20 percent of the air we breathe) into the body, to provide a mechanism for transferring the oxygen over to the circulatory system, and then to rid the body of unwanted carbon dioxide and water.

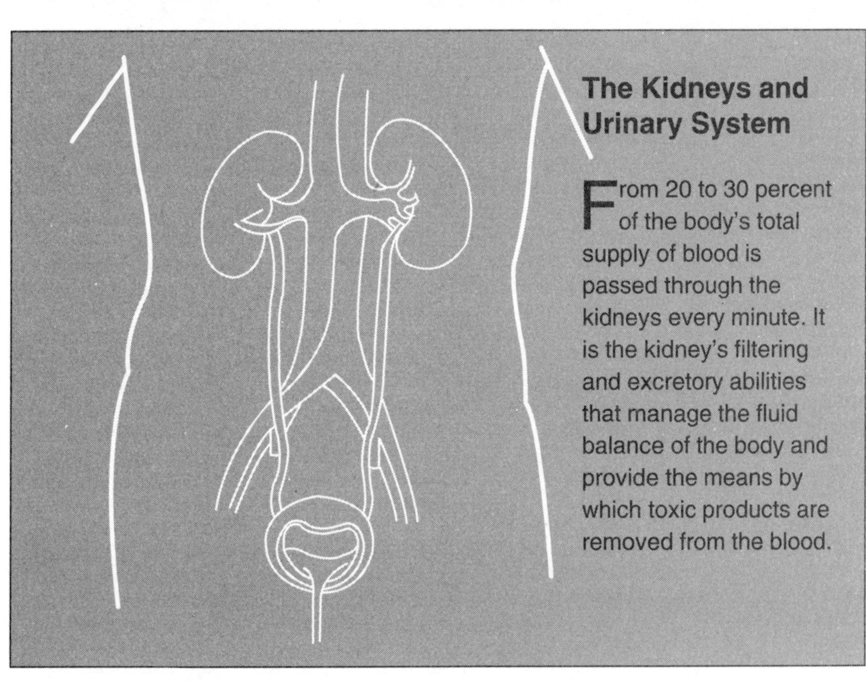

The Kidneys and Urinary System

From 20 to 30 percent of the body's total supply of blood is passed through the kidneys every minute. It is the kidney's filtering and excretory abilities that manage the fluid balance of the body and provide the means by which toxic products are removed from the blood.

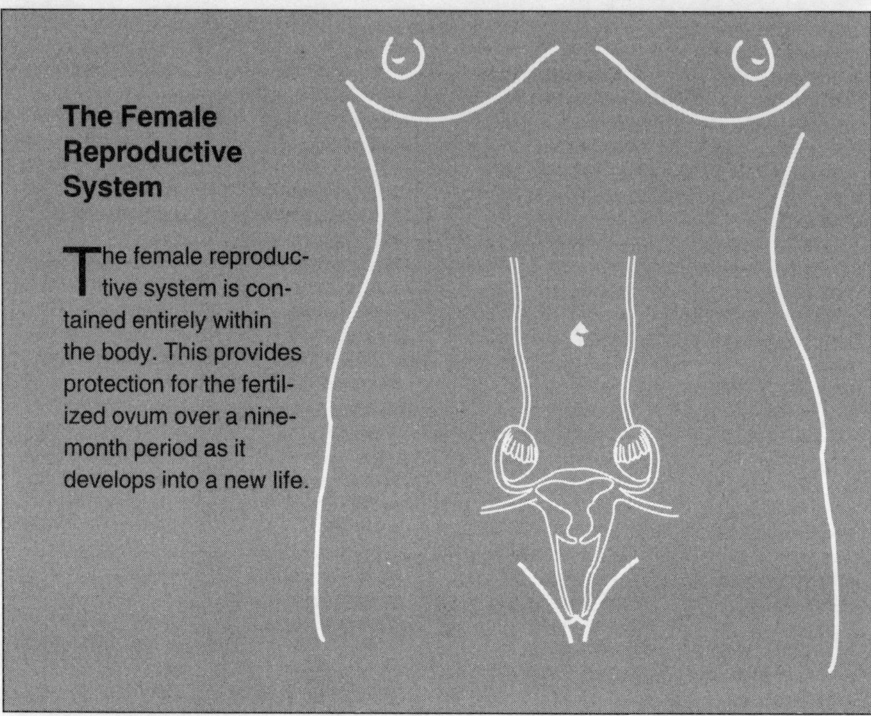

The Female Reproductive System

The female reproductive system is contained entirely within the body. This provides protection for the fertilized ovum over a nine-month period as it develops into a new life.

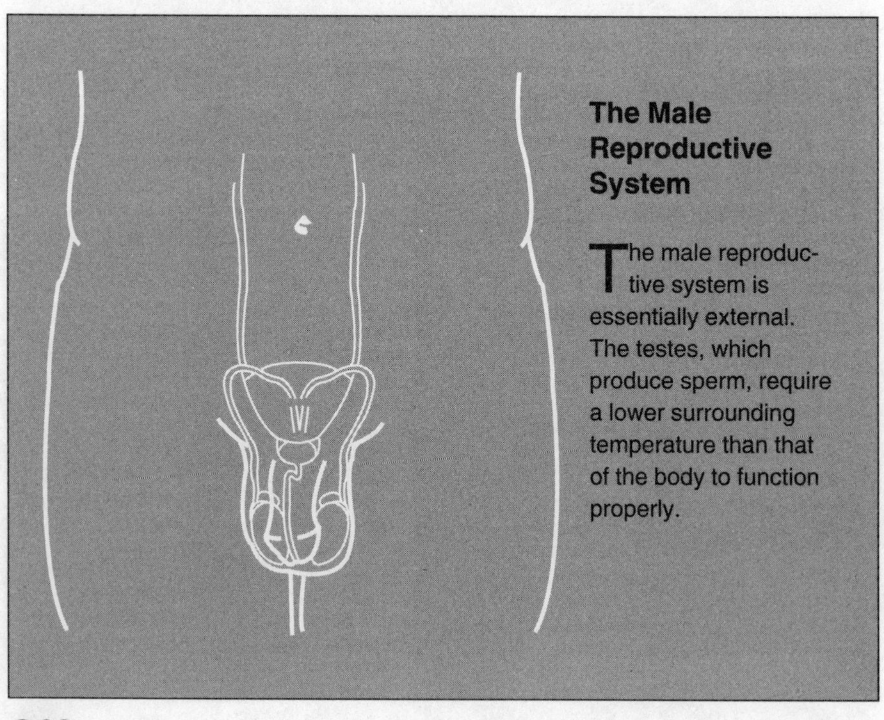

The Male Reproductive System

The male reproductive system is essentially external. The testes, which produce sperm, require a lower surrounding temperature than that of the body to function properly.

Directory of Symptoms
(by Question Number)

The following alphabetized list contains symptoms, problems and diseases covered in this book. Each entry is followed by one or more numbers indicating which questions and answers discuss that particular entry. Referring to this list will give you an overview of the various causes that can result in a particular symptom.

Directory of Symptoms (by Question Number)

Index

Index (by Page Number)

Index (by Page Number)

Index (by Page Number)

Index (by Page Number)